Traditional Chinese Medicine

Diagnosis Study Guide

TRADITIONAL CHINESE MEDICINE

Diagnosis Study Guide

Qiao Yi, M.D. (China), M.P.H., L.Ac.

Al Stone, L.Ac., D.A.O.M.

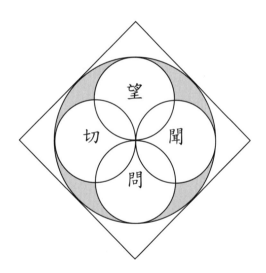

EASTLAND PRESS ▶ SEATTLE

Published by Eastland Press, Inc.
P.O. Box 99749
Seattle, WA 98139, USA
www.eastlandpress.com

Library of Congress Control Number: 2008934266
ISBN: 978-0-939616-64-0
Printed in the United States of America

8   10   9

Book design by Gary Niemeier

TABLE OF CONTENTS

INTRODUCTION 概論

■ CONTENTS

Introduction 概論

Diagnosis in traditional Chinese medicine (TCM) involves the examination of the body for the purpose of diagnosing disease and differentiating patterns under the guidance of the basic theories of TCM. It is a bridge that connects the fundamental studies of TCM with all branches of clinical medicine and includes inspecting the manifestations, analyzing the changes, understanding the pathomechanisms, and predicting the transformation of diseases.

■ The Main Studies in TCM Diagnosis

TCM diagnosis consists of two major areas of study, "examination and testing" (診 *zhěn*) and "decision and judgment" (斷 *duàn*). Examination and testing techniques are used to collect information from the patient. Decision and judgment uses this information, which is sorted, analyzed, synthesized, and reasoned on the basis of TCM theory.

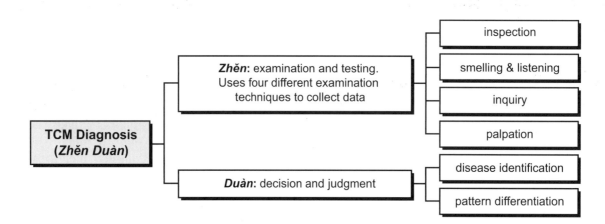

Chart 1 Scope of TCM diagnosis

The processes in TCM diagnosis include: examination and testing, disease identification, and pattern differentiation.

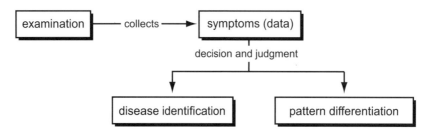

Chart 2 Diagnosis process

I. Examination and Testing

The process of examination uses various methods to inspect the patient in order to collect information relating to changes in health. These methods include inspection, inquiry, listening and smelling, and palpation, which are generally known as the "four pillars".

(1) Inspection utilizes the practitioner's visual sense to observe abnormal changes in the patient's spirit, complexion, appearance of the tongue, and secretions and excreta in order to understand and predict pathological changes in the internal organs.

(2) Listening and smelling (auscultation and olfaction) utilizes the practitioner's sense of hearing to assess the patient's physiological and pathological sounds. Smelling odors arising from the patient also informs the diagnostic process.

(3) Inquiry utilizes conversation to gain insight into the patient's condition through the responses of the patient or their representative. The patient's symptoms, the cause or predisposing factors of disease, the history (onset, development, and treatment) of the disease, the patient's living environment (social and geographic), and personal relationships are all collected to assist in the naming of the disease or differentiation of the pattern.

(4) Palpation utilizes the sense of touch to feel, press, or palpate areas of the patient's body, including the pulse, in order to obtain information regarding the patient's physiological and pathological condition.

II. Disease Identification

Disease identification is the process by which a more exacting assessment of a patient's condition can be made based on the patient's signs and symptoms. After further analysis and judgment, disease identification can be made.

(1) Disease (病 *bìng*) is a deviation from or interruption of the normal structure or function of any body part, organ, or system that is manifested by a characteristic set of signs and symptoms whose etiology, pathology, anatomical location, and prognosis may be known. A disease is a summary of the distinct features of a disorder including the process and life cycle of pathologic development.

When a pathogenic factor (邪气 *xié* qi) attacks the body, the antipathogenic qi (正氣 *zhèng* qi) will struggle against it. At this point, the normal physiology and relative equilibrium of the body's qi, blood, *zàng fǔ* organs, channels and collaterals are disrupted. Manifestations of reduced vitality, limited or total loss of activity, and a series of signs and symptoms may appear. During this process, the antipathogenic qi will always give rise to a struggle between impair and repair, dysfunction and accommodation, in a dynamic manner that reflects the relative strength of the pathogenic factor and the antipathogenic qi.

(2) Disease name. The name of the disease itself represents an additional specificity. It is a summary of the pathology and an abstract of the disease process that may include its etiology, pathomechanism, and signs and symptoms. The name of the disease may also provide insight into the nature of the disease, such that its incidence, evolution, outcome, and prognosis may be further inferred.

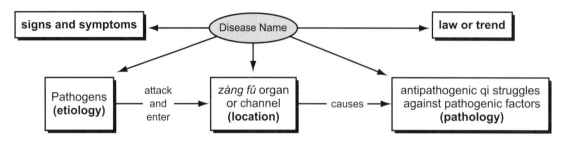

Chart 3 Disease definition

In the history of traditional Chinese medicine, more than 4,000 disease names have been documented. Naming a disease is valuable not only for the purpose of diagnosis, but also for classification. Some diseases are named on the basis of their pathological shape or symptoms, such as edema, jaundice, cough, or asthma. Others are named for the pathology, such as restless organ disorder (*zàng zào*). Some diseases are named for the *zàng fǔ* organ or structure that is involved, such as Lung abscess, or chest painful obstruction (*bì*); and some are named for their etiology, such as sunstroke or "fright wind" (*jīng fēng*).

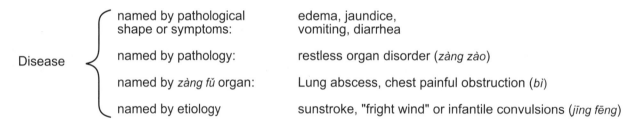

Chart 4 Disease name etymology

III. Pattern Differentiation

Pattern differentiation is the process by which clinical information (obtained from the examination) is analyzed, synthesized, and inferred, leading to a clear representation of a particular phase of a disease in a TCM pattern.

(1) Pattern (證 *zhèng*) is a combination of signs and/or symptoms that forms a distinct clinical picture indicative of a particular disorder. It is the summary of environment, pathogens, pathological location, pathogenesis, condition of the antipathogenic qi, signs and symptoms, and the constitution of a patient. It is based on the information obtained by the four examination methods. The pattern comprehensively and concretely reflects the nature and features of a disease at a given stage. Thus, the pattern reflects the essence of a disease at the moment of the assessment.

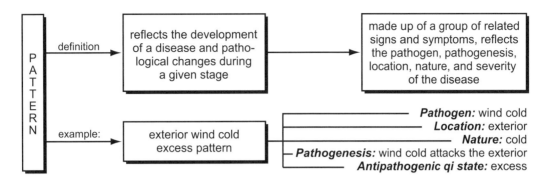

Chart 5 Pattern definition

(2) Signs and symptoms (症狀 *zhèng zhuàng*) are the abnormal phenomena which deviate from the normal physiological range that are associated with a disorder, such as fever, cough, or headache. Signs and symptoms reflect the body's pathological changes. They include 1) symptoms, which are defined as subjective feelings of discomfort; and 2) signs, which are objective data obtained by the practitioner through examination. The signs and symptoms reflect the presence and stage of pathological change and are important indicators for the identification of disease and the differentiation of patterns.

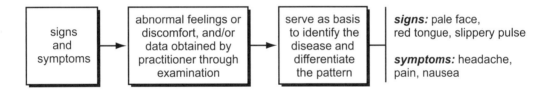

Chart 6 Signs and symptoms

(3) Pattern differentiation. Over the course of thousands of years of clinical practice, practitioners developed many methods of differentiation, such as eight-principle differentiation, six-stage differentiation, four-level differentiation, and etiology differentiation. These methods are a summary of the pathological tendencies and the understanding of patterns from different perspectives. Each method has its special emphasis, and they are related to and supplemented by each other. The following chart summarizes the most commonly used methods of differentiation and their relationships.

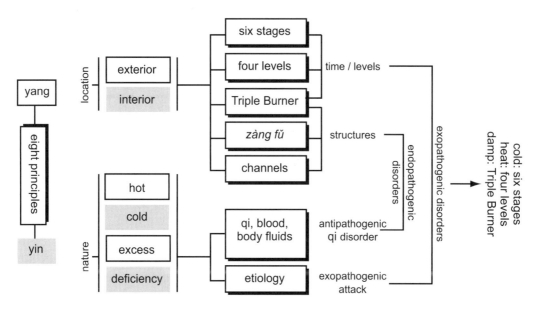

Chart 7 Different methods of pattern differentiation and their relationships

The Principles of TCM Diagnosis

Diseases are very complex processes. Clinical manifestations can be true or false, mild or severe, or latent or active. Disease symptoms can be primary or secondary. Sometimes there may be two disease processes unrelated to each other. Some symptoms may appear early while others only appear later in the disease process. Given all of these variables, the practitioner must be very vigilant to discover the root or essence of the disease. Application of the following three principles is necessary to make an accurate diagnosis for an effective treatment strategy.

I. Holistic Approach

Holism is a fundamental concept of TCM. The holistic approach in diagnosis refers to the comprehensive consideration of the human body and its natural surroundings. This has two aspects:

The human body as a whole. The human body is an organic whole. The internal *zàng fǔ* organs are the center of the body. The outer parts such as the limbs, five sensory organs, nine orifices, skin, muscles, vessels, and tendons and bones are all linked to the *zàng fǔ* organs through channels and collaterals. During the diagnostic process, special attention is paid to the interrelation and interaction between local pathological changes and the maladjustment of the whole body. Local pathological changes may affect the whole body and pathological changes of the whole body may, in turn, be reflected locally. External disorders may penetrate into the interior or pathological changes of the internal organs may manifest externally.

The unification of the human body and its surroundings. Human beings are affected by such natural conditions as weather and other environmental influences. When there are abnormal changes in the natural environment, or when the human body fails to adapt itself to such changes, pathological change will certainly occur in the body.

II. Application of the four examination methods in combination

During the clinical examination, the four diagnostic methods should be used together in order to arrive at a reliable diagnosis, since each of these methods plays its special part in assessing health and gathering clinical information. Each of the sensory organs has a unique function in the diagnostic process. Inspection (observation), listening and smelling, and palpation are applied to the examination of the patient by means of the practitioner's visual sense, hearing, smelling, and tactile sensation. Additionally, inquiring summarizes the patient's feelings and allows them to describe the onset and development of a disease. In other words, each of the four examination methods supplements the others.

III. Combining Disease Identification with Pattern Differentiation

Differentiating the pattern after a disease has been identified is an intrinsic part of the practice of TCM. In order to make an accurate diagnosis, one should first determine the disease and then differentiate the pattern on the basis of the patient's signs and symptoms. Both the disease and the pattern represent a summary of the environment, pathogens, pathological location, pathogenesis, the strength of the antipathogenic qi, signs and symptoms, and constitution of the patient based on the information gathered during the four examinations. However, disease and pattern are two different diagnostic concepts.

The *disease* represents the entire course of pathological changes associated with an illness. Over the course of a disease, the pathogenic qi battles with the antipathogenic qi, however this process is dynamic and the presentation will therefore undergo continuing changes in accordance with certain rules. By contrast, the *pattern* describes the pathology at a particular stage of the disease, where there is a certain configuration in the battle between the pathogenic factor and antipathogenic qi that can be treated. A single disease can evolve through multiple patterns, and the same pattern can be found in multiple diseases.

For this reason, the full course of pathological and predictable changes of a disease cannot be grasped through pattern identification alone. On the other hand, if one identifies only the disease, but not the pattern, treatment cannot be undertaken since the treatment principle is based on the differentiation of the particular pattern, and not the overall disease.

Identification of the disease combined with pattern differentiation enables one to grasp the essentials of the disease more comprehensively in order to make an accurate diagnosis and thereby establish an effective treatment principle and make an accurate prognosis.

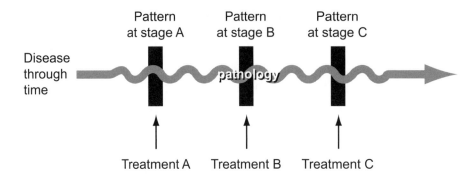

Chart 8 Relationship of disease to pattern through time

Chapter One

Inspection 望診

■ CONTENTS

Inspection 望診

Inspection is the very first assessment used when the initial patient/practitioner contact occurs. This process continues through the diagnostic process: the way in which a patient answers questions or responds is an important aspect of her spirit, as are the actual answers that diagnostic interactions may provide.

I. Definition

Inspection is an examination method which employs the practitioner's visual sense to observe abnormal changes in the patient's spirit, complexion, body, tongue, secretions and excreta in order to understand and predict pathological changes of internal organs.

II. Fundamental Theory of Inspection

In the human body, internal organs and the exterior of the body are closely connected and related through the channels and collaterals, and through the qi and blood. The face and tongue have an especially close relationship with the *zàng fǔ* organs, because all channels and collaterals pass through or connect in the tongue and face. In addition, all five *zàng* organs open to an orifice in the head. Excreta and secreted substances are produced by activities of the internal organs. As such, they can manifest pathological changes of the internal organs. Therefore, through inspection of the external changes of the body, one can know the condition of the internal organs and understand their pathological changes. This process is described in *The Divine Pivot*, Chapter 47 (靈樞。本臟) which states that "Observing the outside manifestations in order to understand the organs inside, so as to identify the diseases."

III. Clinical Significance

Inspection allows one to assess the essence and qi, the state of pathological change, transformation of the illness, prognosis, thermal nature of the pathogenic factor, state of antipathogenic qi, and the *zàng fǔ* organs involved.

IV. The Scope of Inspection

Inspection includes five major areas:

1) **inspection of the whole body,** which includes inspection of spirit, facial complexion, and body appearance

2) **inspection of local areas,** which include the head, face, five sense organs, body, skin, and extremities

3) **inspection of the infant's index finger**

4) **inspection of excreta and secretions**

5) **inspection of the tongue,** which includes inspection of the tongue body and its coating.

Section 1

Inspection of the Whole Body

■ One: Inspection of Spirit (神 *Shén*)

Inspection of spirit means to observe whether the patient's mental state is normal, whether the consciousness is clear, the movements harmonious, and whether reactions are timid in order to determine whether there is a state of excess or deficiency in the *zàng fǔ* organs, yin, yang, qi and blood; and the prognosis of disease.

I. DEFINITION

Spirit: spirit is the general manifestation of the vital activities of the human body, and the outward sign of the relative strength of qi and blood of the *zàng fǔ* organs. The vital activities are divided into two meanings:

- *broad sense:* describes the total external manifestations of the life activities of the human body which are the reflections of *zàng fǔ* organ functions. This may be thought of as general vitality and can be seen in the pulse, tongue, complexion, etc.
- *narrow sense:* describes mental activities, including consciousness and cognition.

II. THEORY OF INSPECTION OF SPIRIT

(1) The Origin of Spirit

The Divine Pivot states: "The combination of two kinds of essences (essence [精 *jīng*] of the father and mother) forms the spirit." "Spirit is the essence of qi and fluids." This means that spirit is formed from a combination of two kinds of congenital essences. Afterwards, spirit is supported and enriched by acquired essence.

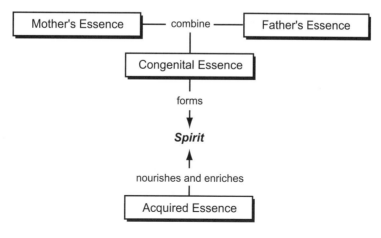

Chart 1.1.1 Origin of Spirit

(2) The Manifestation of Spirit

Spirit dominates the entire body's activity. It can be seen in various manifestations such as facial expression, eye movement, mental state, physical activity and reactivity, voice, tongue, and pulse.

(3) The relationship between essence, qi, and spirit

Essence is the original substance (source) of human life. It makes up the human body. Essence is composed of

- *congenital essence*, which is inherited from the parents, and *acquired essence*, which is produced from food by the Stomach and Spleen.

Qi denotes

- the essential substances of the human body which maintain its vital activities
- the functional activities of the *zàng fǔ* organs and other tissues.

Spirit is the manifestation of all life activities.

- *broad sense:* describes the total external manifestation of vital activities which reflect the functions of the viscera
- *narrow sense:* describes mental activities including consciousness and cognitive activities.

Essence, qi, and spirit are called the "three treasures." Essence is the source of life, qi is the force of life, and spirit is the controller and manifestation of life. They work as a single whole, physically and functionally, and are inseparable. The coitus of parental essences produces life. Then the mental and physical activities (spirit) manifest. After spirit is formed, it is enriched and nourished by qi and blood, and in turn generates and supplies acquired essence.

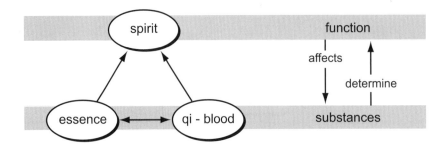

Chart 1.1.2 Relationships between Spirit and Essential Substances

In general, essence is the source of life, one has the essence first and then spirit. Qi and blood maintain life, and spirit is the manifestation of life. Qi, blood, and essence are the material basis of spirit. When there is sufficient qi, blood, or essence, the person will have spirit; if there is insufficient qi, blood, or essence, the person will lack or lose spirit.

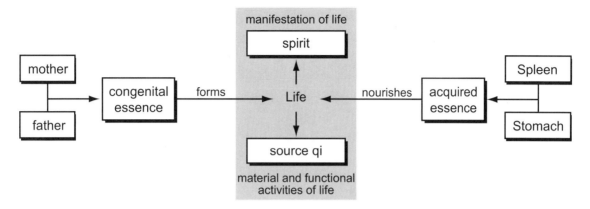

Chart 1.1.3 Relationships between Essence, Qi, and Spirit

III. NORMAL SPIRIT

Normal spirit refers to being full of vigor, which is reflected in sufficiency of both essence and qi. Normal spirit gives one bright and vivid eyes, clear consciousness and speech, quick responses, resonant voice, radiant complexion with natural expressions, and a freely movable and flexible body.

IV. CLINICAL SIGNIFICANCE OF INSPECTION OF SPIRIT

Observation of spirit plays an important role in TCM diagnosis. It can help the practitioner understand:

- the condition of the essence and qi
- the state of the pathological changes
- the transformation of the illness
- the prognosis.

Clinical Significance	Having Spirit	Lack of Spirit
Essence and Qi	sufficient	insufficient or failure
State of Disease	mild	severe
Transformation	from having to lacking: worse	from lacking to having: better
Prognosis	good	poor

Table 1.1.1 Clinical Significance of Inspection of Spirit

V. METHOD OF INSPECTION OF SPIRIT

In order to observe spirit, attention should be placed on the patient's facial expression, mental state, physical activity, language, breathing, reactivity, etc.

Special emphasis should be put on eye movement because of the following:

- the eye is regarded as the window of the Liver
- the eye is the messenger of the Heart
- all the essence and qi of the five *zàng* and six *fǔ* organs rise and pour into the eyes.

VI. Clinical Manifestation of Spirit

Clinically, spirit can be manifested as having spirit, fatigued spirit, and lack of spirit, which can be further divided into subcategories based on the severity of the lack of spirit. These categories include loss of spirit, false spirit, and spirit disturbance.

(1) Having spirit (有神 *yǒu shén*)

DEFINITION: the normal physiological state when the patient is full of vigor, reflected in a sufficiency of both essence and qi.

MANIFESTATION: patient is alert with bright and vivid eyes, clear consciousness and speech, quick responses, resonant voice, radiant complexion with natural expressions, and a freely movable and flexible body.

INDICATION: patient's essence has not been exhausted and the condition of the *zàng fǔ* organs has not fallen into severe disorder, even though there may be illness.

CLINICAL SIGNIFICANCE: the illness is not serious and the prognosis is favorable.

(2) Fatigued spirit (神疲 *shén pí*)

DEFINITION: a mild manifestation of lacking spirit. Fatigued spirit and lacking spirit differ only in degree of severity. Fatigued spirit is between having spirit and lacking spirit.

MANIFESTATION: listlessness, lassitude, poor memory, weak and low voice, aversion to speaking, fatigue, slow and awkward actions. The main symptom of fatigued spirit is poor memory.

INDICATION: deficiency pattern, usually caused by Heart and Spleen deficiency or Kidney yang deficiency.

CLINICAL SIGNIFICANCE: allows one to judge whether the state of qi is in a state of excess or deficiency.

(3) Lack of spirit (少神 *shǎo shén*)

A pathological state wherein deficiencies or disturbances undermine the calm or fullness of the spirit, which manifests in any of the following three presentations:

— A. Loss of Spirit (失神 *shī shén*)

DEFINITION: the patient's loss of spirit, which reflects an exhaustion of the essence, deficiency of qi, and weakness of vitality.

MANIFESTATION: patient has dull eyes, slow and awkward action, blurred vision, dull complexion and facial expression, heaviness of the body, obtuse actions and responses, mental confusion or even unconsciousness, delirium and hallucinations.

INDICATION: patient's qi has been exhausted, essence has declined, functional activities are insufficient, and the disease is severe.

CLINICAL SIGNIFICANCE: the disease is severe and the prognosis is unfavorable.

— B. False Spirit (假神 jiǎ shén)

DEFINITION: an apparent indication of improvement in which the patient suddenly improves during the terminal stage when the patient's essence and qi are extremely debilitated because of chronic disease or serious illness. The sudden appearance of apparent health is a transitory state that precedes death of the patient.

MANIFESTATION: the extremely weak patient in a critical condition is listless, unconscious, with dull eyes; has a dislike of speaking, low and feeble voice, dull complexion, and anorexia. Yet the patient suddenly feels better, has clear consciousness, bright eyes, louder voice, flushed cheeks, and improved appetite.

INDICATION: exhaustion of antipathogenic qi and impending failure of yin and yang, in which yin fails to restrain yang, and the yang is separating from the yin.

CLINICAL SIGNIFICANCE: imminent death.

— C. Spirit Disturbance (神亂 shén luàn)

The spirit disturbance is also a manifestation of lack of spirit but the pathogenesis is totally different from the type caused by essence, blood, or antipathogenic qi exhaustion. Spirit disturbance means that consciousness is obscured or lost. This condition is usually found in one of the following patterns. These patterns are caused by unique etiologies and pathogenesis. Although these patterns are manifestations of 'lack of spirit,' they are not necessarily critical conditions.

⋯ a) Irritability and restlessness (煩躁 fán zào)

SYMPTOMS: (fán) irritability, restlessness, hot and heavy sensations in the chest; (zào) feverish sensation and irritability causes the patient to prefer nudity and even drives the patient to jump into water

PATHOGENESIS: pathogenic heat in the Heart, Lung, or Kidney

⋯ b) Restless organ disorder (臟躁 zàng zào)

SYMPTOMS: mental depression, possible hallucinations, disorientation, frequent attacks of melancholy and crying spells, frequent bouts of yawning, no loss of consciousness

PATHOGENESIS: Heart and Liver blood deficiency

··· c) Hysteria (百合病 *bǎi hé bìng*)

SYMPTOMS: chronic depression, apathy with aversion to speaking, mumbling to one's self, insomnia, anorexia, sleepwalking

PATHOGENESIS: Heart and Lung yin deficiency

··· d) Yin madness (癲 *diān*)

SYMPTOMS: chronic depression, aversion to speaking or mumbling to one's self, laughing, or crying inappropriately

PATHOGENESIS: stagnant phlegm misting the Heart orifices, or Spleen and Heart deficiency

··· e) Yang madness (狂 *kuáng*)

SYMPTOMS: raving with obscenities, madness and restlessness, singing loudly and favoring high places, wandering naked, hitting people or destroying things

PATHOGENESIS: phlegm fire disturbs the mind

··· f) Epilepsy (癇 *xián*)

SYMPTOMS: sudden syncope with drooling saliva and spasms of the limbs. There is a short blackout or period of confused memory, odd changes in the way things look, sound, smell or feel. After the symptoms pass, the patient manifests no abnormality.

PATHOGENESIS: Liver wind with phlegm or phlegm fire disturbing the Heart

Signs	Having Spirit	Loss of Spirit	False Spirit
Complexion	bright hues and moist sheen	dim hues and dull sheen	dull sheen with sudden flushed cheeks
Eyes	alertness, vivid colors, twinkling eyes	dull colors with blurred vision	dull colors but suddenly lustrous
Mental Status	clear speech and consciousness, agile responses	unconsciousness or delirium	unclear consciousness with a sudden change for the better
Motion and Response	freely movable, quick responses	slow movements and responses	suddenly responsive
Respiration	even	rapid, feeble, or with difficulty	feeble, but suddenly strengthening
Diet	good	poor	poor, but suddenly improving

Table 1.1.2 Comparison of Having Spirit, Loss of Spirit and False Spirit

VII. SUMMARY OF INSPECTION OF SPIRIT

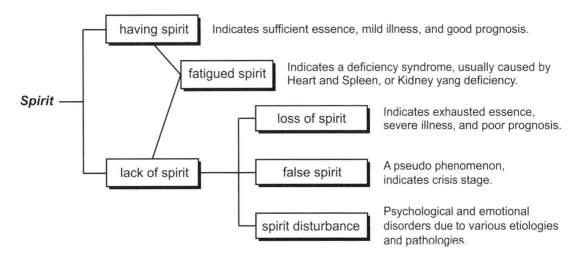

Chart 1.1.4 Summary of Clinical Manifestation of Spirit

▨ Two: Inspection of Facial Complexion

Inspection of the facial complexion means to inspect and examine the color and sheen of the facial skin in order to understand the condition of the qi, blood, and *zàng fǔ* organs.

I. INTRODUCTION

(1) Definition:

Facial color: the color of the skin. Skin color is associated with blood and yin. Color on the face can directly reflect the ebb and flow of the blood and the condition of the blood circulation. Under pathological circumstances, it can reflect the different characteristics of the *zàng fǔ* organs and their pathological changes.

Facial sheen: the luster of the skin. Skin luster is associated with qi and yang. Luster is the exterior manifestation of the essence qi of the *zàng fǔ* organs.

(2) Theories of Facial Complexion Diagnosis

The Heart dominates the blood vessels; its luster is reflected on the face. *The Divine Pivot* states that "the qi and blood of the twelve primary channels and the three-hundred-sixty-five connections ascend to the face." All six yang channels rise up to the face, especially the foot *yáng míng* Stomach channel. Therefore, there are abundant channels and blood vessels on the face. Thus facial colors not only manifest the Heart's condition but also the functions of all other organs.

Facial color is derived from yin blood and facial luster from the spirit. Complexion is the outward manifestation of the condition of the five *zàng* organs.

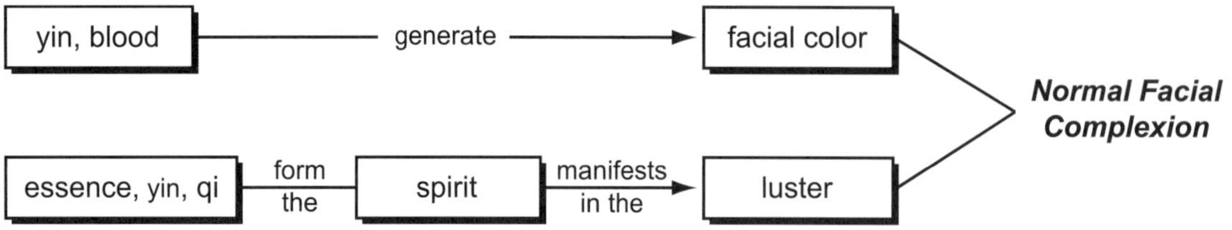

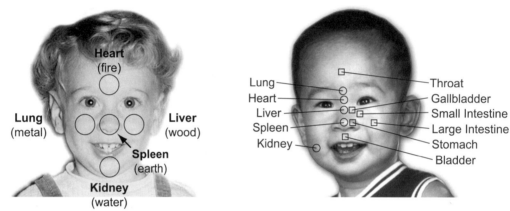

Chart 1.1.5 Physiology of Normal Facial Complexion

(3) The Correspondence of Portions of the Face with the *Zàng Fǔ* Organs

Each of the *zàng fǔ* organs has a corresponding location on the face. Observation of the facial complexion should be integrated with inspection of localized facial regions. There are two different arrangements, one according to *Basic Questions* (素問) and the other according to *The Divine Pivot* (靈樞).

Chart 1.1.6 Portions of the Face Corresponding to the *Zàng Fǔ* Organs According to *Basic Questions* (left) and the *Divine Pivot (*right)

(4) Normal Facial Complexion

DEFINITION: normal facial complexion refers to the facial color and luster of a person in a healthy physical condition. Because of different genetic pools, facial color and skin color have many variations.

CHARACTERISTICS: bright, moist, and lustrous.

INDICATION: qi and blood are sufficient and the functional activities of the *zàng fǔ* organs are in good condition.

CLINICAL MANIFESTATION AND PHYSIOLOGICAL VARIATION: the color and texture of the complexion can vary in accordance with different constitutions, geographic environments, seasons, weather, and profession. Normal facial skin color can be classified as follows:

- *host or governing (zhǔ) color:* the normal facial skin color of one's race, it remains unchanged during life.
- *guest or visitor (kè) color:* the slight change of facial skin color, which follows seasonal changes.

Seasons	Spring	Summer	Late Summer	Autumn	Winter
Origin	channels	collaterals	muscles	skin	marrow
Complexion	blue-green	red	yellow	white (pale)	black (dark)

Table 1.1.3 Guest Complexions

- *transient normal complexion:* changes in the complexion due to different working conditions, climates, living environments, diet, sexual activity, and emotions.

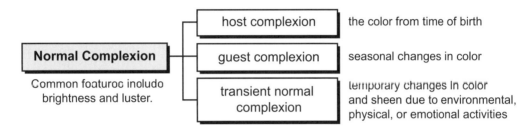

Chart 1.1.7 Normal Complexion and its Manifestations

(5) Clinical Significance of Inspection of Complexion

Observation of the complexion will help the practitioner:

- recognize the location of pathological change and judge the condition of the pathogenic and antipathogenic qi
- differentiate the thermal nature of the pathological change
- identify the organs and channels involved
- make a prognosis

(6) Method of Facial Complexion Diagnosis

In order for the practitioner to obtain the most accurate data from the patient, one must pay attention to the following variables:

- time: early morning is the best, or at a time after the patient has calmed down
- environment: quiet and without stimulation
- light: natural light

II. CLINICAL MANIFESTATIONS OF PATHOLOGICAL FACIAL COMPLEXIONS

(1) Definition: the facial complexion of a sick person. It may be said to include all the abnormal colors, as well as a pathological brightness and sheen.

(2) Scope of Abnormal Facial Complexion

Abnormal facial complexion includes abnormal facial color and sheen.

— A. Abnormal facial color

··· A) SINGLE COLOR DOMINATES: in different races, facial color and skin color have many variations, although in general, the normal facial color should be a harmonized mixture of the five different colors. When a single color dominates, it indicates a pathological change.

··· B) OBVIOUS EXPOSURE OF COLOR: normal facial color should be subtle and gentle. A sharply contrasting color on the skin indicates a disorder of the qi, blood, or *zàng fǔ* organs.

··· C) COLOR CHANGES ARE INCONSISTENT WITH CHANGES IN THE SEASONS: facial colors should change slightly following the changes of the seasons. Color changes inconsistent with the seasons indicate pathology.

— B. Abnormal facial sheen

Withered and dim is a pathological change of the facial sheen. This indicates a deficiency or failure of the essence qi.

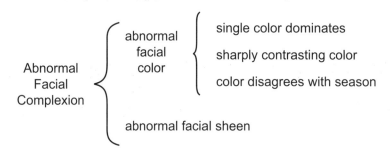

Chart 1.1.8 Scope of Abnormal Facial Complexions

(3) Pathological Facial Complexion and Indications

— A. The five colors and their associated diseases

··· A) BLUE-GREEN is ascribed to wood. It governs in spring, is the color of wind, and is related to the Liver and Gallbladder organs.

Distinguishing Features	Blue-Green Complexion		
	Indications	Pathogenesis	
blue-green	wind	Blood doesn't fill up the vessels (which are naturally blue-green) in the face due to obstruction or contraction of the blood vessels.	
dark blue-green (black)	cold		
sudden appearance blue-green	pain		
blue-green-purple	stasis		

Table 1.1.4 Blue-green Facial Color and its Indications

··· B) RED is ascribed to fire. It governs in summer, is the color of heat, and is related to the Heart and Small Intestine organs.

Red Complexion		
Distinguishing Features	**Indications**	**Pathogenesis**
red over entire face	excess heat	heat accelerates the flow of blood and fills vessels leading to the appearance of the red color
red cheeks	deficiency heat	
superficial zygomatic flush with pale face beneath	floating yang	

Table 1.1.5 Red Facial Color and its Indications

··· C) YELLOW is ascribed to earth. It governs in late summer, is the color of dampness, and is related to the Spleen and Stomach organs.

Yellow Complexion			
Distinguishing Features	**Indications**		**Pathogenesis**
bright orange yellow	jaundice	yang type	damp heat obstructs and steams the bile to the surface
smoky hazy yellow		yin type	
dim luster yellow	dampness		dampness accumulates which limits Spleen's transportation function leading to a lack of blood rising to the face, a slightly pale or yellow color ensues.
dull pale color yellow	cold damp in middle burner		
pale color yellow	Spleen qi deficiency		
puffy pale color yellow	Spleen qi deficiency with water accumulation		

Table 1.1.6 Yellow Facial Color and its Indications

··· D) WHITE (PALE) is ascribed to metal. It governs in autumn, is the color of dryness, and is related to the Lung and Large Intestine organs.

White (Pale) Complexion		
Distinguishing Features	**Indications**	**Pathogenesis**
pale blue-green	cold	cold contracts blood vessels which prevents color from appearing on face
pale white	qi deficiency	qi or blood deficiency gives rise to a loss of nourishment of the face which causes the pale color
bright white	yang deficiency	
pale white and withered yellow	blood deficiency	
pale white without sheen	bleeding	

Table 1.1.7 Pale Facial Color and its Indications

··· E) BLACK (DARK) is ascribed to water. It governs in winter, is the color of cold, and is related to the Kidney and Bladder organs.

Distinguishing Features	Black (Dark) Complexion	
	Indications	Pathogenesis
dark black	internal cold	channels and blood vessels spasm and contract causing the blood to stagnate and thus darken
dark black	Kidney yang deficiency	channels and blood vessels spasm and contract causing the blood to stagnate and thus darken
dry scorched black	Kidney yin deficiency	channels and blood vessels spasm and contract causing the blood to stagnate and thus darken
black eye sockets, swollen lower eyelid	phlegm damp	channels and blood vessels spasm and contract causing the blood to stagnate and thus darken
purple black	blood stasis	channels and blood vessels spasm and contract causing the blood to stagnate and thus darken

Table 1.1.8 Dark Facial Color and its Indications

— B. *Qualities of abnormal color*

When pathological colors manifest on the face, besides differences in color, there are also differences in such qualities as location, brightness, thickness, and concentration.

Quality		Description	Indications
Location	deep	color hidden inside skin	internal pattern
Location	floating	color visible superficially	exterior pattern
Brightness	bright (clear)	color is clear and distinct	yang pattern
Brightness	dull (dim)	color is dark and dim	yin pattern
Thickness	thin (faint)	color is shallow and light	qi deficiency
Thickness	thick (extreme)	color is deep and thick	excess pattern
Concentration	scattered	color is dispersed or scanty	new or mild disease
Concentration	concentrated	accumulated color	enduring or serious disease

Table 1.1.9 Qualities of Abnormal Facial Color and their Indications

— C. *Abnormal sheen*

CLINICAL MANIFESTATION: withered ("perishing"), dim, lusterless, and dry.

INDICATIONS: exhaustion of essence, loss of spirit, imminent death, and poor prognosis.

III. SUMMARY OF INSPECTION OF FACIAL COMPLEXION

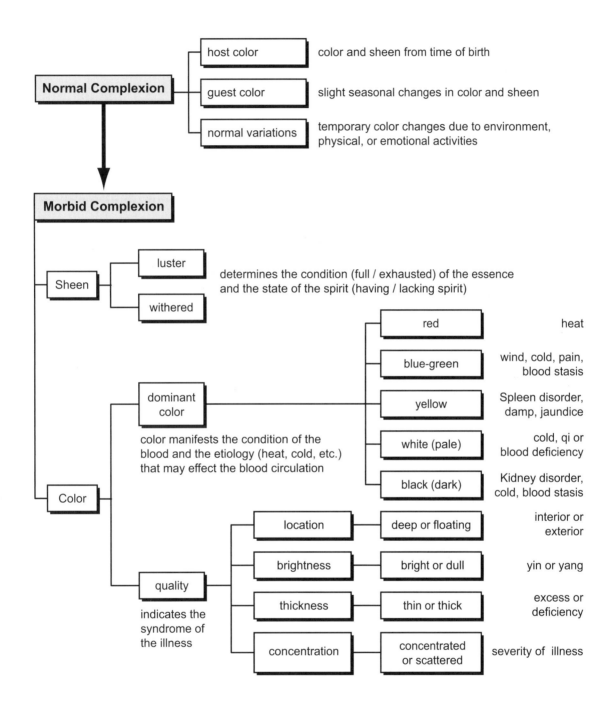

Chart 1.1.9 Summary of Inspection of Facial Complexion

■ Three: Inspection of Body Appearance

Inspection of the body appearance includes observing the body and its bearing. Body shape and bearing reflect the condition of the *zàng fǔ* organs, the status of yin and yang, and the state of qi and blood.

I. INTRODUCTION

(1) Definition

Form of the body or "body shape": This refers to the external form and constitution of the individual which can be described as robust (strong), weak, corpulent (fat) or emaciated (skinny).

Bearing or "movement": This refers to the posture and movements of the body, both the entire body, and also the individual parts such as eyes, face, mouth, limbs, or fingers.

(2) Physiology of the Body Appearance

Body appearance includes body form and body bearing. Bones, muscles, sinews, skin, and visible blood vessels are the basic elements for inspection of body form as well as the bearing of movement.

Kidney produces marrow and controls the bones. Spleen dominates the muscles and the four limbs. Liver dominates the sinews. Lung dominates the skin and hair. Heart dominates the blood vessels and houses the spirit. This is how TCM connects the body appearance to the condition of the internal organs. Hence, when the functions of *zàng fǔ* organs are sound, the physical body is strong and replete. When *zàng fǔ* organs are damaged, the physical body is weak.

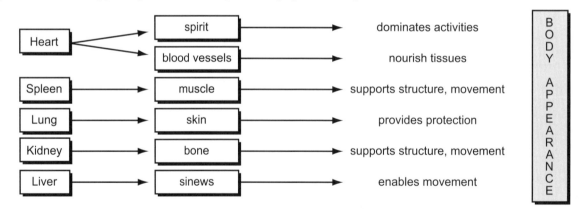

Chart 1.1.10 Internal Organs and Body Appearance

(3) Normal Body Appearance

Body appearance includes the form (figure, shape) and the bearing (posture and movement). The normal body form should be neither too tall nor too short, neither too fat nor too slim. There should be no swelling, distension, or deformation. The normal bearing should be natural and relaxed, flexible in movement, and quick in response.

(4) Clinical Significance of Body Appearance Inspection

Inspection of the body's appearance helps the practitioner:

- understand the function of *zàng fǔ* organs
- know the condition of yin and yang
- know the condition of qi and blood

II. INSPECTION OF THE BODY FORM

The body form refers to the exterior form and to the constitution of an individual. Every individual is born with a certain constitution and consequently a certain body shape. There is a tremendous variety of body shapes.

There are three aspects to consider when examining the physical appearance of a patient: constitution, long-term changes, and short-term changes.

(1) Constitutional Body Shapes according to the Five Phases

Constitution means the fundamental physical and mental make-up of the individual. Five constitutional types can be identified, each referring to one of the five phases. According to *The Divine Pivot*, Chapter 64 (靈樞。陰陽二十五人), identifying a particular type can be useful in determining the character and prognosis of any disease.

Body Type and Bearing	Phase	Facial Color	Characteristics	Strength
tall, thin body; fairly broad shoulders, strong and straight back	wood	green	hard workers, tendency to over think or worry	bones and sinews
small pointed head, or pointy chin, curly hair, or little hair, small hands, walks fast	fire	red	quick, energetic, and active; tend to be unconcerned about material wealth, fond of beauty, have short lives	blood vessels and blood
broad and square shoulders, triangular white face, strongly built body, walks slowly and deliberately	metal	white	meticulous, rational, independent and strong willed, a capable leader and manager	lungs and voice
large head and rounded body, large abdomen, strong thighs and wide jaws, walks without lifting feet	earth	yellow	calm and generous, not very ambitious, good interpersonal skills	muscles
round face and body, long spine	water	soft white	sympathetic and slightly lazy, loyal to their work colleagues; aware, sensitive, and sometime psychic	digestive system

Table 1.1.10 Constitutional Body Shape and Five Phases

(2) Long-term Changes in Physical Appearance

Long-term changes in physical appearance are usually related to the constitution of the individual, the condition of congenital essences, and acquired essence (nutrition).

— *A. Weight:* fatness and thinness can reflect the relative exuberance or debilitation of the yin, yang, qi, and blood of the body. Generally speaking, the obese patient will have excessive phlegm while the thin patient will have abundant fire.

	Body Form	Indications
overweight	obese, moves slowly	phlegm damp accumulation with qi deficiency
underweight	thin and dry body, muscles are emaciated	qi and blood deficiency, or yin deficiency with fire
emaciation	muscles are emaciated, bones are thin, skin is dry and shriveled, muscles have wasted away	critical condition, qi and essence exhausted, *zàng fǔ* organ failure

Table 1.1.11 Inspection of the Body Weight and its Indications

— *B. Height:* tallness and shortness can reflect the condition of the congenital and acquired essences. One must also remember to compare "normal" height and weight to the genetic pool from which the observed patient comes.

	Body Form	Indications
tall	tall and strong	sufficient essence
short	short, delayed development	insufficiency of congenital or acquired essence

Table 1.1.12 Inspection of the Body Height and its Indications

— *C. Deformation:* joints, spine, or other parts of the body structure. Usually indicates congenital insufficiency and/or poor nourishment after birth, and manifests as Spleen/Kidney depletion and softness of the bones.

(3) Short-term Changes in Physical Appearance

Short-term changes in the physical appearance are usually related to pathological changes in the body. Changes are the result of the struggle between the pathogenic factors and antipathogenic qi. These short-term changes reflect the condition of the *zàng fǔ* organs.

— A. Swelling

DEFINITION: enlargement due to accumulation of water, blood, or pus.

edema: subcutaneous retention of fluid which leads to puffiness of the head, face, eyelids, limbs, abdomen, or even the whole body. It usually happens bilaterally, but can also be unilateral.

swelling: to grow larger; to dilate or extend the exterior surface or dimensions. Usually happens unilaterally, or just local areas with pain or skin color change; occasionally may arise bilaterally.

PATHOMECHANISM: the pathogenesis of swelling is due to the dysfunction of water metabolism. This dysfunction can be related to *zàng fǔ* organ disorders or obstruction caused by blood stasis or phlegm accumulation.

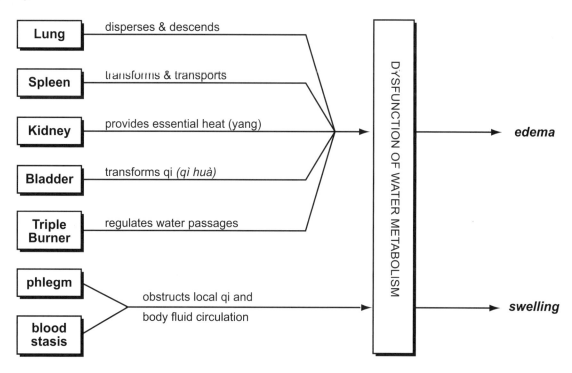

Chart 1.1.11 Pathogenesis of Edema and Swelling

SYMPTOMS AND INDICATIONS:

	Symptoms	Indications
Swelling	usually unilateral, or highly localized with pain and change in skin color	blood stasis or phlegm stagnation
Edema	abrupt onset, starts from the upper portion of the body, puffy face and eyelids	wind damp attack
	slow onset, usually found in the lower portion of the body	Spleen and/or Kidney yang deficiency

Table 1.1.13 Swelling, Edema, and their Indications

— B. Joint deformities

DEFINITION: joint shape changes characterized by swelling with or without redness; deformity, and limited range of motion; accompanied by soreness, pain, numbness and heavy sensations.

PATHOMECHANISM: when bone loses strength, joints deform. Kidney governs the bones, so Kidney deficiency is the major cause of joint deformities. Healthy bones need the nourishment of qi, blood, and marrow. If qi, blood, or marrow is insufficient, the bones can weaken and cause joint deformities. There are two causes for qi, blood, or marrow deficiency. One is pathogenic wind, cold, or damp invasion which obstructs the channels and collaterals. The second is a *zàng fǔ* organ deficiency, especially of the Kidney.

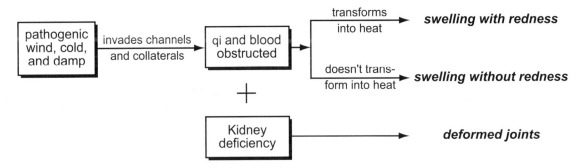

Chart 1.1.12 Pathogenesis of Joint Deformation

SYMPTOMS AND INDICATIONS:

	Symptoms	Indications
swelling	one or multiple joints with redness	damp heat, or wind damp heat
	usually involves lower limbs, bilateral, swollen without redness	damp, or cold damp
deformity	usually involves multiple small joints on the hands and feet	Kidney deficiency with cold damp

Table 1.1.14 Swelling, Deformity, and their Indications

III. Inspection of Bearing and Movement

Inspection of bearing includes observing the body's posture (static) and movement (dynamic). Normal bearing should be natural and relaxed, with flexible movement and quick responses.

(1) The Yin and Yang of Eight Pathological Bearings

Bearing or movements can be described in terms of yin and yang. Generally speaking, yang governs movement; yin governs stillness. Observation of the patient's movement or lack thereof can provide insight into the nature of their condition.

	Animation	Movement Strength	Lying Position	Posture
yang	movement	strong	face up	extended
yin	stillness	weak	face down	flexed

Table 1.1.15 Organization of Bearing by Yin and Yang

(2) Pathological Bearing and Movement

— A. Internal Wind Pattern

DEFINITION: involuntary movements such as convulsions, tremors, shaking, spasms, twitching, quivering, deviation of the mouth or eyes, and hemiplegia.

PATHOMECHANISM: internal wind is a spasm of the muscles and tendons. Movement and posture is the coordinated function of the muscle, sinews, and bones. Under healthy conditions, muscles and sinews are nourished by body fluids and blood. Any condition that results in the loss of nourishment to the muscles and sinews can give rise to contractions or spasms. Conditions that cause this lack of nourishment include excessive heat injuring the body fluids; yin or blood deficiency due to dysfunction of *zàng fǔ* organs; and pathogens such as phlegm or blood stasis obstructing the channels and collaterals.

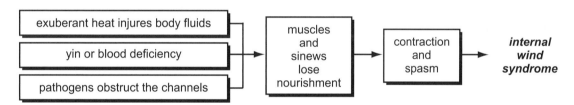

Chart 1.1.13 Pathomechanisms of Interior Wind Pattern

SYMPTOMS AND INDICATIONS:

Body Bearing and Movement	Indications
convulsive spasms, hypertonicity of the limbs, tremors, shaking, clenched jaw, opisthotonus in severe cases	damp heat toxin, or wind damp heat
deviated eyes and mouth, facial paralysis or hemiplegia	phlegm damp obstructing channels
twitching, quivering	Kidney deficiency with cold damp

Table 1.1.16 Pathological Body Bearing and Movement and their Indications

— B. Atrophy Disorder (痿症 *wěi zhèng*)

DEFINITION: limpness, weakness and lack of strength of the limbs; or inability to lift limbs, but not due to pain. In severe cases, muscle atrophy may occur.

PATHOMECHANISM: normal movement and posture depend on the strength of the bones and contraction of the muscles and sinews. Pathomechanisms for atrophy disorder include Spleen and Stomach deficiency in which the muscles lose their nutrition; Kidney deficiency where the bones become desiccated and the marrow is reduced; or when the Kidney fails to nourish the Liver giving rise to sinews that are deprived of nourishment. Pathogenic factors that obstruct the flow of qi and blood in the channels can also deprive structures of nourishment, leading to atrophy disorder.

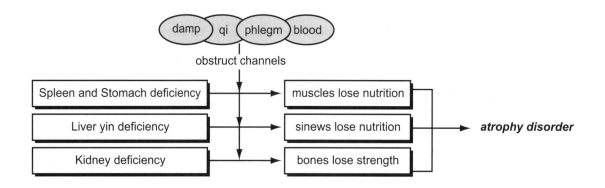

Chart 1.1.14 Pathomechanisms of Atrophy Disorder

SYMPTOMS AND INDICATIONS:

Body Bearing and Movement	**Indications**
heavy, cumbersome limbs that are limp & lack strength, they may be slightly swollen or numb with sensations of heaviness, more likely occurring in the lower limbs	damp heat
gradually worsening weakness and wilting of the limbs, over time muscles lose strength or even atrophy	Spleen and Stomach deficiency
usually effecting the lower limbs, bilateral or unilateral, chronic and gradual onset, numbness, without pain	Liver and Kidney yin deficiency

Table 1.1.17 Atrophy Disorder and its Indications

IV. Summary of Inspection of Body Appearance

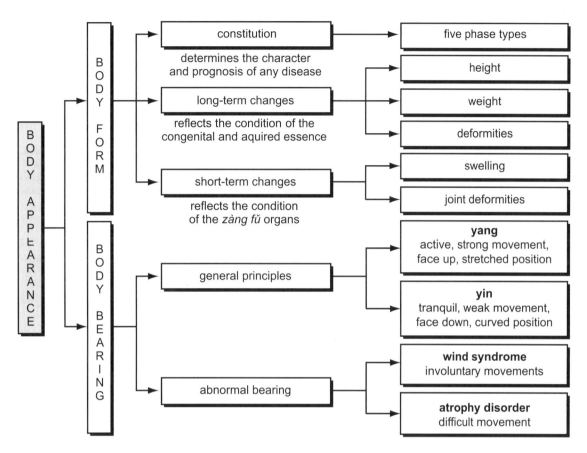

Chart 1.1.15 Summary of Body Appearance

Section 2

Inspection of Local Areas

■ One: Inspection of Eyes

Inspection of the eyes means to observe and examine the spirit, color, shape, and bearing of the eyes in order to assess the patient's spirit, the thermal nature of any pathogens, and the condition of the *zàng fǔ* organs.

I. INTRODUCTION

(1) Eye Inspection Theories

— A. Eye and Zàng fǔ Organ Relationship

The eye is the gathering place of essence qi (精氣 *jīng qì*) from the five *zàng* and six *fǔ* organs. *The Divine Pivot*, Chapter 80 (靈樞。大惑论) says "The essence from the five *zàng* and six *fǔ* flows upwards to irrigate the eyes." The Heart houses the spirit, and the capability to identify and visually distinguish items depends on the normal activities of the spirit. The Heart is also the organ that governs the blood. It is the Heart qi that provides the power to maintain normal blood circulation, which supplies nourishment to the eye. The eyes are the orifice of the Liver. The function of the Liver is to store the blood and control the sinews to maintain the eyes' normal vision and movement. Blood is the nutritive resource for the eyes, therefore the Spleen's function of generating blood and the Kidney's function of storing essence are directly related to the normal functioning of the eyes. The dispersing and descending function of the Lung maintains smooth qi circulation, which provides the power to maintain blood circulation. Because of this, the Lung is also indirectly related to the eyes.

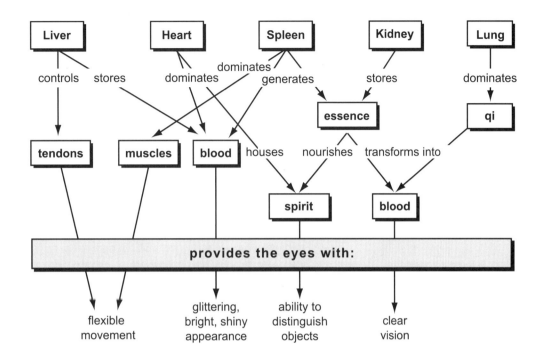

Chart 1.2.1 Eye and *Zàng Fǔ* Organ Relationships

— B. Five Wheels Theory

The theory of five wheels describes the relationship between the *zàng fǔ* organs and the eyes. It divides the eyes into five different parts or "wheels" in which each part is related to a different organ. These relationships not only describe anatomical and physiological connections, but also serve to reflect the pathological changes which make the five wheels diagnostically significant.

This theory was originally documented in *The Divine Pivot*: "The refined energies of the five *zàng* and the six *fǔ* of the human body pour upward to the eyes to enable one to see. The nest of the refined energy is the eye, the essence of the bone is the pupil, the essence of the sinews is the iris, the essence of blood is in the superficial veinules of the two canthi and the eye sockets, the essence of the breathing air of the body is the white of the eyes, the essence of the muscle is in the eyelid and surrounding flesh; when the refined energies of the sinews, bone, blood, and qi combine in the channels and collaterals of the eye, it forms the ocular system."

Five Wheels	**Corresponding Part of Eye**	***Zàng Fǔ* Organs**
blood wheel	inner and outer canthus	Heart / Small Intestine
qi wheel	sclera	Lung / Large Intestine
wind wheel	iris	Liver / Gallbladder
water wheel	pupil	Kidney / Urinary Bladder
flesh wheel	eyelids and surrounding muscle	Spleen/Stomach

Table 1.2.1 Five Wheels

— C. Eye and Channels Relationship

The connection between the eyes and *zàng fǔ* organs is dependent on the channels and collaterals. All twelve channels and collaterals are in direct or indirect connection with the eyes.

Eye Areas	Channels	Channel and Collateral Pathway
Originates at eyes	Foot *Shào Yáng*	arises from the outer canthus
	Foot *Tài Yáng*	arises from the inner canthus
	Foot *Yáng Míng*	originates lateral to the ala nasi (LI 21), ascends to inner canthus, meets BL channel at BL 1
Terminates at eyes	Hand *Shào Yáng*	a branch emerges anterior to the ear and reaches the outer canthus to link with the Gallbladder channel
	Hand *Tài Yáng*	a branch reaches the inner canthus to link with the BL channel, a branch passes through the outer canthus to enter the ear
	Foot *Yáng Míng*	divergent channel of the Stomach runs upward lateral to the nose and connects wtih the eye before joining the Stomach channel
	Rèn Mài	curves around the lips, passes through the cheek, and enters the infraorbital region.
	Yáng Qiào channel	ascends along the neck to the corner of the mouth, from which it then enters the inner canthus
	Yīn Qiào channel	from the zygoma, it reaches the inner canthus and communicates with the *yáng qiào* channel
Passes through eye region	Hand *Shào Yīn*	ascending portion of "Heart system" runs alongside the esophagus to connect with the "eye system"
	Foot *Jué Yīn*	ascends along the posterior aspect of the throat to the nasopharynx and connects with the "eye system"
Musculo-tendon meridian	Hand *Shào Yáng*	musculo-tendon meridian joins with the foot *tài yáng* to form a muscular net around the eye
	Foot *Yáng Míng*	musculo-tendon meridian joins with the foot *tài yáng* to form a muscular net around the eye

Table 1.2.2 Eye and Connected Channels and Collaterals

(2) Eye and Corresponding Parts of *Zàng Fǔ* Organs

As a further development of the five wheels theory, in modern times we associate specific parts of the eye structure with internal organs. The two canthi are associated with the Heart. The sclera corresponds to the Lung. The iris is associated with the Liver. The pupil corresponds to the Kidney. The eyelids and tissues immediately surrounding the eye are associated with the Spleen.

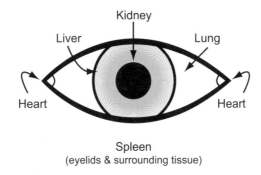

Illustration 1.2.1 Eye and Corresponding *Zàng Fǔ* Organs

(3) Normal Eyes

The normal eye should glitter and shine with clear and sharp vision, as well as flexible movement of the eyeballs. There is no swelling or ulcers on the eyelids; both eyes are the same size, and the eyelids freely open and close.

(4) Scope of Eye Inspection

Inspection of the eyes includes observing their spirit, color, shape, and bearing.

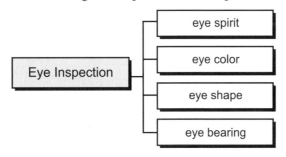

Chart 1.2.2 Scope of Eye Inspection

(5) Clinical Significance of Eye Inspection

Eye inspection enables the practitioner to:

- identify pathogenic factors and their thermal nature
- identify involved *zàng fǔ* organs
- understand the conditions of *zàng fǔ* organs
- make a prognosis.

II. Eye Inspection

(1) Inspecting the Spirit of the Eyes

DEFINITION: the spirit of the eyes is the external manifestation of the *zàng fǔ* organs. The spirit manifests in the vision, shape, and bearing (movement) of the eyes. It reflects the condition of the *zàng fǔ* organs and indicates the severity of the illness.

CLINICAL SIGNIFICANCE: inspecting the spirit of the eyes can assist in making a prognosis.

PATHOMECHANISM: under normal circumstances, essence qi from the five *zàng* and six *fǔ* all flow upward to nourish the eyes, which allows them to clearly distinguish things, appear bright and shiny, and move flexibly. When there is a *zàng fǔ* organ disorder, especially of the Kidney and Liver, essence and blood are unable to nourish the eyes. The eyes then lose their spirit and look dull and dim; eyesight is diminished, and the eyes move sluggishly.

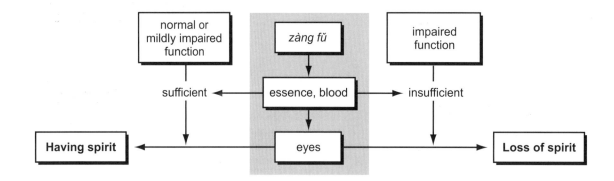

Chart 1.2.3 Pathomechanism of the Eye Spirit

Physiological and Pathological Eye Spirit and its Indications

	Manifestation	Indications	Prognosis
Having spirit	clear vision; bright and shiny luster, distinguishable iris, pupil, and sclera, flexible movement, little tear or eye secretion	sufficient Liver and Kidney qi, mild illness	good prognosis, curable disease
Loss of spirit	poor vision; dull luster, turbid hue in the sclera, iris and pupil borders are indistinguishable, dull luster, no tears or eye secretion	insufficient Liver and Kidney qi, severe illness	poor prognosis, disease difficult to cure

Table 1.2.3 Inspecting Eye Spirit and its Indications

(2) Inspecting the Color of the Eye

DEFINITION: in general, this refers to the colors found on the sclera. Eye color may also be extended into the iris and pupil. The normal color of the eyes should be white in the sclera; slightly red at the inner and outer canthi; brown (or blue, green, gray, etc.) in the iris; and black in the pupil. All colors should be clearly distinguishable.

CLINICAL SIGNIFICANCE: changes in eye color often signify pathogenic factors and their pathogenesis.

PATHOMECHANISM: redness in the eyes indicates pathogenic heat invading the body. Heat injures the blood vessels and causes bleeding. It also pushes blood upward to fill the blood vessels, giving rise to a red color.

White eye color indicates a lack of blood to fill the vessels. This can be due to qi or blood deficiency, or yang deficiency with cold, which obstructs the blood vessels and leads to insufficient blood.

Yellow eye color indicates that the Liver and Gallbladder channels are obstructed by dampness, qi, or blood stasis. In each case, the stagnation generates heat, which steams bile in the Liver and Gallbladder, which rises up to the eyes.

Black eye color is caused by extreme heat consuming the body fluids and concentrating the blood, which gives rise to the darker color. The color black is associated with Kidney failure by virtue of its five phase correspondence.

Blue-green indicates wind or Liver dysfunction. The blue-green color is associated with wind and the Liver by virtue of its five phase correspondence.

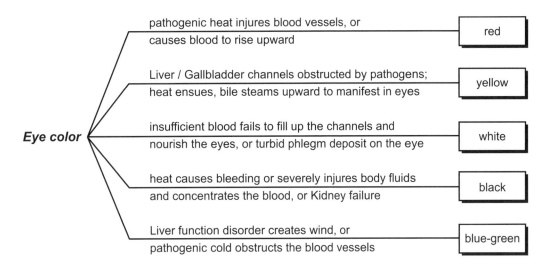

Chart 1.2.4 Pathomechanisms of Eye Color

Pathological Changes of Eye Color and their Indications

— *A. Yellow:* yellow on the sclera that may extend to the iris and pupil. Yellow signifies dampness.

Yellow Color	Other Symptoms	Indications
pale yellow, gradually becoming bright yellow orange	yellow urine, yellow tongue coating	damp heat
pale yellow, sometimes effects the vision	fatigue, loose stools	blood deficiency
dull yellow color, chronic	abdominal bloating, cold limbs	cold damp
golden yellow color of the eye and body, acute onset	fever, irritability, constipation	toxic heat
dim dull yellow	difficult urination, abdominal distention	qi / blood stagnation

Table 1.2.4 Yellow Eye Color and its Indications

— *B. Red:* excessive redness on the inner or outer canthus, or on the sclera; red vessels may also appear over the entire eye. Red signifies heat.

Red Color	Other Symptoms	Indications
red in the canthus area	excessive tearing, irritability, red tongue, dark urine	heat in the Heart
redness and swelling in the entire eye	headache, easily angered	rising of Liver fire or exterior wind heat
red in the sclera of the eyes	sore throat, cough	heat in the Lung
red in the iris and pupil of the eye	eye pain, headache, dark urine	excess heat in the Bladder
red that may extend into the pupils	dizziness, tinnitus, scanty tongue coating	yin deficiency with heat
blue-green or purple red vessels on the sclera	pain from physical trauma	traumatic injury
red eyes upon awakening that clear up later	bleeding, thirst	blood level heat

Table 1.2.5 Red Eye Color and its Indications

— C. *Blue-green:* blue-green on the sclera or iris. Blue-green signifies wind and cold.

Blue-Green Color	Other Symptoms	Indications
blue-green color in the sclera	severe headache, nausea, irritability, restlessness	wind fire attacking the eyes
	vertex headache, aversion to cold, desires warmth	cold stagnation, pain
blue-green on pupil, dry and dim sclera	dizziness, tinnitus, insomnia, poor memory	Kidney yin deficiency

Table 1.2.6 Blue-green Eye Color and its Indications

D. *Black:* black on the sclera. Black signifies water.

Black Color	Other Symptoms	Indications
black on the sclera which resembles crab eyes	severe pain, bitter taste in the mouth	accumulation of excess heat
black eye sockets	dizziness, poor memory, tinnitus, irritability, scanty coating	Liver and Kidney deficiency
black on the sclera, dim and dull eyeball	feeble respiration, profuse sweating of oily sweat	*zàng fǔ* organ qi depletion

Table 1.2.7 Black Eye Color and its Indications

— E. *White:* white on the inner or outer canthus is pale; the iris or pupil may also be white. White signifies deficiency.

White Color	Other Symptoms	Indications
white ring around iris	obesity, dizziness, stifling sensation in chest	turbid phlegm
iris color gradually lightening	dim vision, cold limbs, loose stools and frequent urination	yang deficiency with cold
cloudy white iris	dizziness, tinnitus, irritability, red tongue body, thirst	Liver and Kidney deficiency
pale white blood vessels in the canthus of the eyes	fatigue, dizziness, dry skin, pale tongue and face	qi and blood deficiency

Table 1.2.8 White Eye Color and its Indications

(3) Inspecting the Shape of the Eye

DEFINITION: also called "appearance" of the eyes. This refers to the outward appearance of the eyes' shape. The normal eye shape should be the same size on both sides. There is no swelling or ulcers on the eyelids. The eyelids open and close easily and flexibly.

CLINICAL SIGNIFICANCE: changes in the shape of the eye usually reflect the state of the qi (excess/deficiency) and the pathogenic factor (heat, dampness, etc.)

PATHOMECHANISM: normal eye shape requires the nourishment of qi, blood, and body fluids, as well as the normal functioning of the muscles and sinews to support the eyes' position in the skull. If qi, blood, or body fluids are insufficient due to an attack of exogenous pathogens or *zàng fǔ* organ deficiency, then the eyes, and the muscles and sinews around the eyes, will lose nourishment and support, which will cause the eyes to sink inward. If an accumulation of excessive pathogens fights with exuberant antipathogenic qi, this can push the eyeballs outward, leading to exophthalmia. Dampness may also accumulate around the eyes, giving rise to local swelling.

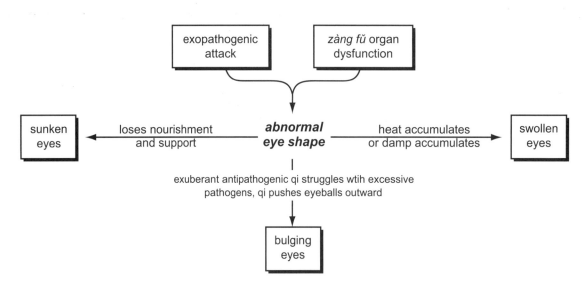

Chart 1.2.5 Pathomechanisms of Pathological Eye Shape

Pathological Changes of Eye Shape and their Indications

— A. Exophthalmia:

Also called "bulging eyes," this refers to the protrusion of the patient's eyeball on one or both sides. Exophthalmia usually indicates a condition of excess.

Description		Indications
protruding eyeballs, headache, red tongue, yellow greasy tongue coating		Liver yang rising
protruding eyeballs with dyspnea or asthma with an inability to lie flat, palpitations		Lung qi stagnation
protruding eyeballs with swellings in the neck	distention headache and dizziness, irritability, easily angered	qi stagnation with heat
	dizziness, tinnitus, five center heat, red tongue, scanty coating	yin deficiency with relative yang excess
	headache, diplopia (double vision), purple tongue body with spots on the lateral margins	qi and blood stagnation

Table 1.2.9 Bulging Eyes and their Indications

— B. Sunken Eyes

Sunken eyes means that the eyeball has sunken deeper into the eye socket. It usually indicates a condition of deficiency.

Description	Indications
following severe or chronic illness, the eyeball gradually sinks deeper into the eye socket	qi deficiency
sudden onset of sunken eyes, follows severe vomiting, diarrhea, or loss of blood	Spleen deficiency with Liver excess
chronic or critical condition, the eyeball sinks inward relatively deeply, suggests unfavorable prognosis	yin and yang depletion

Table 1.2.10 Sunken Eyes and their Indications

— C. Swollen Eyes

Swollen eyes means that the eyelid (upper, lower, or both) is swollen; it may be accompanied by redness and wet skin. It usually indicates dampness or water retention.

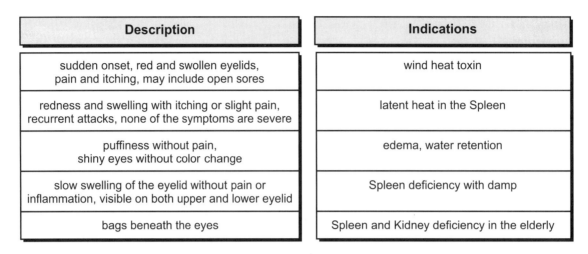

Description	Indications
sudden onset, red and swollen eyelids, pain and itching, may include open sores	wind heat toxin
redness and swelling with itching or slight pain, recurrent attacks, none of the symptoms are severe	latent heat in the Spleen
puffiness without pain, shiny eyes without color change	edema, water retention
slow swelling of the eyelid without pain or inflammation, visible on both upper and lower eyelid	Spleen deficiency with damp
bags beneath the eyes	Spleen and Kidney deficiency in the elderly

Table 1.2.11 Swollen Eyes and their Indications

(4) Inspecting the Bearing of the Eye

DEFINITION: also called the state of the eye, this refers to the movement and bearing of the eyeball and eyelid. Normal eye bearing means that the pupils are of equal size, 3–5 mm in diameter, and are responsive to light. In general, movement of the eyeballs should be flexible and agile.

CLINICAL SIGNIFICANCE: inspection of the eye bearing can help to identify the thermal nature of the pathogens and their pathogenesis.

PATHOMECHANISM: normal eye bearing depends on the normal functioning of the muscles and sinews. Therefore abnormal functioning of the muscles (spastic or flaccid) and sinews (spasms) are the pathomechanisms of pathological eye bearing. Spasms of the muscles or sinews can be due to either exopathogenic attack (wind or heat) or to qi and blood deficiency, where the muscles and sinews lack nourishment. Flaccidity of the muscles and sinews is usually due to *zàng fǔ* organs dysfunction, especially the Kidney and the Liver.

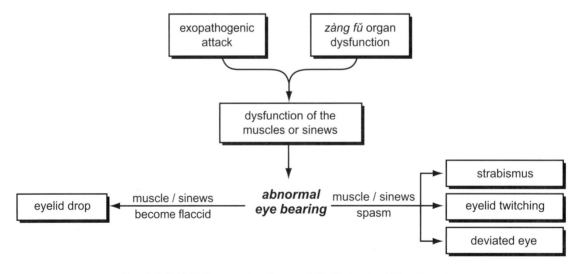

Chart 1.2.6 Pathomechanisms of Pathological Eye Bearing

Pathological Changes of Eye Bearing and their Indications

— *A. Strabismus*

The eye cannot look straight, or deviates to one side or the other. This can happen in one eye or both eyes.

Description	Indications
sudden onset, usually upon arising from sleep, eyeball deviated to one side, no redness or swelling, usually happens in only one eye, may be accompanied by deviated mouth, headache, dizziness, and aversion to wind	wind attack in the collaterals
sudden onset, eyeball deviates to one side and is difficult to move, usually happens in one eye, accompanying symptoms include nausea, vomiting, fatigue, tightness in chest, greasy tongue coating, slippery pulse	damp phlegm obstructing the collaterals
both eyeballs deviate to one side or upward, high fever, headache, possible coma, convulsion, red tongue, wiry rapid pulse	wind heat flaring upwards
unilateral or bilateral deviation of the eyeball, red color in sclera, accompanying symptoms include headache, bitter taste in mouth, irritability, numbness in the limbs, wiry pulse	Liver wind
onset following traumatic injury	blood stagnation
congenital onset, unilateral or bilateral, sometimes with delayed development and mental retardation	benign birth defect or essence deficiency

Table 1.2.12 Strabismus and its Indications

— *B. Eyelid spasms*

Also described as "eyelid twitching," this refers to the involuntary unilateral spasms of the eyelid. It may also radiate to the eyebrow.

Description	Indications
frequent involuntary spasm, dry and itchy eyes, pale face and lips, thready pulse	blood deficiency
eyelid spasms with frequent blinking, eyelid feels heavy and tired, poor appetite, fatigue, flabby tongue	Spleen and Stomach qi deficiency
occasional eyelid spasm; red, painful, or itchy eyes, may have sores surrounding eye; may be accompanied by headache, fever, chills, and floating pulse	wind heat attack

Table 1.2.13 Eyelid Spasms and their Indications

— C. Eyelid Drop

Also known as "blepharoptosis," this refers to the drooping of the upper eyelid and difficulty in keeping the eye open completely. The upper eyelid may block half or more of the eye.

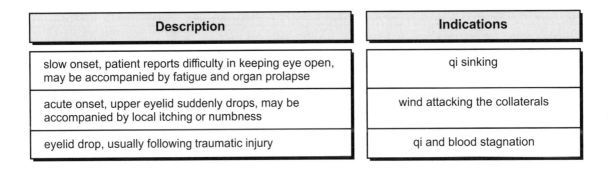

Description	Indications
slow onset, patient reports difficulty in keeping eye open, may be accompanied by fatigue and organ prolapse	qi sinking
acute onset, upper eyelid suddenly drops, may be accompanied by local itching or numbness	wind attacking the collaterals
eyelid drop, usually following traumatic injury	qi and blood stagnation

Table 1.2.14 Blepharoptosis and its Indications

— D. Platycoria

Platycoria refers to dilation of the pupils, where the diameter increases to more than 5 mm. It usually indicates exhaustion of the Kidney essence, which fails to pour upward to the eyes to contract the pupils. It is usually a sign of the terminal stage of a disease. It is sometimes seen in glaucoma patients as well.

— E. Myosis

Myosis refers to contraction of the pupils, the diameter of the pupils decreases to less than 2 mm. It usually indicates flaring-up of Liver and Gallbladder fire. Myosis may also indicate an overdose of *chuān wū tóu* (Aconiti Radix Preparata), *cǎo wū tóu* (Aconiti Kusnezoffii Radix), *zhì fù zǐ* (Aconiti Radix lateralis preparata), or poisonous mushrooms.

III. Summary of Inspection of the Eyes

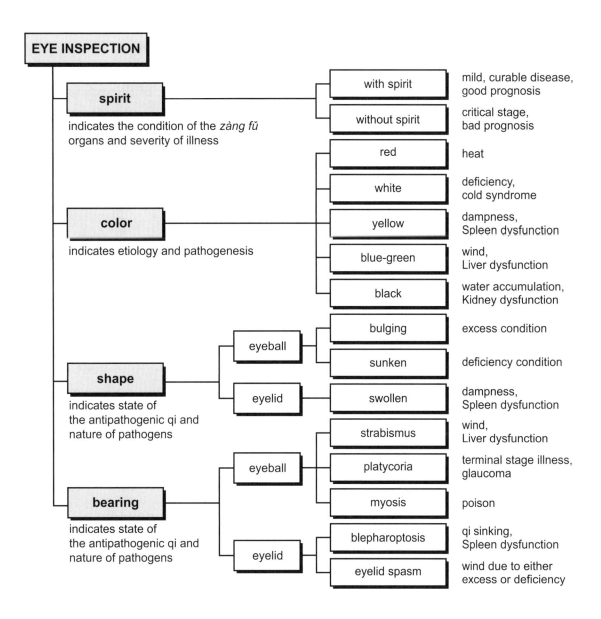

Chart 1.2.7 Summary of Eye Inspection

■ Two: Inspection of Ears and Nose

I. INSPECTION OF THE EARS

The Kidney opens to the ears. All six yang channels travel into or around the ears. They are a gathering place for the channels and collaterals. Through the channels and collaterals, the ears connect with the five *zàng*, the six *fǔ*, and the entire body. Therefore, inspection of the ears not only helps one to know the pathological changes of the Kidney and Gallbladder, but the condition of the entire body.

(1) Inspection of Ear Shape

The normal ear shape should be of average size without dryness or scaling. Healthy ears are also free of sores, boils, or swellings.

Ear Shape	Indications
small and thin ear	insufficient congenital essence or Kidney qi
dry helix with scales	blood stasis
sores, boils, or swelling and redness on the helix	wind heat or Liver and Gallbladder fire

Table 1.2.15 Pathological Changes of Ear Shape and their Indications

(2) Inspection of Ear Discharge

The appearance of a small amount of ear wax is considered normal, however the appearance of yellow or white pus, or blood, are considered pathological.

Ear Discharge	Indications
ear wax	normal discharge
yellow or white pus	Kidney yin deficiency fire with damp heat in the Liver and Gallbladder channels
blood	heat in blood

Table 1.2.16 Pathological Changes in Ear Discharge and their Indications

(3) Inspection of Ear Color and Sheen

The normal ear color and sheen should not favor any of the five colors or appear withered, parched, or burnt.

Ear Color and Sheen		Indications
withered and parched helix		exhaustion of Kidney qi
five colors	white	sudden onset of wind cold, or cold
	green-black	excruciating pain
	black	Kidney failure
	red	excess heat or damp heat
	red collateral on the back of the ear that feels cold to the practitioner's touch	prodrome of measles
	yellow	damp heat accumulation in Kidney

Table 1.2.17 Pathological Changes in the Color and Sheen of the Ear and their Indications

II. INSPECTION OF THE NOSE

The Lung opens to the nose. The nose is the sense organ for smelling and is the passageway of inhalation and exhalation. It is located in the center of the face (analogous to the middle burner) and is associated with earth; for these reasons, it is governed by the Spleen. Air is inhaled into the body, and stored in the Heart and Lung. When there is a disorder of the Heart and Lung, the nose will be congested. The *yáng míng* channels of hand and foot, as well as the hand *tài yáng* channel, all directly connect to the nose.

Inspection of the nose will not only help us understand the pathological changes of the Lung, Spleen, and Stomach, but also to judge the excess or deficiency of the *zàng fǔ* organs and the condition of the Stomach qi. Knowing the condition of the Stomach qi can ultimately inform the prognosis.

(1) Inspection of Nose Shape

The normal nose shape should be neither swollen nor sunken or shrunken. There should be no sores or missing nasal tissues. Flaring nostrils can arise in the presence of pathological changes to the Lung.

Nose Shape	Indications
swollen nose	excess condition
sunken	insufficient antipathogenic qi, deficiency condition
nasal polyp	stagnated heat in *yáng míng* channel
ulcerous and sunken nasal septum	syphilis
sunken nasal septum with loss of eyebrows	leprosy
flaring nostrils with high fever	wind heat or phlegm heat accumulation in the Lung, or asthma
flaring nostrils during critical stage of illness	Lung failure

Table 1.2.18 Pathological Changes of Nose Shape and their Indications

(2) Inspection of Nasal Discharge

The normal nose should lack any particular discharge. When there is discharge, its color and consistency can provide insight into pathological changes of the Lung.

Nasal Discharge		Indications
epistaxis (nosebleed)		heat injury to the Lung and Stomach
nasal discharge	clear and thin	wind cold attack
	yellow or turbid	wind heat attack
	chronic and turbid	internal damp

Table 1.2.19 Pathological Changes of Nasal Discharge and their Indications

(3) Inspection of Nasal Color and Sheen

The normal color and sheen of the nose should be supple and moist without a predominance of any of the five colors listed below.

Nasal Color and Sheen		Indications
withered		exhaustion of Spleen and Stomach qi, severe disease
five colors	white	Lung disorder, bleeding, or qi and blood deficiency
	blue-green	abdominal pain or excess cold
	black	water retention due to Kidney deficiency
	red	heat in the Spleen and Lung channels, if deep red or purple with acne, it indicates alcoholism
	yellow	internal damp heat, or constipation due to Spleen yang deficiency

Table 1.2.20 Pathological Changes in the Color and Sheen of the Nose and their Indications

■ Three: Inspection of Teeth, Gums, and Throat

Teeth are the surplus of bone, and bone is governed by the Kidney. Therefore, the growth, changes, and failure of the teeth are all directly related to the function of the Kidney. The *yáng míng* channels of hand and foot pass through the gums. Hence, inspection of the teeth and gums contributes to understanding Kidney, Stomach, and Intestinal disorders.

I. INSPECTION OF TEETH

Normal teeth should be bright, moist, and clean without tartar. All the teeth should be present.

Teeth Inspection		Description	Indications
color	white	white with a moist sheen, bright and clean	Kidney qi flourishing
		white, dry, without sheen	Kidney yin exhaustion
	yellow	gradually yellows with age	normal physiology
		sudden change to yellow	Kidney deficiency
		dull yellow, like soy bean	Kidney failure
	black	purplish black, like black bean	exhaustion of both yin and yang
tartar		grimy yellow	evaporated Stomach turbidity
		burnt and dry	Kidney & Stomach yin exhaustion
shape		delayed appearance of baby or adult teeth in children	essence deficiency
		teeth grow at deviated angles, or missing teeth	insufficient *yáng míng qi*
		loss of teeth among adults, receding gums with exposure of the roots of the teeth	flaming upward of deficiency fire due to Kidney yin deficiency

Table 1.2.21 Pathological Changes of the Teeth and their Indications

II. INSPECTION OF THE GUMS

Normal gums should be moist, pink, and free of bleeding, ulcers, or swellings.

Gums Inspection		Description	Indications
color	red	red with moist sheen	normal
		deep red with swelling	excess heat in the *yáng míng*
	pale	pale gums	blood deficiency
		pale, atrophied gums	Kidney deficiency
	blue	line between teeth and gums	mercury poisoning
shape		swollen gums	Stomach fire flaming upwards
		ulcerations or bleeding	
bleeding		bleeding with pain & swelling	Stomach fire flaming upwards
		chronic bleeding without pain	deficiency fire flaming upwards
			Spleen qi deficiency

Table 1.2.22 Pathological Changes of the Gums and their Indications

III. INSPECTION OF THE THROAT

The throat is the gateway to the Lung and Stomach and the passageway for breath and food. The throat is also the structure that produces the voice. The Liver channel ascends along the posterior aspect of the throat to the nasophrynx; the Gallbladder channel rises up the throat; and the Kidney channel enters the Lung, runs along the throat, and terminates at the root of the tongue. In addition, the Stomach, Heart, Small Intestine, Spleen, Lung, Large Intestine, Pericardium, Conception Vessel *(rèn mài)*, Governing Vessel *(dū mài)*, and Penetrating Vessel *(chōng mài)* are all directly or indirectly connected to the throat. Hence, changes in the throat can reflect internal *zàng fǔ* organ disorders.

The normal throat should be pink to red in color, moist with normal breathing sounds, and permit smooth swallowing.

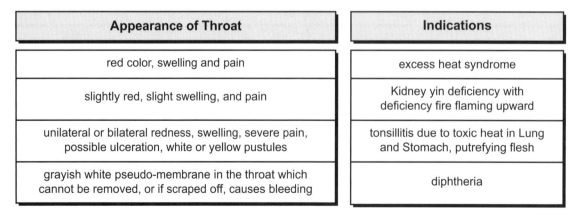

Appearance of Throat	Indications
red color, swelling and pain	excess heat syndrome
slightly red, slight swelling, and pain	Kidney yin deficiency with deficiency fire flaming upward
unilateral or bilateral redness, swelling, severe pain, possible ulceration, white or yellow pustules	tonsillitis due to toxic heat in Lung and Stomach, putrefying flesh
grayish white pseudo-membrane in the throat which cannot be removed, or if scraped off, causes bleeding	diphtheria

Table 1.2.23 Pathological Changes of the Throat and their Indications

◼ Four: Inspection of Lips and Mouth

Inspection of the lips involves examining their color, moisture, shape, and bearing, which reflect the state of the qi and blood and the body fluids. This will enable the practitioner to identify pathogenic factors and to make a prognosis.

I. INTRODUCTION

(1) Lip Inspection Theory

The Spleen opens to the mouth and manifests externally on the lips. The Stomach channel encircles the lips, the Large intestine channel curves around the upper lip, the Liver channel curves around the inner surface of the lips, and the Governing Vessel *(dū mài)* circulates inside the lips. Hence, the condition of the lips not only reflects the functioning of the Spleen, but also of the Stomach, Large Intestine, Liver and Governing Vessel *(dū mài)*.

The appearance of the lips is supported by the Heart, Spleen and Stomach, whose relationship to the blood gives rise to the lustrous red color of the lips. The Kidney, Lung, and Spleen all provide the body fluids which are necessary to moisturize the lips; and the Spleen and Liver govern the muscles and tendons, which enable the lips to move flexibly.

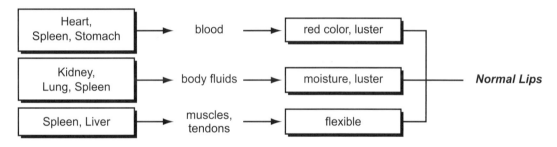

Chart 1.2.8 Physiology of the Lips

(2) Normal Lips

Normal lips are red, lustrous and moist, neither swollen, nor atrophied, and neither deviated, nor shaking. Their movement is free and flexible. Normal lip appearance reflects Stomach qi sufficiency, harmonized qi and blood, and no disturbing pathogenic factor.

(3) Clinical Significance of Lip Inspection

Inspection of the lips can help the practitioner:

- identify pathogenic factors, and their thermal nature
- understand the condition of the Spleen, Stomach, and other *zàng fǔ* organs
- understand the condition of the body fluids
- predict a disease prognosis.

(4) Scope of Lip Inspection

When looking at the lips, the practitioner should assess the color, luster, moisture, shape, and bearing (movements) of the lips.

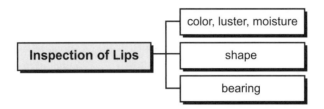

Chart 1.2.9 Scope of Lip Inspection

II. Clinical Manifestation of Pathological Changes of the Lips

(1) Lip Color

DEFINITION: normal lips should have a lustrous, moist, fresh red color. This indicates sufficient Spleen and Stomach qi as well as blood and yin. Lip color usually depends on the quantity and quality of the blood.

CLINICAL SIGNIFICANCE: to assess the condition of the qi and blood, and the thermal nature of any pathogenic factors.

PATHOMECHANISM: color of the lips depends on the condition of the qi and blood. When qi and blood are sufficient to fill the lips, the color is red and bright. If the lips are overfilled, the color will be a deep red. When there is not enough blood to fill the lips, they will look pale.

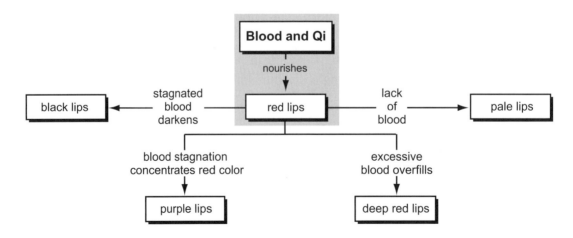

Chart 1.2.10 Pathomechanisms of Pathological Lip Colors

Pathological Changes in Lip Color and their Indications

— A. *Pale lips:* the color is much more pale than normal.

Description	Indications	Pathomechanism
pale lips and tongue	blood deficiency	red is the color of blood, when blood deficiency fails to fill the lips, or qi deficiency cannot push the blood up to the lips, they'll lose red color
pale lips with fatigue	qi deficiency	
pale withered lips, usually seen in critical conditions	qi depletion	
pale lips and face, with sensations of cold	deficiency cold	blood lacks the power to push or cold causes vessels to contract

Table 1.2.24 Pale lips and their Indications

— B. *Deep Red lips:* the color is more red than normal.

Description	Indications	Pathomechanism
dry and crimson lips	interior heat	the color of heat and fire is red; heat injures and concentrates the yin and blood
bright red lips	heat toxin	
crimson lips	deficiency heat	
cherry colored lips	gas poisoning	toxin damages the blood cell changing its color

Table 1.2.25 Deep Red Lips and their Indications

— C. *Purple lips:* the color is purple.

Description	Indications	Pathomechanism
pale purple lips	Heart yang deficiency cold	cold causes the vessels to constrict and blood to stagnate, when blood stagnates locally, the purple color ensues
bluish purple lips	excess cold	
purple lips with dark spots or greenish purple lips	blood stagnation	
deep red purple lips	heat in the nutritive or blood levels	heat consumes blood or body fluids which causes blood to accumulate

Table 1.2.26 Purple Lips and their Indications

— D. *Blackish lips:* the color looks greenish or blackish, with a dull intensity.

Description	Indications	Pathomechanism
greenish black lips	extreme cold	cold causes the vessels to constrict and blood to stagnate, when blood stagnates locally, the purple color ensues
gray lips	qi depletion	
purplish black lips with dark spots	qi and blood stagnation	
deep purple with green tint	excessive Stomach heat	heat consumes the body fluids and causes blood to concentrate

Table 1.2.27 Blackish Lips and their Indications

(2) Lip Shape

DEFINITION: lip shape refers to the general appearance of the lips. Normal lip shape should be free of swelling, atrophy, peeling, or erosion. The surface of the lips should be smooth and moist.

CLINICAL SIGNIFICANCE: the lip shape can help identify the pathogens and reflect the condition of the qi and blood.

PATHOMECHANISM: normal shape of the lips requires sufficient qi, blood, and body fluids for nourishment, and normal functioning of the muscles and sinews for support. Hence, if qi, blood, or body fluids are insufficient due to an exogenous pathogenic attack or dysfunction of internal organs, the lips will become dry and peeled. If the muscles or sinews are impaired by exogenous factors or suffer a loss of nourishment due to internal organ dysfunction, the lips may become swollen or eroded.

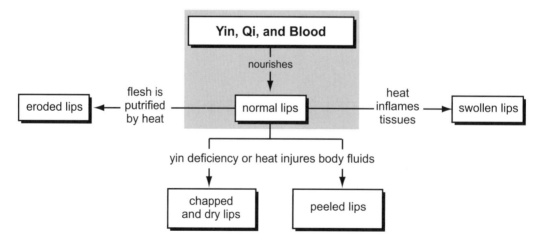

Chart 1.2.11 Pathomechanisms of Lip Shape

Pathological Changes of Lip Shape and their Indications

— A. *Swollen lips:* the lips are swollen, and their color is red or overly shiny.

Description and Symptoms	Indications
red swollen lips with a dry mouth, red tongue, dry yellow coating	toxic heat in Spleen and Stomach
red swollen lips with poor appetite, red tongue, yellow greasy coating	damp heat
itching and swollen lips; with clear discharge and burning pain after broken	"lip wind" due to Stomach fire
pale swollen lips, lips that are dim and lusterless; cold limbs, thready and weak pulse	qi depletion

Table 1.2.28 Swollen Lips and their Indications

— B. *Chapped and dry lips:* the lips are very dry, even cracked.

Description	Indications	
chapped lips, thirst with desire to drink	excess interior heat	Lung / Stomach
chapped lips, no thirst		Spleen / Large Intestine
chapped lips, thirst but with little desire to drink		nutritive or blood levels
chapped lips, thick yellow coating, belching		food stagnation
dry mouth and throat, dry nose, red and dry lips, red tongue with scanty coating	yin deficiency with dryness	
dry mouth and lips, dark purple lip color, thirst with no desire to swallow, black or purple spots on the lips or tongue	blood stagnation	
dry and cracked lips, no thirst, pale lips and tongue, cold limbs	deficiency cold	

Table 1.2.29 Chapped Lips and their Indications

— C. *Peeled lips:* the lips are peeled and dry, and slightly swollen with cracks; mostly seen in the lower lip.

Description and Symptoms	Indications
peeled lips without color change, red tongue, yellow coating	Spleen heat
peeled red lips, dry mouth and thirst, irritability, red tongue, scanty coating	yin deficiency

Table 1.2.30 Peeled Lips and their Indications

— *D. Erosion:* marked by white tissue in mouth sores. There is a stabbing pain when the white tissue is removed, beneath which is raw tissue with a reddish color.

Description and Symptoms	Indications
eroded lips, irritability, red tongue body, yellow coating	excess interior heat
usually arises after febrile disease, erosion of the lips, dry red tongue, scanty coating	yin deficiency with heat
eroded lips, anorexia, red tongue, greasy yellow coating	damp heat in the Spleen

Table 1.2.31 Eroded Lips and their Indications

(3) Lip Bearing

DEFINITION: lip bearing is also called the state of the lips. It refers to the movements and relaxed state of the lips. Normal lips should open and close flexibly and voluntarily, without deviation or twitching, tightness or drooling. The lips are relaxed and flexible.

CLINICAL SIGNIFICANCE: the bearing of the lips can help identify the pathogens and reflect the condition of the *zàng fǔ* organs.

PATHOMECHANISM: the bearing of the lips is dependent upon the muscles and sinews. When the muscles around the mouth are flaccid, it can lead to a drooping mouth, drooling, or a mouth that cannot close. If the sinews and muscles around the mouth spasm due to malnutrition or a pathogenic attack of wind, there could be tightness, lockjaw, twitching, or deviation of the mouth.

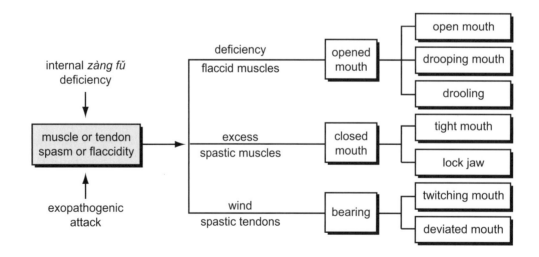

Chart 1.2.12 Pathomechanisms of Lip Bearing

Pathological Changes of Lip Bearing and their Indications

— A. *Tight mouth:* the lips are rigid and spastic, causing tightly pouting closed lips which impede the ability to eat and drink.

Description and Symptoms	Indications
usually seen in neonatal patients, tight mouth with spasm of limbs and opisthotonus	excess wind ("umbilicus wind")
usually seen in the late stage of a critical condition, tight mouth, cold limbs	deficiency wind

Table 1.2.32 Tight Mouth and its Indications

— B. *Lockjaw:* the mouth and teeth close tightly, and cannot open.

Description and Symptoms	Indications
lockjaw, opisthotonus, limb spasms, chills and fever	exterior wind toxin (tetanus)
usually associated with a high fever, limb spasms, may be accompanied by dysentery	wind due to excess heat
hemiplegia, lockjaw, coma in some cases	wind stroke
sudden attack, twisted limbs, recovers after a few minutes	wind phlegm (epilepsy)
neonatal patient, bluish face color, cold body	excess cold

Table 1.2.33 Lockjaw and its Indications

— C. *Deviated mouth:* the mouth is twisted to one side, usually accompanied by deviation of the eye.

Description and Symptoms	Indications
mouth or eyes twisted to one side, usually no other symptoms	wind attack in the collaterals
sudden loss of consciousness, deviated eyes, mouth, or tongue, hemiplegia	wind stroke
deviated mouth and eye, burning pain, earache accompanied by headache, bitter taste in the mouth, red face	heat toxin injures collaterals

Table 1.2.34 Deviated Mouth and its Indications

— *D. Open mouth:* the mouth remains open and cannot close.

Description and Symptoms	Indications
patient's mouth remains open with high fever, red face, thirst, canker sore	excess heat
open mouth breathing, shortness of breath, cough with foamy sputum	Lung deficiency with phlegm stagnation
sudden attack, open mouth, drooling with mucus, loss of consciousness	wind phlegm (epilepsy)

Table 1.2.35 Open Mouth and its Indications

— *E. Lip droop:* the lips hang down and cannot close.

Description and Symptoms	Indications
drooping lips, fatigue, pale tongue with white coating	middle qi sinking
lips droop or excessive flaccidity, usually occurring after chronic diarrhea or dysentery, cold limbs, low back pain	Spleen/Kidney yang deficiency

Table 1.2.36 Lip Droop and its Indications

— *F. Lip twitching:* the lips tremble, twitch, or shake involuntarily.

Description and Symptoms	Indications
lips shake or tremble; pale lips, face, tongue; weak pulse	Spleen qi deficiency
lips twitching or shaking, pale lips and nails, thin pulse	wind due to blood deficiency

Table 1.2.37 Lip Twitching and its Indications

— *G. Involuntary drooling:* there is copious saliva, mucus in the corner of the mouth, or drooling.

Description and Symptoms	Indications
involuntary drooling, profuse watery saliva, aggravated by cold	Spleen deficiency
profuse saliva in the mouth with occasional drooling, cough with foamy sputum, pale tongue	Lung deficiency with cold
mostly seen in children, involuntary drooling, red lips and tongue, possible canker sores	Spleen heat
deviated mouth and tongue, drooling, hemiplegia	wind stroke
sudden attack, drooling, loss of consciousness	wind phlegm (epilepsy)

Table 1.2.38 Involuntary Drooling and its Indications

III. SUMMARY OF LIP INSPECTION

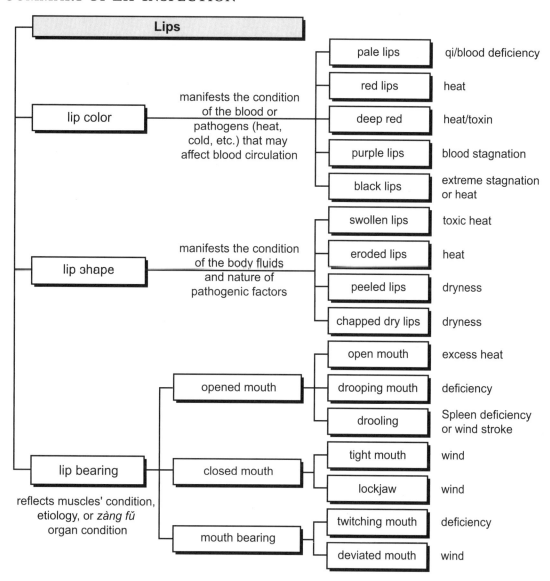

Chart 1.2.13 Summary of Lip Inspection

▦ Five: Inspection of Skin, Hair, and Nails

I. INSPECTION OF SKIN

The skin covers the entire surface of the body. It is irrigated by the body's blood vessels and collaterals, and correlates with the Lung internally. Skin is the external manifestation of qi and blood. Defensive qi circulates beneath the skin, and acts as a protective shield for the human body. Attack by exogenous factors, or disorders of the qi, blood, and body fluids, can all cause pathological changes in the skin.

Inspection of the skin not only helps us understand the pathological changes of the Lung, but also helps us assess the excess or deficiency of the *zàng fǔ* organs or other pathological changes, the condition of qi and blood, and the thermal nature of the pathogens. Inspection of the skin can also reveal the severity of the illness and its prognosis.

The scope of inspection of the skin includes its color, moisture, edema and distention, and lesions.

(1) Skin color: normal skin color should be bright, lustrous, and a harmonious blend of all five colors.

Skin Color	Indications
red	internal heat
yellow: entire body has a yellow hue	jaundice due to cold damp or damp heat
black (dark): skin color is dark and dim	Kidney yang failure
white: white patches gradually appear with clear margin	vitiligo due to wind damp attack which causes qi and blood disharmony

Table 1.2.39 Abnormal Skin Colors and their Indications

(2) Skin Moisture

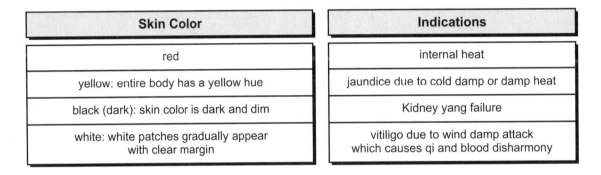

Skin Moisture		Indications
moist skin		exuberance of Lung qi, sufficient body fluids
dry skin	generalized dry skin	decline of Lung qi or insufficient body fluids
	dry skin with scales	blood stasis or internal carbuncle

Table 1.2.40 Skin Moisture and its Indications

(3) Edema and Distention

edema: subcutaneous retention of fluid which leads to puffiness, usually caused by water retention due to a disorder of the Lung, Spleen, or Kidney.

distention: abdominal expansion and bulging, usually caused by qi stagnation due to a disorder of the Spleen and Stomach.

Edema and Distention		Indications
edema	starts from face or upper part of body, then gradually involves entire body	yang edema
	starts from feet or lower limbs, then involves entire body, but lower part is more severe	yin edema
distention		qi stagnation or dampness in the middle burner

Table 1.2.41 Edema, Distention and their Indications

(4) Inspection of Skin Lesions

— *A. Papule (疹 zhěn):* also called a "rash," with an eruption roughly the size and shape of a seed. It has a red color, distinct borders, and is raised above the skin. It can be felt by touching and may be scattered or accumulated in patches. Its red color will disappear with pressure.

Description	Indications and Pathogenesis
Papules first appear on forehead, then spread downward over face, neck, body, and finally down to the feet. Red to red-brown blotchy appearance, raised with a distinct border.	**Measles** due to invasion of exogenous factors that stagnate in the Lung and enter the blood which then erupts on the skin through the collaterals. Measles are usually seen in children.
A rash appears first on the face and then spreads downward. As it spreads downward it often clears up on the face. The rash is either pink or light red spots that are tiny and sparse but may merge to form evenly colored patches. The rash can itch and last up to three days. As the rash passes, the affected skin occasionally sheds fine flakes.	**Rubella or German Measles**, also called "three day measles". In TCM, this is a wind rash. It is due to wind heat that attacks the Lung, defensive level, and space between the skin and muscles. Because the qi and blood combat the pathogens, they are pushed outward into the skin where the wind rash is visible.
Severe itching; upon scratching, the skin swells at once with a slightly red color and irregular shape. These rashes appear intermittently.	**Urticaria**, hives, or "obscure rash", usually caused by exogenous wind attack on the channels due to deficiency of nutritive qi and blood.

Table 1.2.42 Skin Papules and their Indications

— *B. Macule (癍 bān):* also called "plaque," this is a kind of skin rash appearing during a disease process. It is characterized by red patches, spots, or connected in a network pattern. It is flat, and has a clear edge with no swelling on the skin. Its red color does not disappear with pressure.

Description	Indications and Pathogenesis
Large interwoven patches with a red or purple color that does not change with pressure.	*Yang macule* which indicates heat in the nutritive and blood levels. Heat compels blood to overflow to the surface where it causes the macule.
Sparse irregular macules in different sizes with a reddish or purple black color that changes with pressure.	*Yin macule* is due to a deficiency of qi and blood or *zàng fǔ* organ disorder.

Table 1.2.43 Skin Macules and their Indications

— *C. Blister (疱 pào):* the skin surface rises, in a variety of sizes, as small as the tip of a needle or as big as a coin. Blisters contain clear or turbid fluids. Their walls may be thin or thick.

Description	Indications and Pathogenesis
Arising from what look like bug bites, it grows into a blister that spreads from the face, back or abdomen to the rest of the body. The blister is filled with a watery liquid. After fully expressing, there is no scar left behind.	*Chicken pox* is due to an exogenous factor entering the Lung through the nose or mouth, dampness stagnates in the Lung and Spleen giving rise to dampness filled blisters appearing on the skin, commonly seen in children.
Seed-sized transparent vesicles on the skin. Usually appearing on the neck and chest, sometimes the limbs, but rarely on the face. May appear repeatedly.	*Miliaria Alba* is commonly seen in damp warm (*wēn bìng*) disease. It is due to damp heat attacking the body and accumulating on the surface.
Millet-sized blister appears on the lips or corner of the mouth giving rise to a burning sensation or pain.	*Cold sore, fever blister, oral herpes* or "heat qi blister" in TCM. It is due to an attack of exogenous wind heat that accumulates in the Lung and Stomach.
First symptom is intense itching followed by the appearance of a rash. It is patchy and starts out as flaky or scaly dry skin on top of reddened inflamed skin. Some people develop red bumps filled with a clear fluid that look "bubbly" and when scratched add wetness to the overall appearance.	*Eczema* or "damp rashes" in TCM. This condition is due to damp heat that accumulates internally which is then brewed to the exterior when attacked by wind.

Table 1.2.44 Skin Blisters and their Indications

— *D. Boils and sores (癰疽疔癤 yōng jū dīng jié):* the skin is red, with a raised surface. Boils and sores come in a variety of sizes, and are usually limited in locale. They are due to subcutaneous inflammation.

Description	Indications and Pathogenesis
Redness, swelling, and pain with a scorching sensation on the skin in specific localized areas with a distinct border.	**Yōng** is a yang-type carbuncle. It is caused by internal accumulation of fire toxin which leads to local necrosis of flesh.
Swelling without clear boundaries, changes in skin color, or fever; there may be some pain, the pus is thin.	**Jū** is a yin-type carbuncle. It is caused by an insufficiency of qi and blood or internal stagnation of yin cold.
Seed-sized boil with a white top and a deep hard root. Initially arises with local numbness, itching, and pain. Most appear on the face, hands, & feet.	**Dīng** are boils or furuncles due to exogenous wind, fire toxin attack, or toxic heat accumulation on the surface.
Tiny round boils with slight red swelling and pain. They are shallow, mild, and soft. Rupturing the pustule will lead to healing.	**Jiē** are furuncles caused by stagnation of qi and blood due to damp heat retention in the skin.

Table 1.2.45 Skin Boils, Sores and their Indications

— *E. Nodule (結節 jiē jié):* these are palpable, solid, and round lesions.

Description	Indications
Bright red in color, though eventually they can turn dark red to purple. There is swelling, but no suppuration even with pressure.	blood stagnation
No change in skin color.	qi stagnation, phlegm nodule, cold damp

Table 1.2.46 Nodules and their Indications

II. INSPECTION OF THE HAIR

Hair is the surplus of blood and the external manifestation of the Kidney qi. Abnormal changes in the hair are also closely related with the functions of the Spleen. Inspection of the hair can help one recognize excess or deficiency of qi and blood as well as the health of the Kidney and Spleen.

Normal hair should be thick, luxuriant, evenly distributed, and with a natural color.

Inspection of the hair includes its color, sheen, texture, thickness, and loss.

Quality	Description	Indications
color	original color	sufficient blood and Kidney essence
	premature graying hair	deficiency of Kidney essence
sheen	shining, lustrous, and moist	sufficient blood and Kidney essence
	withered, lusterless, easily broken	deficiency of blood and Kidney essence
	pediatric cases: dry and withered, sparse, hair sticks together in spikes	malnutrition syndrome (疳積 *gān jī*)
thickness	thick and lusterous	sufficient Lung qi, or Kidney essence
	thin and sparse	insufficient Kidney essence or Kidney deficiency
	pediatric cases: sparse, coarse, light colored hair	insufficiency of pre-natal essence or constitutional deficiency
hair loss	hair thinning or falling out	blood deficiency
	hair falling out in patches (alopecia areata)	blood deficiency with wind attack

Table 1.2.47 Inspection of the Hair

III. INSPECTION OF THE NAILS

The nails are the surplus of the sinews. Their healthy growth and appearance depends on nourishment from qi and blood. They are the external manifestation of the Liver. Hence, abnormal changes in the nails reflect pathological changes in the qi, blood, or Liver function.

Normal nail color is pink and shiny. The nails should be appropriately thick without roughness, ridges, or breaks.

Inspection of the nails includes their color, bed, texture, and shape.

(1) Inspection of the Color of the Nails and Nail Beds

Description	Indications
normal pink color with luster	sufficient qi and blood
dark red	exuberant heat
crimson	yin deficiency
pale	cold syndrome
yellow	blood deficiency, damp heat
nail bed color turns white with pressure, color returns immediately upon removing pressure	sufficient qi and blood, favorable prognosis
nail bed turns white with pressure, but color returns slowly when removing pressure	exhaustion of qi and blood, unfavorable prognosis

Table 1.2.48 Abnormal Nail Colors and their Indications

(2) Inspection of the Texture and Shape of the Nails

Description	Indications
withered and dry	insufficiency of Liver and Kidney yin, or chronic painful obstruction (*bi*) with deficiency of qi and blood
atrophy of the nails	Heart yin deficiency with blood stagnation, or epidemic disease
soft and thin nails (onychomalacia), nails so thin as to lose their protective function	qi and blood deficiency or chronic painful obstruction (*bi*)
rough and thick, lusterless, dim color, loss of transparency	qi and blood deficiency with wind attack, or damp invasion causing qi and blood stagnation
striped (horizontal or vertical)	blood loss, Liver blood deficiency, trauma, or tinea (fungal infection)
brittle, chipped	blood deficiency with wind, trauma, or tinea
hook shaped	qi & blood stagnation or wind painful obstruction
spoon shaped	qi & blood stagnation, malnutrition, Spleen deficiency, or chronic painful obstruction (*bi*)
pediatric cases: flat shaped	qi and blood circulation disorder due to excessive sucking or biting fingers
ridges	Kidney yin deficiency with Liver yang rising, or qi and blood deficiency
horizontal and vertical stripes together	dry heat attacking the Lung, Liver qi stagnation, or qi deficiency with blood stagnation
twisted and bent	Liver qi deficiency (qi stagnation with Spleen qi deficiency), or Liver blood deficiency

Table: 1.2.49 Abnormal Nail Shapes and their Indications

Section 3

Infant Finger Examination

Infant finger examination is a diagnostic method based on observation of the vein in the index finger. This is a commonly used diagnostic technique for children under three years of age.

I. INTRODUCTION

(1) Theory of Index Finger Vein Inspection

The examination of the finger veins has considerable clinical value in diagnosing children below the age of three. It provides supplementary diagnostic data that is particularly useful in judging the severity of a disease.

First, the vein on the palmar aspect of the index finger lies on a branch that separates from the main channel at a point proximal to the wrist, and provides diagnostic data that is consistent with that of the radial pulse. *The Divine Pivot*, Chapter 10 (靈樞.經脈) states that "The hand *tài yīn* channel of the Lung ... runs along the inner side of the forearm and the lower end of the radius to reach the radial artery pulse, and then runs along the thenar eminence to reach the tip of the thumb; its branch starts from the rear of the wrist and runs to the tip of the inner side of the forefinger..."

Second, the skin in children below the age of three is thinner, which affords greater visibility of the vein in the index finger than is the case in adults.

(2) Location of the Three Bars (Gates)

The index finger is divided into three segments, known as "bars" or "gates."

- wind bar: from the metacarpophalangeal joint to the proximal interphalangeal joint
- qi bar: from the proximal interphalangeal joint to the distal interphalangeal joint
- life bar: from the distal interphalangeal joint to the fingertip.

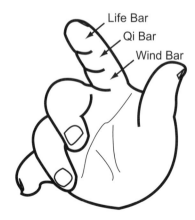

Illustration 1.3.1 Infant Index Finger and its Segments

(3) Normal Condition

In healthy children (under the age of three), the veins on the palmar aspect of the index finger are dimly visible and appear as pale purple or reddish brown lines. Generally, they are only visible inside the wind bar. If they can be seen beyond the wind bar, a pathological process is indicated.

(4) Inspection Method

The examination should be conducted in good light. The practitioner uses the left hand to hold the child's hand and wrist. With the right thumb, the practitioner lightly rubs the network vessels on the palmar aspect of the index finger. The blood is pushed out of the finger toward the palm from the life bar toward the qi and wind bars; this should be repeated several times to make the veins stand out more clearly.

Traditionally, the left index finger is examined on boys and the right finger on girls.

(5) Scope of Index Finger Vein Inspection

The scope of inspection of the index finger vein includes its length, depth, color, and the "flow" or speed at which it refills.

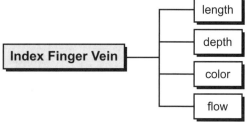

Chart 1.3.1 Scope of Inspection of Index Finger Vein

II. Clinical Manifestation of Pathological Changes in the Index Finger Vein

(1) The Length of the Index Finger Vein

The length of the index finger vein reflects the severity of the illness. The longer the visible vein, the more severe the illness. Three bars are used to measure the length of the index finger vein.

Length of Index Finger Vein	Indications	Location of Pathogen
vein distinct only into the wind bar	mild illness	network vessels (or collaterals)
vein distinct also in qi bar	stronger illness	channels
vein extends into the life bar	severe illness	*zàng fǔ* organs
vein extends through all bars to the fingertip	critical condition	

Table 1.3.1 Length of the Infant Index Finger Vein and its Indications

(2) The Depth of the Index Finger Vein

The depth of the index finger vein reflects the location of the pathogen.

Depth	Description	Indications
shallow	vein is particularly distinct and close to the surface	exterior pattern
deep	vein appears deep and is only dimly visible	interior pattern

Table 1.3.2 Depth of the Infant Index Finger Vein and its Indications

(3) The Color of the Index Finger Vein

The normal color of the index finger vein should be pale purple or reddish brown. When pathogens attack the body and cause pathological change, the color of the vein will change. In general, the color of the index finger vein reflects the thermal nature of the pathogen (heat/cold) and certain other disease patterns.

Color	Indications
bright red	exterior pattern, usually wind cold
blue-green purple	exterior wind heat
purple	interior heat
green-blue	Liver pattern, fright wind and pain patterns
pale red	deficiency cold
white	food stagnation, malnutrition
pale yellow	Spleen deficiency
purple black or dark purple	blood stasis
black	severe or critical condition

Table 1.3.3 Abnormal Color of the Infant Index Finger Vein and its Indications

(4) The Flow of the Index Finger Vein's Refill

The practitioner uses the thumb of her right hand to lightly rub the palmar aspect of the index finger several times, from the life bar toward the wind bar. She then observes how quickly the vein reappears. The rate of return can help differentiate whether the pattern is one of excess or deficiency.

Refill Flow	Description	Indications
normal refill	index finger vein refills quickly and smoothly	normal or deficiency pattern
stagnated refill	index finger vein refills slowly or unsmoothly	excess patterns: phlegm damp, food stagnation, blood stagnation

Table 1.3.4 Rate of Refill of the Infant Index Finger Vein and its Indications

III. Summary of Infant Index Finger Vein Inspection

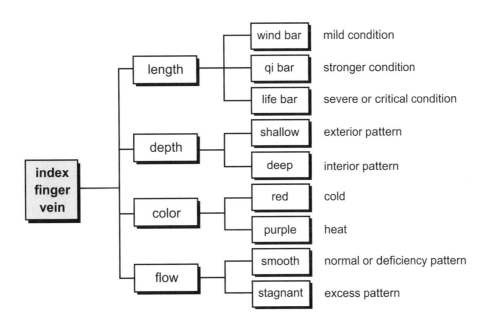

Chart 1.3.2 Summary of Inspection of Infant Index Finger Vein

Section 4

Inspection of Excreta and Secretions

Excreta and secretions are the products of physiological and pathological changes in the human body. Under normal circumstances, these excreta are secreted regularly and in certain expected forms. When there is pathology, excreta may change in color, shape, texture, quantity, and frequency.

I. Introduction

(1) Definition:

excreta (排泄物 *pái xiè wù*): waste matter that is expelled from the body, such as sweat, urine, and stools. This is the result of the metabolism of the body.

secretions (分泌物 *fēn mì wù*): lubricating fluids that are secreted from orifices, such as tears, saliva, nasal discharge, spittle, etc.

five humors (五液 *wǔ yè*): the Heart, Lung, Liver, Spleen, and Kidney are associated with the production of sweat, snivel (nasal mucus), tears, drool, and spittle, respectively.

(2) Physiology of Excreta and Secretions

Under normal circumstances, the Stomach receives and absorbs food and water. The Spleen transforms it into fluid essence and transports it to the Lung where it is distributed to the entire body to nourish the organs and tissues. Fluid that is not absorbed by the Stomach will descend to the Small Intestine. The Small Intestine separates the clear from the turbid, reabsorbs the clear, and transports it to the Spleen where it will then rise to the Lung. The turbid in the Small Intestine pours down to the Bladder and Large Intestine where it is eliminated. The dispersing and draining functions of the Liver, and warming function of the Kidney, also play important roles in this process.

The five *zàng* organs form the humors: the Heart forms sweat, the Lung forms snivel, the Liver forms tears, the Spleen forms drool, and the Kidney forms spittle.

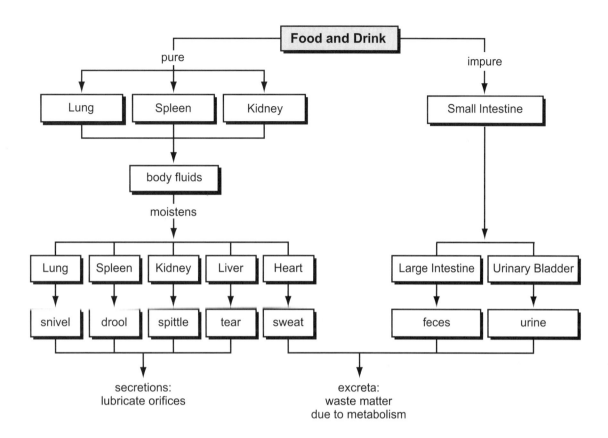

Chart 1.4.1 Physiology of Excreta and Secretions

(3) Clinical Significance of the Excreta and Secretions

Inspection of excreta allows the practitioner to:

- identify the pathogen and pathogenesis
- identify the associated organs and understand the condition of any excess or deficiency within those organs
- make a prognosis for the disease.

(4) Cautions for Inspection of Excreta and Secretions

- Observation of excreta and secretions must be combined with other diagnostic methods, such as inquiry and smelling. The odor and accompanying symptoms are very important for differentiation.
- Changes in the excreta and secretions can be caused by external factors or internal pathological changes. Many external factors may affect excreta and secretions which are not pathological changes, especially the urine and stool. For example, the intake of fluids, medications, diet, etc. may affect the color and quantity of the urine.

(5) Scope of Inspection of Excreta and Secretions

Inspection of the excreta and secretions includes the color, quality, quantity, forms, and odors of excreta, which includes sweat, nasal discharge, saliva, urine, phlegm, feces, pus, and blood. (Sweat, urine, and feces will be discussed in Chapter Three: Inquiry.)

Observation		Indications
Color	white	cold
	yellow	heat
Quality	thin	deficiency and/or cold
	thick	excess and/or heat
Quantity	profuse	cold
	scanty	heat
Form	formed	excess and/or heat
	formless	deficiency and/or cold
Odor	no odor	cold and/or deficiency
	strong odor	excess and/or heat

Table 1.4.1 Scope of Excreta Inspection and its Indications

II. CLINICAL MANIFESTATION OF PATHOLOGICAL CHANGES IN EXCRETA AND SECRETIONS

(1) Phlegm

— *A. Definition:*

phlegm *(痰 tán):* a viscous substance

sputum*:* mucus that is expectorated from the Lung and trachea

rheum *(飲 yǐn):* thin and clear fluids

concrete phlegm*:* substance that is visible, palpable, or audible (can be phlegm or thin mucus)

formless phlegm*:* phlegm that is evident through its symptoms such as dizziness, vertigo, or nausea, but has no concrete form and can be cured by methods of eliminating phlegm

— *B. Phlegm in Chinese Medicine*

In TCM, phlegm means more than what sputum is conceived of in biomedicine. It is both the product of pathological change as well as a cause (pathogen) of additional pathological change. After phlegm is formed due to the dysfunction of the *zàng fǔ* organs, it can accumulate anywhere in the body, leading to further pathological change.

There are two different forms of phlegm in Chinese medicine: concrete phlegm and formless phlegm. Concrete phlegm is that which is visible, palpable, and/or audible. Based on its consistency, it, too, can be further divided into rheum and phlegm. Formless phlegm causes symptoms that are treated by the method of resolving phlegm, even though there is no observable mucoid substances.

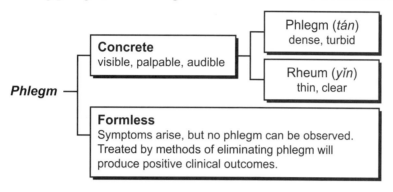

Chart 1.4.2 Types of Phlegm

— C. Pathomechanism of Phlegm Formation

Fluids are brought into the body through the mouth. The Spleen transports and transforms the fluids, after which they are sent to the Lung to be distributed and dispersed. The Kidney steams and generally governs the water in the body, transforming the water into body fluids, which are then distributed systemically in order to moisten and provide nourishment to the body.

When any of the organs involved in water metabolism (Spleen, Lung, or Kidney) are in a state of disharmony, fluids that are consumed may not be transformed into body fluids. Instead, these fluids will accumulate inside the body and form dampness. When dampness condenses or concentrates, it is called phlegm. When phlegm forms, it can circulate with the qi and cause a variety of illnesses.

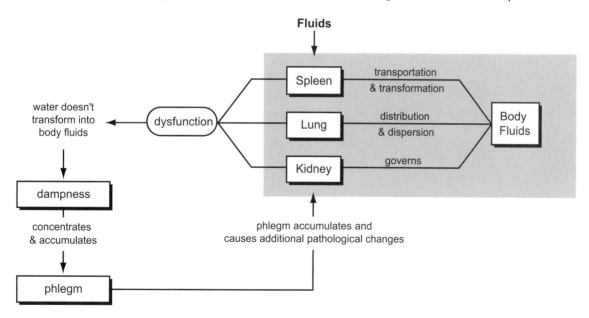

Chart 1.4.3 Pathomechanisms of Phlegm Formation

— D. Symptoms and Indications

Depending on the accompanying pathogenic factors, phlegm can present with different symptoms.

Phlegm Description	Indications	
Profuse white thin sputum that is easy to expectorate, worse at night and late summer. Damp phlegm is mostly encountered in obese patients.	damp phlegm	
White thin sputum that may appear with gray to black spots or a greenish white color. It is easy to expectorate, worse at night and in the winter, mostly encountered in the elderly.	cold phlegm	
Yellow sticky sputum that may accumulate as clots, difficult to expectorate.	heat phlegm	
Scanty white thick sputum or white clots. This phlegm is very difficult to expectorate and may ultimately appear blood streaked. It is worse during the fall. It is mostly encountered in the elderly or yin deficient patients.	dry phlegm	
White copious and foamy sputum that is easy to expectorate. It arises with cough, chills and fever.	wind phlegm	external
White copious and foamy sputum with dizziness and vertigo.		internal
This phlegm looks like dirty cotton balls. It can have a dark black color or be sticky like glue. It is difficult to expectorate.	old phlegm	

Table 1.4.2 Phlegm and its Indications

(2) Saliva: Drool and Spittle

— A. Definition:

saliva (唾液 *tuò yè*): fluids in the mouth which are secreted by the parotid gland, submaxillary glands, and sublingual glands. Saliva keeps the mouth moist and assists in digestion. It includes both drool and spittle.

drool (涎 *xián*): the clear fluids in the mouth, drool can flow out from corners of the mouth during sleep and is associated with the Spleen.

spittle (唾 *tuò*): the foamy fluids in the mouth, spittle is often spat out of the mouth. Spittle is associated with the Kidney.

— B. Saliva in Chinese Medicine

Saliva in Chinese medicine includes drool and spittle. Drool is the humor of the Spleen, and spittle is the humor of the Kidney.

Drool is secreted into the mouth from the cheeks, and can flow out from the corners of the mouth during sleep. Spleen opens to the mouth, hence drool is the humor of the Spleen. Drool is the fluid that enters the mouth when you encounter something that you would like to eat.

The Kidney channel rises to the root of the tongue to communicate with CV-23 *(lián quán)* and CV-18 *(yù táng)*, where spittle is secreted from beneath the tongue. Spittle is the fluid of the Kidney.

— C. Pathomechanisms of Pathological Saliva Formation

As with all body fluids, many organs are involved in the creation of saliva. Because saliva is made up of both drool and spittle, both the Kidney and Spleen are involved. The Spleen transforms liquids into body fluids, which then ascend and enter the mouth, while the Kidney assists in the production of body fluids at a different stage of fluid metabolism. The Kidney's fluids also rise and enter the mouth in the form of spittle. Together, these two fluids make up saliva, which moistens the mouth and assists with digestion.

When there is a deficiency in the Spleen or an attack by an exogenous factor, the Spleen's ability to carry out its function of transforming liquids into body fluids is compromised, giving rise to excessive or sticky drool. In the case of Kidney deficiency or excess cold, one can expect compromised functions to cause profuse, thick, or sticky spittle.

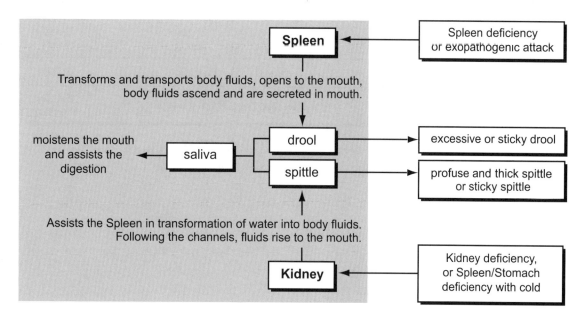

Chart 1.4.4 Pathophysiology of Saliva

— D. Symptoms and Indications

··· a) Drool

Description	Indications
watery drool	Spleen cold
sticky drool	Spleen heat
drool drips out of the mouth consistently and unconsciously, and is aggravated at night	Spleen qi deficiency
inconsistent involuntary drooling with deviated mouth and eyes	wind phlegm
drooling with manic behavior	phlegm heat disturbing Heart

Table 1.4.3 Drooling and its Indications

··· b) Spittle

Description	Indications
profuse and thick spittle, sticky spittle with bloating, poor appetite, fatigue, loose stools	Spleen and Stomach deficiency with cold
profuse and thick spittle, sticky spittle with dizziness, palpitations, and shortness of breath	Kidney deficiency

Table 1.4.4 Spittle and its Indications

··· c) Comparison of Phlegm, Drool, and Spittle

Excretion	Common	Definition	Organ
phlegm	fluid excreta exits the mouth	expectorated mucus, originates in the Lung and trachea	Spleen Lung
drool		clear fluids in the mouth	Spleen
spittle		foamy mucus spit from the mouth	Kidney Stomach

Table 1.4.5 Comparison of Phlegm, Drool, and Spittle

(3) Snivel (Nasal Mucus)

— A. Definition:

nasal mucus: small amounts of clear fluid produced by the membranes lining the nose which function to moisten the nasal passages and to clear away extraneous material. It is a physiological product.

nasal discharge: the excessive thicker or stickier nasal secretions. Nasal discharge may arise from post-nasal drainage and be expelled from the mouth. It is a pathological product, resulting from an exogenous invasion of the Lung or dysfunction of the internal organs.

— B. Snivel (Nasal Mucus) in Chinese Medicine

The nose is the outer opening of the respiratory tract, through which air enters the Lung. The nose is the opening of the Lung, hence nasal mucus is the humor of the Lung.

— C. Pathomechanism of Pathological Nasal Discharge Formation

Body fluids are distributed by the Lung to the entire body through its dispersing and descending functions. Body fluids appear in the nose as nasal mucus which moistens the nose and the air that enters the Lung, and clears away extraneous material. When exogenous pathogenic factors attack the Lung, or a disorder of any of the other *zàng fŭ* organs affects the Lung, its function of dispersing and descending body fluids is compromised. The fluids which fail to descend back up and flow from the nose.

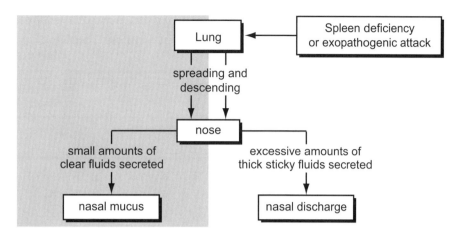

Chart 1.4.5 Pathophysiology of Nasal Mucus and Nasal Discharge

— D. Symptoms and Indications

Description	Indications
clear and copious discharge	external cold
yellow and copious discharge, intermittent nasal congestion	external heat
copious turbid, dark yellow or green yellow, foul smell, may include pus	damp heat
scanty yellow discharge, may be blood streaked or include pus	dry heat
clear copious discharge, frequent attacks, induced by wind and cold, color ranges from white to green to light yellow	qi deficiency
scanty thin white discharge, induced by cold, discharge may be yellow, chronic, and difficult to cure	Kidney qi deficiency

Table 1.4.6 Nasal Discharge and its Indications

(4) Vomitus

— A. Definition:

vomiting: ejection of food through the mouth.

nausea: the prodromal sensation to vomiting.

retching: dry vomiting. The patient produces the sound of vomiting, but without the expression of expelled matter.

— B. Vomiting in Chinese Medicine

The Chinese term for vomiting is composed of two characters, 呕 *(ǒu)* and 吐 *(tù)*. *Ou* is the ejection of food through the mouth with sound, and *tù* is the ejection of matter (food, water, phlegm, spittle, etc.) through the mouth without sound. Because they commonly occur together, we call it *ǒu tù*.

Sometimes, vomiting is a protective reaction for ejecting harmful substances from the Stomach, a physiological phenomenon. It is also a treatment method in Chinese medicine to quickly remove toxic substances from the Stomach.

— *C. Pathomechanism of vomiting*

Under normal circumstances, the Stomach qi should flow downward. Stomach qi sends transformed food to the Small Intestine. However sometimes the Stomach qi fails to descend but instead moves upward to push food out through the mouth. This can be due to exogenous factors such as cold, heat, or dampness invading the Stomach, or to the Liver attacking the Stomach, or to Stomach deficiency. Hence, vomiting is due to the disharmony and rebellion of Stomach qi.

By observing the form, color, quality, and quantity of the vomitus, one can understand the cause of the Stomach qi rebellion.

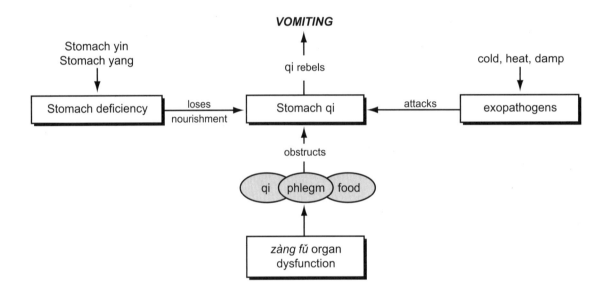

Chart 1.4.6 Pathophysiology of Vomiting

— *D. Symptoms and Indications*

Vomitus	Other Symptoms	Indications
thin, scanty vomitus without strong odor	vomiting undigested foods and fluids together	Spleen and Stomach yang deficiency
	vomiting clear fluids first and then vomiting undigested food	pathogenic cold attacking Stomach
turbid vomitus with strongly acidic or foul odor	acid regurgitation, belching, thirst	heat in Stomach
turbid vomitus with acidic or foul odor, and undigested food	induced by overeating, discomfort relieved by vomiting	food stagnation
vomitus is undigested food with mild odor	mild, intermittent attack, induced by emotional stress	qi stagnation
vomitus is yellow-green or green-blue fluids, bitter or sour taste	bitter taste in mouth, irritability	Liver and Gallbladder fire
severe vomiting, food first then clear or green fluids	often found during the late stage of a febrile disease or after a surgery	Stomach yin deficiency
vomitus is clear fluids	thirst with desire to drink, vomiting immediately after drinking	water retention
vomitus includes blood clots or fresh blood	epigastric pain	blood stagnation

Table 1.4.7 Vomitus and its Indications

(5) Pus and Blood

— *A. Definitions:*

pus: the excreta from a carbuncle or furuncle. It is the result of the struggle between the pathogenic factor and antipathogenic qi.

blood: the red fluid in the body. It flows through the vessels carrying nourishment.

bleeding: blood leaving its vessels and flowing out of the body.

— *B. Pus in Chinese Medicine*

Pus is the result of the struggle between pathogenic factors and antipathogenic qi. It is caused by excessive heat lodged between the skin and flesh. The heat putrefies the flesh. The *Huáng Dì Nèi Jīng* (黃帝內經) states that "Excessive heat can putrefy flesh, then pus is formed." Hence, observation of pus can help us assess the health of the antipathogenic qi. The antipathogenic qi is the active aspect of the organs, blood, fluids, essence, and qi. Qi and blood are the major components so it is said that pus is generated by qi and blood.

— C. Pathomechanism

··· a) Pus

When exogenous factors attack the body, the antipathogenic qi will fight them. This fight brings qi and blood into the infected area, which generates pathogenic heat. The heat becomes lodged between the skin and flesh where it putrefies the flesh and forms pus.

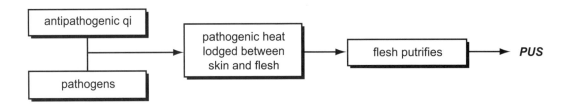

Chart 1.4.7 Pathomechanism of Pus Formation

··· b) Blood

Under normal circumstances, the Spleen qi maintains the circulation of blood inside the blood vessels. There are two major pathomechanisms that cause bleeding: damage to the blood vessels, and qi failing to control the blood. Blood vessel damage can be caused by external injury or by pathogenic factors such as heat and blood stasis.

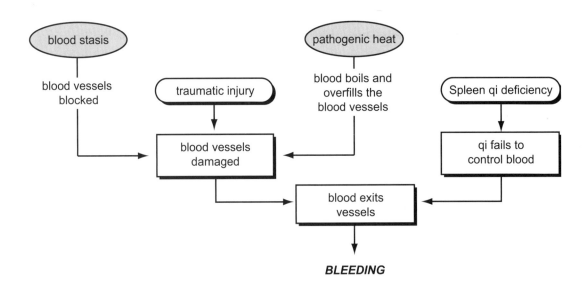

Chart 1.4.8 Pathomechanisms of Bleeding

— D. Symptoms and Indications

··· a) Pus

Pus	Indications
yellow, thick, bright color, slightly fishy odor	excess
white, thin, watery, dim color, no odor	deficiency
white, thick	half excess, half deficiency
pus changing from thin to thick	prognosis: good
pus changing from thick to thin	prognosis: bad

Table 1.4.8 Pus and its Indications

··· b) Blood

Blood	Indications	
thick, red	excess / deficiency	blood sufficiency
thin, pale red		blood deficiency
bright red color	yin / yang	yang syndrome
dark purple color, like pig's liver		yin syndrome
bright color	new / old	new blood
dark color		old blood
thick blood with bright purple color	state of qi	sufficient
thin and watery pale blood		deficient
greenish color	pathogenic factors	wind syndrome
dark and opaque		cold syndrome
very red		heat syndrome
slightly dark		dampness syndrome

Table 1.4.9 Abnormal Bleeding and its Indications

III. Summary of Inspection of the Excreta

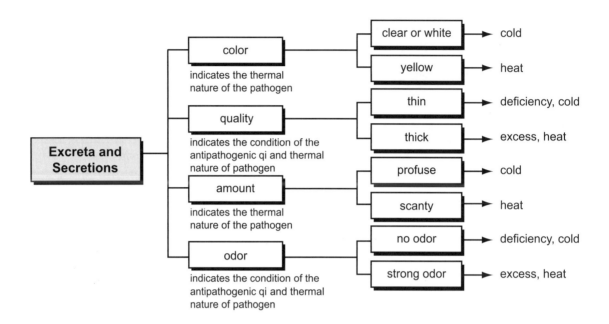

Chart 1.4.9 Summary of Inspection of the Excreta

Section 5

Tongue Inspection

Tongue inspection is a unique and important diagnostic method in TCM. It is used to observe the abnormal changes in the tongue body and coating in order to analyze and diagnose disease.

I. INTRODUCTION

The tongue is the large bundle of muscles on the floor of the mouth that manipulates food for chewing and swallowing. It is the key organ of taste, as the surface of the tongue is covered in taste buds. The tongue also assists in forming the sounds of speech.

(1) Structures and functions of the tongue

— A. Anatomical Structure

The tongue is a muscular organ in the mouth which is covered by a mucous membrane. It extends from the hyoid bone at the back of the mouth upward and forward to the lips. Its upper surface, borders, and the anterior part of the lower surface are free; elsewhere it is attached to the floor of the mouth. The intrinsic muscle fibers, which run vertically, transversely, and longitudinally, allow great range of movement. The upper surface is covered with small projections called papillae which give it a rough texture. The color of the tongue is usually pink-red but can be discolored by various diseases, which makes it an excellent indicator of health.

⋯ a) Lingual papillae

There are many papillae on the tongue surface. According to their shape, size, and distribution, papillae can be divided into four categories:

FILIFORM PAPILLAE: the most numerous and smallest papillae on the tongue; distributed over the tongue tip, body, and sides

FUNGIFORM PAPILLAE: mostly seen on the tip of the tongue and scattered among the filiform papillae; newborn babies have more fungiform papillae than adults

CIRCUMVALLATE PAPILLAE: the largest papillae, seven to nine in number, arranged in a V-shaped distribution anterior to the sulcus terminalis, which separates the tongue body from the tongue root

FOLIATE PAPILLAE: three to six in number, these papillae are found only in a small percentage of the general population and are considered a remnant of past evolutionary stages

— B. Functions

The functions of the tongue include:

- differentiating tastes
- mixing food: chewing and swallowing
- modulating the voice: speaking

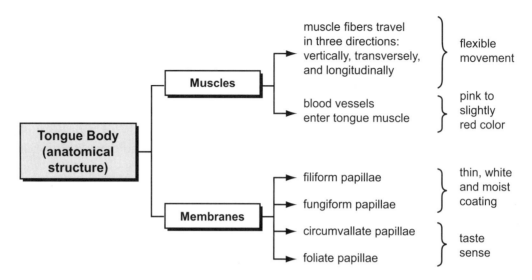

Chart 1.5.1 Tongue Anatomical Structure

(2) The Relationship between the Tongue and the *Zàng Fǔ* Organs

— A. Connections to channels and collaterals

All channels and collaterals are directly or indirectly connected to the tongue. The following are the major connections to the channels.

Three yin channels of foot: *The Divine Pivot*, Chapter 10 (靈樞。經脈篇) states: "The Spleen channel of foot *tài yīn* ... connects with the root of the tongue and scatters over the bottom; the Kidney channel of foot *shào yīn* ... harbors the tongue root; the Liver channel of foot *jué yīn* ... has a channel network in the tongue root."

Yang channels of foot: *The Divine Pivot*, Chapter 13 (靈樞。經筋篇) states: "The Bladder channel of foot *tài yáng* ... muscle region ... a branch enters the root of the tongue."

Yin channels of hand: *The Divine Pivot*, Chapter 13 (靈樞。經筋篇) states: "... the divergent channel of the hand *shào yīn* ...follows the channel into the Heart, and then to the root of the tongue."

— B. Relationship with zàng fǔ organs

All of the *zàng fǔ* organs are directly or indirectly related to the tongue.

Heart: The tongue is the sprout of the Heart. "The Heart opens to the tongue." The Heart helps to distinguish taste and enables speech.

Spleen: The tongue is the external sign of the Spleen. The Spleen is the root of qi, blood, and body fluids, which nourish the tongue. The Spleen also controls the muscles and affects tongue movement.

Liver: The Liver controls the tendons and affects tongue movement.

Lung: The Lung system passes through the throat and is connected to the tongue. The filiform papillae are associated with the Lung because they depend on the nourishment of body fluids which are distributed by the Lung.

Kidney: Kidney is the root of the congenital essence, stores the yin, and hence affects the shape, size, and moisture of the tongue.

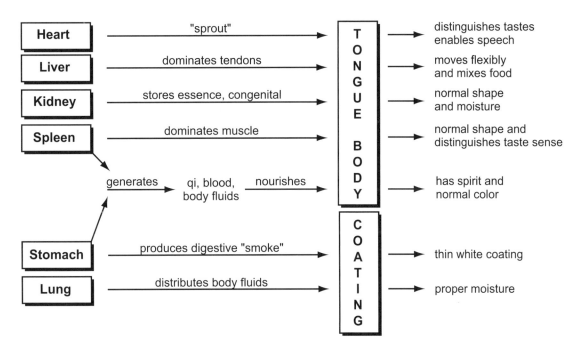

Chart 1.5.2 Relationships between *Zàng Fǔ* Organs and the Tongue

— C. Divisions of the Tongue and their Corresponding Zàng Fǔ Organs

The tongue is divided into several parts that correspond to each of the individual *zàng fǔ* organs. The posterior third (closest to the throat) is associated most closely with the organs of the lower burner, such as the Kidney and Bladder. The middle of the tongue is analogous to the middle burner and hence reflects the state of the Spleen and Stomach. The anterior third of the tongue is most closely associated with the upper burner organs including the Lung and Heart. Finally, the lateral portions of the tongue are associated with the lateral aspect of the abdomen, which is dominated by the Liver and Gallbladder and thus reflects their health.

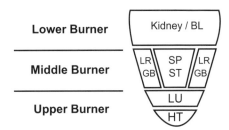

Chart 1.5.3 Tongue Divisions and their Correlations with *Zàng Fǔ* Organs

— *D. The fundamentals of tongue diagnosis*

The tongue serves as a mirror of the *zàng fǔ* organs. This is because:

- The channels and collaterals of the *zàng fǔ* organs are all connected directly or indirectly to the tongue.
- The mucosa on the tongue is thin and transparent with a rich supply of blood, and the tongue papillae are sensitive to changes. Therefore, being a sensitive marker of internal changes, the tongue serves as an indispensable tool when differentiating patterns.
- The taste sense of the tongue can affect the appetite. The Spleen and Stomach functions are related to the tongue function. The Spleen and Stomach are the source of qi and blood. Appetite and taste are related, and both are functions of the qi of the Spleen and Stomach.

(3) Clinical Significance of Tongue Inspection

Changes in tongue appearance usually follow changes in the antipathogenic qi, pathogens, and the location of the illness. Therefore, inspecting the tongue can help to:

- judge the exuberance or decline of the antipathogenic qi
- distinguish the thermal nature of a disease
- detect the location of a disease
- predict the prognosis of a disease

(4) Method of Tongue Inspection and Cautions

The patient's posture: The patient should sit or lie down, open her mouth wide, and allow the tongue to naturally hang outward without pointing the tip.

Sequence: Tongue inspection benefits from a habitual sequence that favors the tongue body first (see the Q&A section to this chapter), as follows:

Observe the tongue body → then the tongue coating → then the hypoglossal vessels. Observe the tip of the tongue → then the middle of the tongue → then the root of the tongue.

Lighting: The source of light can have a big influence on the color of the tongue. When possible, observation of the tongue should be made under natural light.

Diet and medications: Food, drink, and medications can change the color of the tongue body and coating, as well as affect its moisture.

Seasons and time: The normal tongue condition will change slightly in accordance with the seasons. The tongue coating is usually thicker in the morning before the first meal. The color of the tongue body may also appear dim ("dusky") when one first awakens.

	Spring	Summer	Autumn	Winter
Tongue Coating	normal	slightly thick and yellow	thin and dry	moist

Table 1.5.1 Tongue Coating Changes correlated with Seasonal Change

Age and constitution: In children under two years of age, it is easy to find a white membrane or blisters with yellow mucus, or a swollen tongue. Over three or four years of age, the tongue condition will be similar to that of an adult.

Gender: In females, preceding menstruation one may find that the tip or sides of the tongue is slightly more red; after the menstrual period, there may be a slightly pale color to the tongue body. A black tongue coating in a female is not a critical sign, though it is in the male. In the female, a black tongue coating caused by extreme heat will usually not have prickles.

Elderly: Scanty tongue coating, or the absence of a coating, are commonly seen in the elderly, as are multiple cracks.

Dark complexions: The darker the skin, the lighter or more pale the tongue body may appear. This is due to the greater contrast between the color of the tongue and the skin on the face. Among those of African ancestry, blotches of darker pigmentation are sometimes evident on the tongue body. This is not a pathological sign.

Hobbies or habits: smoking, drinking or other lifestyle choices may affect the condition of the tongue.

(5) Scope of Tongue Inspection

The areas that require the most attention in tongue diagnosis can be divided into two large categories: the tongue body and the tongue coating. While inspecting the tongue body, attention should be paid to the spirit, color, shape, bearing, and hypoglossal veins of the tongue. When inspecting the tongue coating, attention should be paid to the color and qualities of the coating.

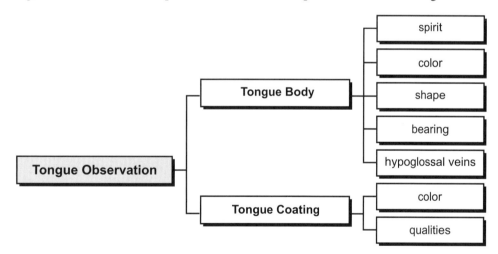

Chart 1.5.4 Scope of Tongue Inspection

(6) Normal Tongue

The normal tongue is described as having a medium-sized body, soft, neither tough nor tender, which moves freely, is pink in color, and covered by a thin, even, white coating that is moderately moist. One should not be able to scrape off the coating; rather, it should be well-rooted to the tongue surface. A briefer description of the normal tongue is "pink with a thin white coating."

II. Inspection of the Tongue Body

DEFINITION: The tongue body encompasses the entire musculature system of the tongue. The normal tongue body is pink in color, bright and moist, and of moderate size; it is soft and flexible.

CLINICAL SIGNIFICANCE OF TONGUE BODY INSPECTION

Examining the tongue body enables one to:

- assess the condition of antipathogenic qi and the state of the *zàng fǔ* organs
- differentiate the depth of the disease
- deduce the advance or retreat of the disease process

SCOPE OF TONGUE BODY INSPECTION

Inspection of the tongue body means to look for abnormal changes in the spirit, color, shape, and bearing (movement) of the tongue body.

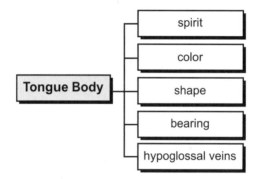

Chart 1.5.5 Scope of Inspection of the Tongue Body

(1) Tongue Spirit (*Shén*)

DEFINITION: Also known as tongue vitality, observation of the tongue spirit is an assessment of the flourishing or withering of the tongue.

CLINICAL SIGNIFICANCE: The spirit of the tongue will reflect the condition of *zàng fǔ* organs, qi and blood, and body fluids.

PATHOMECHANISM: The five *zàng* and six *fǔ* organs are all directly or indirectly connected to the tongue. The tongue needs the nourishment of qi, blood, and body fluids. When the condition of the *zàng fǔ* organs is normal, and the qi, blood, and body fluids are all sufficient, the tongue body will appear pink, bright, and moist, move flexibly, and will be able to taste. When this is the case, the tongue is said to have spirit. If there are *zàng fǔ* disharmonies or failure, the qi, blood, or body fluids may become insufficient and thus unable to nourish the tongue. This will cause the tongue to look dim, dark, withered and dry, and have a sluggish movement. When this is the case, the tongue is said to lack spirit.

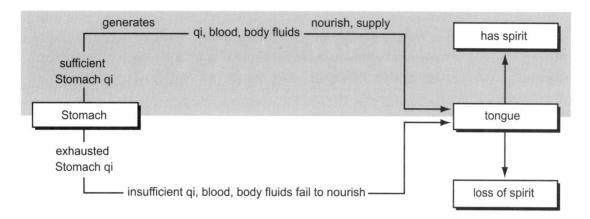

Chart 1.5.6 Pathomechanism of the Tongue Spirit

Pathological Changes in Tongue Spirit and its Indications

— A. Flourishing

DEFINITION: The tongue body is bright, its movement is energetic, and it has enough moisture.

INDICATION: The Stomach qi is normal and the prognosis is good.

— B. Withering

DEFINITION: A dark and dry tongue body with sluggish movement that lacks spirit.

INDICATION: The Stomach qi is exhausted and the prognosis is poor.

	Spirit	**Loss of Spirit**
Tongue Color	light red	dark
Moisture	moist	dry
Impression	flourishing	withering
Movement	energetic	sluggish
Indications	normal Stomach qi	exhausted Stomach qi
Prognosis	good	poor

Table 1.5.2 Comparison of Spirit and Loss of Spirit

(2) Tongue Color

DEFINITION: The tongue color refers to the color of the tongue body. The tongue body color almost always reflects the true condition of the body because it is not easily affected by other short-term factors.

CLINICAL SIGNIFICANCE: Inspection of the tongue body color can help identify the thermal nature of the disease.

PATHOMECHANISM OF TONGUE COLOR: Tongue color depends on the volume of the blood filling the tongue. If the blood overfills, then the tongue will turn red, deep red, or crimson. If the qi and blood are insufficient, the tongue body will become pale. If the blood stagnates inside the channels and/or the blood vessels are contracted due to pathogenic cold, the tongue body will become purple or blue.

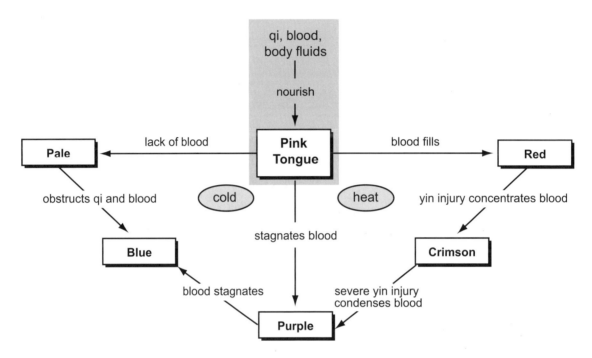

Chart 1.5.7 Pathomechanisms of Pathological Tongue Colors

PATHOLOGICAL CHANGES IN THE TONGUE BODY COLOR

Pathological tongue color can be divided into two general categories: more red or less red.

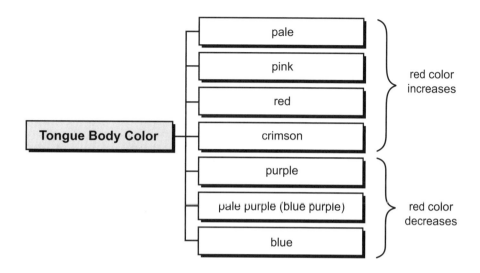

Chart 1.5.8 Pathological Changes of the Tongue Color

— *A. Pale tongue:* The tongue color is lighter than normal.

	Pale Tongue		
Indications	cold syndrome	yang deficiency	qi and blood deficiency
	Biomedicine: Anemia, erythropenia, disturbance of albumin synthesis, lower plasma proteins, and tissue edema.		
Tongue Body	moist	flabby and moist	small and dry
Tongue Coating	thick and white	thin and white	
Pathogenesis	cold causes blood vessels in the tongue to constrict which prevents blood from entering tongue	deficiency of yang fails to lift qi and blood up to the tongue	deficiency of qi and blood fails to fill the tongue vessels and nourish the tongue
	Biomedicine: hypofunction of endocrine glands, contraction of terminal blood vessels, slow circulation of blood, lower basal metabolism, and disorder of digestive function all contribute to the formation of the pale tongue.		

Table 1.5.3 Pale Tongue and its Indications

— *B. Red tongue:* The tongue is redder than normal.

	Red Tongue		
Indications	Heat Syndrome		
	external heat	internal heat	
		excess heat	deficiency heat
	Biomedicine: High fever, deficiency of vitamins or dehydration		
Tongue Body	slightly red or red tip or red tongue edge	red and tough	small red tongue body with or without fissures
Tongue Coating	thin yellow	thick yellow	no coating
Pathogenesis	Heat in body causes qi and blood to overfill the vessels of the tongue with the fresh red color		
	Biomedicine: the red tongue arises from inflammation of the tongue capillaries, dilation of the periglottis proper, or a concentration of blood or state of hypercoagulation in the tongue.		

Table 1.5.4 Red Tongue and its Indications

— *C. Crimson (deep red) tongue:* The crimson tongue evolves from the red tongue, but the color is a deeper red.

	Crimson Tongue		
Indications	exogenous febrile disease	internal diseases	
		yin deficiency or exhaustion	blood stagnation
	Biomedicine: High fever, deficiency of vitamins or dehydration		
Tongue Body	dry	dry and small	with purple hue
Tongue Coating	dry	no coating	thin and moist
Pathogenesis	Pathogenic heat invades the nutritive and blood levels, consumes the blood and body fluids, which concentrates the blood leading to a darker color.	When yin is deficient or exhausted, the blood will become more concentrated which gives it a deeper red color.	Blood stagnation leads to a slower flow of blood which then accumulates and produces a deeper color.
	Biomedicine: the red tongue arises from inflammation of the tongue capillaries or a concentration of blood or state of hypercoagulation in the tongue.		

Table 1.5.5 Crimson Tongue and its Indications

— *D. Purple tongue:* The tongue body looks purple.

	Purple Tongue						
Indications	blood deficency	internal cold	blood stag-nation	extreme heat	phlegm damp	yin exhaus-tion	alcohol toxin
Indications	**Biomedicine:** venous stagnation, slower blood circulation, increase of blood viscosity and hypoxia						
Tongue Body	blue purple (pale purple)			dark red purple			
Tongue Coating	moist and white		can be dry	dry yellow	glossy or greasy	no coating	dry
Pathogenesis	Invasion of exopathogenic heat, cold, or damp; or internal pathogenic changes can both lead to the stagnation of qi and blood which accumulates in or overfills the vessels giving rise to the purple color.						
Pathogenesis	**Biomedicine:** the purple or blue tongue color arises from changes in blood components and their dynamic changes beneath the lower layer of the periglottis.						

Table 1.5.6 Purple Tongue and its Indications

— *E. Blue tongue:* The tongue color is like the blue veins visible through the skin, or it is bloodless, like the tongue of a buffalo.

	Blue Tongue	
Indications	cold accumulation	blood stagnation
Indications	**Biomedicine:** venous stagnation, slower blood circulation, increase of blood viscosity and hypoxia	
Tongue Body	entire tongue body is blue	blue on the sides of the tongue, may include a dry mouth with a dislike of swallowing water
Tongue Coating	glossy	may have dry coating
Pathogenesis	The natural color of the vessels is blue-green. Pathogenic cold attack can cause blood vessel spasms and blood stagnation. With the absence of the flow of red blood, the blue color of the vessels appears.	
Pathogenesis	**Biomedicine:** the purple or blue tongue color arises from changes in blood components and their dynamic changes beneath the layer of the periglottis.	

Table 1.5.7 Blue Tongue and its Indications

(3) Tongue Shape

DEFINITION: This refers to the external form of the tongue. (It is also called the tongue form.) Normal tongue shape is neither too thin nor too wide. It is soft and supple, without being swollen. Its form tapers off toward the tip. There are no cracks on the surface.

CLINICAL SIGNIFICANCE: Tongue shape is the outward manifestation of the tongue body. It reflects the condition of the *zàng fǔ* organs. Observation of the tongue shape can provide more information than can be gleaned from the color of the tongue body alone.

- A change in the shape of the tongue body indicates a more severe condition than if the shape were unchanged.

- The shape of the tongue body helps provide a correct diagnosis when the color of the tongue body has not changed, especially when the tongue shape is grossly abnormal.

PATHOLOGICAL CHANGES IN THE TONGUE BODY SHAPE:

Changes in the tongue body shape include its texture, size, and surface.

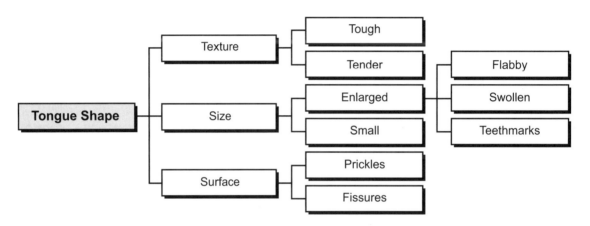

Chart 1.5.9 Pathological Changes in the Tongue Body Shape

— A. Texture

The texture of a normal tongue body should be neither tough nor tender. Identifying the toughness or tenderness of the tongue can help one differentiate whether the pattern is predominantly one of excess or deficiency.

PATHOMECHANISM OF THE ABNORMAL TONGUE TEXTURE: The texture of the tongue body reflects the condition of the tongue muscle and membranes, which require nourishment from qi, blood, and body fluids.

A rough tongue texture arises when excessive pathogens invade the body and there is exuberant antipathogenic qi. The battle between the antipathogenic qi and the pathogenic factors will be strong, causing the muscle fibers to bulge, which causes the striae to become rough and coarse.

A tender tongue is mostly associated with states of deficiency. If the qi and blood are deficient and unable to fill up or nourish the tongue body, causing the muscle fibers to become thin and atrophied, the surface texture of the tongue will appear tender. Or if the yang is deficient and unable to adequately transform the body fluids, then cold-damp can accumulate in the tongue and cause its tender appearance.

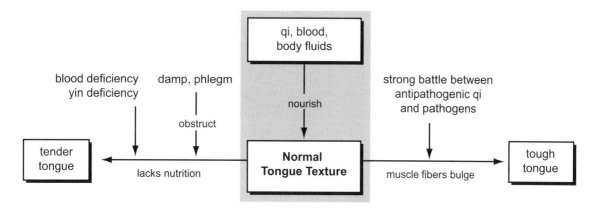

Chart 1.5.10 Pathomechanism of Abnormal Tongue Textures

··· a) Toughness

The muscle fibers of the tongue body are rough and coarse. The tongue is striated like red meat.

	Tough Tongue	
	excess syndrome	
Indications	excess heat	blood stagnation
Tongue Body	red and tough	purple and tough
Pathogenesis	Excessive pathogenic qi invades and struggles with antipathogenic qi, causing the qi and blood to move upwards and the muscle fibers to bulge.	

Table 1.5.8 Tough Tongue and its Indications

··· b) Tenderness

The striae of the tongue are delicate, fine, and smooth. The tongue is smooth like skinless chicken breast.

	Tender Tongue	
	deficiency syndrome	
Indications	qi and blood deficiency	yang qi deficiency
Tongue Body	tender and dry	tender and glossy
Pathogenesis	Qi and blood deficiency can't nourish the tongue body, or a yang deficiency cannot transform body fluids giving rise to their accumulation in the tongue and the tender texture.	

Table 1.5.9 Tender Tongue and its Indications

— B. Tongue size

Tongue sizes often reflect an individual's constitution. If a person doesn't exhibit any signs or symptoms, a larger or smaller tongue would simply be a physiological variation.

PATHOMECHANISM OF ABNORMAL TONGUE SIZES: When the tongue body is overfilled with blood, or dampness accumulates in the tongue body, an enlarged tongue will result. A small tongue is caused by a lack of nutrition due to a deficiency of qi, blood, and/or body fluids.

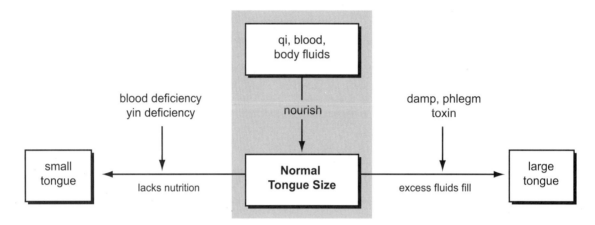

Chart 1.5.11 Pathomechanisms of Abnormal Tongue Size

··· a) Flabby tongue

The tongue body is enlarged horizontally.

	Flabby Tongue	
Indications	damp heat or phlegm heat accumulation	Spleen or Kidney yang deficiency with accumulation of dampness
Tongue Body	red	pale, tender, teethmarks
Pathogenesis	pathogenic heat pushes fluids up to the tongue where they stagnate and accumulate in the tongue	deficiency of yang qi fails to transform and transport fluids which accumulate in the tongue body
Remarks	The flabby tongue may be found in healthy persons, especially in the absence of any other symptoms.	

Table 1.5.10 Flabby Tongue and its Indications

··· b) Swollen tongue

The tongue body is enlarged mostly in a vertical direction. It can fill the mouth, become difficult to retract, and in some cases cause difficulty in closing the mouth. The swollen tongue is a toxic enlargement of the tongue.

Swollen Tongue		
Indications	pathogenic heat invades the Heart and Spleen	alcohol poisoning	blood stagnation due to chemical toxicity
Tongue Body	bright red tongue body, possibly with pain	purple and swollen	dark blue purple or pale blue purple and swollen
Pathogenesis	heat pushes blood into the tongue which causes the swelling	qi, blood stasis leads to blood accumulation in the tongue body resulting in the swollen tongue	
Remark	Unlike the flabby tongue, the swollen tongue is not found in the healthy person and always indicates a pathology.		

Table 1.5.11 Swollen Tongue and its Indications

··· c) Tongue with teeth marks (scalloped tongue)

The tongue with teeth marks refers to the tongue where the indentations of the teeth are visible along the lateral and anterior edges of the tongue body.

Tongue with Teeth Marks		
Indications	dampness	Spleen deficiency
Tongue Body	pale and moist	slightly pale
Pathogenesis	in both cases, water or dampness stagnate in the tongue which causes the tongue to grow wider leading to the edges being compressed by the teeth	
Remark	Teeth marks may also be seen in the healthy person.	

Table 1.5.12 Tongue with Teeth Marks and its Indications

	Flabby	Teeth Marks	Swollen
Tongue Body Enlargement	+	+	+++
Teeth Marks	±	+++	±
Vertical Thickness	+	+	+++
Horizontal Thickness	+++	+	+
Stiffness of Tongue Body	-	-	+++
Physiological or Pathological	±	±	+++
Indications	damp, phlegm with or without Spleen/Kidney yang deficiency		heat, alcohol toxin, blood stasis
Remarks	Teeth marks may occur with either a flabby or swollen tongue, however a flabby or swollen tongue may not have teeth marks. The flabby and swollen tongue may occur simultaneously.		

± = may or may not be present or pathological

Table 1.5.13 Comparison of the Flabby, Teeth-marked, and Swollen Tongues

··· d) Thin and small tongue

The tongue body is thinner (vertically) and smaller (horizontally and vertically) than normal.

	Thin	**Small**
Indications	qi and blood deficiency	yin deficiency with heat
Tongue Body	pale and thin body, with thin coating	red and thin, small body with little or no coating
Pathogenesis	When qi and blood are deficient, the tongue body lacks nourishment and becomes thin.	When there is a deficiency of yin, the tongue body is underfilled and thus the tongue's size will shrink.
Remark	A thin or small tongue without other complaints may prove to be congenital and not indicate a pathology.	

Table 1.5.14 Thin and Small Tongue and its Indications

— *C. Tongue Surface*

The surface of the tongue should be moist, relatively smooth, and have neither prickles, ulcers, nor cracks.

Pathomechanism of abnormal changes of the tongue surface: When the surface of the tongue body is inadequately nourished by qi, blood, and body fluids, cracks may result. The two etiologies are heat, which injures the blood and body fluids, and dampness, which obstructs the upward flow of qi and blood.

Pathogenic heat can also push the qi and blood upward where they overfill the tongue body. This causes the papillae to thrust outward and the appearance of prickles. If pathogenic heat putrefies the muscles, there will be ulcerations.

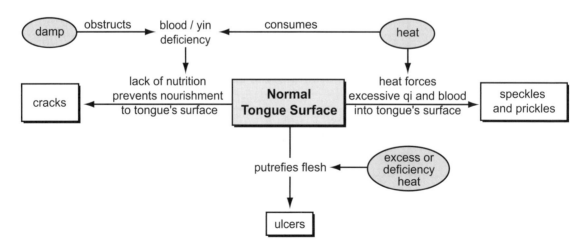

Chart 1.5.12 Pathomechanism of Abnormal Tongue Surfaces

··· a) Tongue cracks (fissures)

These are obvious cracks on the surface of the tongue which are not covered or filled with coating. The size, depth, and shape of cracks vary. They may be found over the entire tongue or be restricted to the anterior or central portion, or the lateral edges of the tongue.

Tongue Cracks				
Indications	excess heat	deficiency syndrome		
		yin deficiency	blood deficiency	Spleen qi deficiency with dampness
Tongue Body	deep red	red body	pale or slight red	pale, flabby, with teethmarks
Tongue Coating	dry coating	no coating	varied	varied
Pathogenesis	excess heat impairs body fluids; or a deficiency of essence, blood, yin, or body fluids; all lead to insufficient nutrition of the tongue body's surface which causes the cracks			damp accumulation in the tongue body obstructs the fluids and blood from nourishing the tongue's surface
Remarks	Cracks in the tongue will occur in 0.5% of healthy people. In this case, there will be no complaints, the cracks are not deep, and they'll persist on the tongue unchanged.			

Table 1.5.15 Tongue Cracks and their Indications

··· b) Tongue speckles and prickles

There are speckles (flat) or prickles (raised) on the surface of the tongue that look like thorns on the skin of a strawberry. Speckles look red, white, or black, while prickles often look red or black. They both tend to appear on the lateral borders of the tongue but can be found scattered over the entire tongue.

Speckled and Prickled Tongue			
Indications	toxic heat	heat in the nutritive or blood level	damp heat accumulation in blood
Tongue Body	bright red tongue body	deep red, red, or dark purple prickles	red prickles
Tongue Coating	yellow coating	little or no coating	thick yellow coating
Pathogenesis	Prickles or speckles are formed when the papillae enlarge. Pathogenic heat pushes blood to excessively fill the fungiform papillae.		
Remarks	Speckles (flat) are generally considered to be due to blood stagnation, while the prickles (raised) prickles are most likely due to pathogenic heat.		

Table 1.5.16 Speckles and Prickles on the Tongue and their Indications

··· c) Tongue sores

Tongue sores vary in size. They can form a yellow head. After some time, they erode and create ulcerations. The area is red and painful.

Tongue Sores		
Indications	heat toxin in the Heart channel	deficiency heat rising up from the lower burner
Tongue Body	red	red with fissures
Tongue Coating	yellow	scanty yellow
Pathogenesis	Heat (toxic or deficiency) flames upward, accumulates in the surface of the tongue and then putrefies the tissues.	
Remark	Sores have yellow dimples, in time they erode and create ulcerations. They are red and painful.	Sores do not protrude from the tongue. The red color and pain is relatively mild.

Table 1.5.17 Tongue Sores and their Indications

(4) Tongue bearing (movement)

DEFINITION: Tongue bearing is also called tongue movement or the tongue state. The normal tongue can be extended outward easily and neither trembles nor quivers uncontrollably. It is neither involuntarily stiff nor immobile. It is flexible and moves smoothly.

CLINICAL SIGNIFICANCE: Abnormal tongue bearing usually indicates severe conditions in the interior.

PATHOLOGICAL CHANGES IN THE TONGUE BODY BEARING: Changes to the bearing of the tongue body include changes to its flexibility, movement, and length.

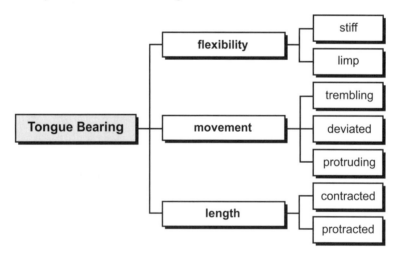

Chart 1.5.13 Abnormal Tongue Bearing

— *A. Flexibility of the Tongue Body*

Flexibility refers to how the tongue moves. The normal tongue should move freely and smoothly.

Pathomechanisms of abnormal changes in flexibility of the tongue: Flexibility in the movement of the tongue depends on the condition of its muscles and sinews. A sinew can spasm due to a loss of nourishment, which arises either from deficiency of the internal organs, or from phlegm or blood stasis that obstructs the flow of qi and blood. In either case, there is a lack of nutrition reaching the muscles and sinews of the tongue. The tongue will stiffen and its movement will lack flexibility. If the sinews lack the nourishment of qi, blood, or body fluids, the tongue may also become limp.

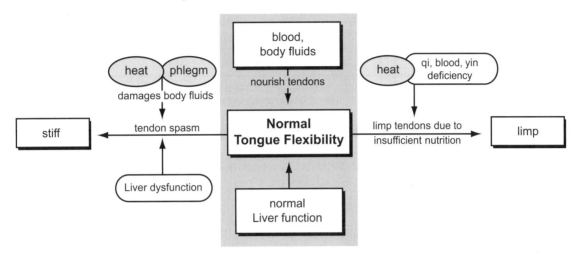

Chart 1.5.14 Pathomechanisms of Abnormal Tongue Flexibility

··· a) Stiff tongue

The stiff tongue is inflexible, making it difficult to move or turn. It causes slurred speech and makes it difficult to take in food.

	Stiff Tongue		
Indications	external heat invades the Pericardium	internal wind	turbid phlegm
Tongue Body	crimson	slightly red or green-purple	flabby
Tongue Coating	yellow	varied	thick and greasy
Pathogenesis	excess heat exhausts body fluids leading to tongue's malnutrition	Liver dysfunction gives rise to wind leading to spasm of the tongue	phlegm obstructs qi and blood leading to tongue's malnutrition

Table 1.5.18 Stiff Tongue and its Indications

··· b) Limp (flaccid) tongue

This refers to a tongue that is so weak that its muscles atrophy and it is unable to protrude or curl up. In severe cases, it has a crumpled look with many wrinkles on its surface.

	Limp Tongue		
Indications	severe qi and blood deficiency	exhaustion of yin and body fluids	excess heat
Tongue Body	pale	crimson	red
Tongue Coating	varied	dry with no coating	yellow
Pathogenesis	extreme deficiencies lead to malnutrition of the tongue muscles		heat injures body fluids leading to tongue malnutrition

Table 1.5.19 Limp Tongue and its Indications

— B. Abnormal Movement of the Tongue Body

Under normal circumstances, the tongue should be stable, without trembling, quivering, involuntary or uncontrolled movements. It should have symmetry without deviation.

Pathomechanisms of abnormal movements of the tongue: Spasms of the sinews and muscles cause abnormal movements of the tongue. The Liver controls the sinews and the Spleen controls the muscles. Spasms can be caused either by internal wind, which is often due to hyperactivity of the Liver, internal excessive heat, or by malnutrition due to insufficient qi, blood, or body fluids.

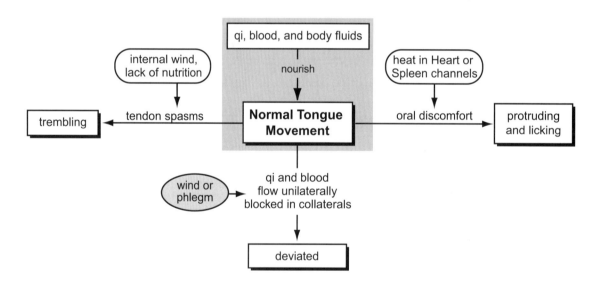

Chart 1.5.15 Pathomechanisms of Abnormal States of the Tongue

··· a) Trembling tongue (quivering tongue)

When the tongue is extended or retracted, the tongue body shivers or quivers uncontrollably.

Trembling Tongue			
Indications	deficiency of qi and blood, or yang depletion causes body fluid impairment	internal wind due to extreme pathogenic heat	alcohol intoxication
Tongue Body	pale, or pale and limp	red and dry	deep red and swollen
Pathogenesis	qi and blood, or yang deficiency fails to nourish tongue	internal pathogenic heat gives rise to internal wind and injures body fluids which fail to nourish and moisten the tongue's tendon and muscle	

Table 1.5.20 Trembling Tongue and its Indications

··· b) Deviated tongue

When the tongue protrudes from the mouth, the tongue tip is inclined to one side.

Deviated Tongue				
Indications	wind stroke			
	internal wind due to...			external pathogenic wind entering collaterals
	Liver yang rising	blood deficiency	wind phlegm	
Tongue	purple red body, acute onset	pale body chronic onset	thick coating	red body
Pathogenesis	pathogenic factor (wind or wind phlegm) obstructs one side of the tongue's collaterals causing that side of the tongue to lose circulation of qi and blood			
Remarks	A deviated tongue may also indicate an impending stroke or cranial nerve tumor.			

Table 1.5.21 Deviated Tongue and its Indications

··· c) Protruding and licking

A tongue that remains outside of the mouth is called a protruding tongue. A tongue that sticks out momentarily and then returns to the mouth, like that of a snake, is called a "licking" tongue. (Some translators refer to this as a "worried tongue.")

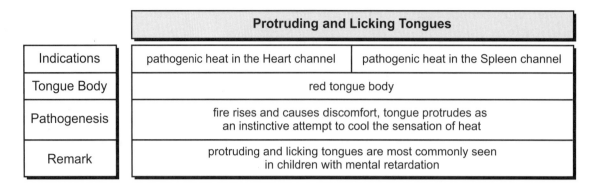

	Protruding and Licking Tongues	
Indications	pathogenic heat in the Heart channel	pathogenic heat in the Spleen channel
Tongue Body	red tongue body	
Pathogenesis	fire rises and causes discomfort, tongue protrudes as an instinctive attempt to cool the sensation of heat	
Remark	protruding and licking tongues are most commonly seen in children with mental retardation	

Table 1.5.22 Protruding and Licking Tongues and their Indications

— C. Abnormal length of the tongue body

Under normal circumstances, the tongue body remains inside the mouth, but is able to extend outward if needed.

Pathomechanism of abnormal length of the tongue: Dysfunction of the tongue muscles and sinews are the causes of the abnormal length of the tongue. When excessive cold attacks, it causes constriction and contraction, thus the muscles and sinews of the tongue contract and spasm. This gives rise to a shortened tongue that is unable to extend. Muscle and sinew spasm and contraction can also be caused by malnutrition arising from turbid phlegm obstructing the channels, excessive pathogenic heat injuring the body fluids, or qi and blood deficiency resulting from Spleen and Kidney function failure.

The loosened tongue doesn't retract easily back into the mouth. This condition arises from excessive pathogenic heat consuming the qi, blood, or body fluids; or from internal organ failure. When these conditions occur, the muscles and sinews will lack nourishment and be unable to contract. When the tongue muscles and sinews are unable to contract, the tongue will become loose.

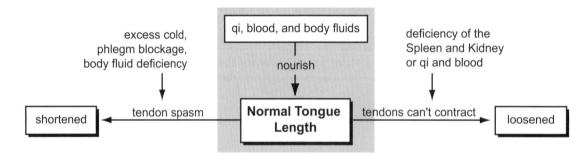

Chart 1.5.16 Pathomechanisms of Abnormal Lengths of the Tongue

··· a) Shortened (contracted) tongue

The tongue contracts and shortens, and is unable to stretch, even to the point that it cannot reach the front teeth.

	Shortened Tongue			
	critical condition			
Indications	excessive pathogenic cold invades tendons and channels	turbid phlegm accumulation	excessive pathogenic heat injures body fluids	Spleen and Kidney failure, deficiency of qi and blood
Tongue Body	pale	flabby	red	pale, tender, flabby
Pathogenesis	cold constricts tongue tendons	phlegm obstructs qi in channels and collaterals	lack of qi, blood, yin, or body fluids leads to atrophy of the tongue muscle	
Remark	In the absence of critical signs and symptoms, the shortened tongue may not indicate a disease process, but rather a congenitally shortened frenulum linguae.			

Table 1.5.23 Shortened Tongue and its Indications

··· b) Loosened (protracted) tongue

The tongue hangs outside the mouth when it is extended, and retracts with difficulty. This may be accompanied by drooling.

	Loosened Tongue		
Indications	interior excess heat	phlegm heat	qi deficiency
Tongue Body	red or crimson color, may be swollen		flabby, possibly numb
Pathogenesis	tongue body lacks nourishment		
	heat injures body fluids and phlegm obstructs qi flow in channels		deficiency of qi leads to atrophy of the tongue muscles
Remark	The loosened tongue is most often seen in critical conditions.		

Table 1.5.24 Loosened Tongue and its Indications

	Limp	Loosened
Mobility	compromised	
Tongue Location	inside the mouth	outside the mouth
Pathogenesis	Excess heat injures the body fluids, or any deficiency syndrome that can give rise to a tongue which lacks nutrition and thus limits the tongue's ability to move.	

Table 1.5.25 Comparison of Limp and Loosened Tongues

(5) Hypoglossal Veins

— A. Normal hypoglossal veins

Under normal circumstances, two thick bluish purple vessels can be seen lateral to the frenulum. Their diameter is no more than 2.7 mm, and their length is no greater thane one-third the distance from the sublingual caruncle (base of the tongue) to the tip of the tongue. They have no branches, varicosities, or bulges.

— B. Abnormal hypoglossal vessels

The following are considered abnormal changes in the hypoglossal veins:

- The shape of the vein is bulging due to varicosities.
- The length of the vein extends past the midpoint of the length of the tongue.
- Branches of the hypoglossal vein are visible or are as filled as the hypoglossal vein proper.
- The color is darker than usual.
- The peripheral ends of the veins are cystic, with thick round processes that may resemble a cluster of grapes.
- The diameter is wider than 2.7 mm.

Indication of hypoglossal vein abnormalities: qi and blood stagnation

III. Inspection of Tongue Coating:

Definition: The superficial layer of material on the tongue that looks like moss or fur. The coating is formed, according to TCM theory, by the rising of "the smoke of digestion" from the Stomach and Spleen.

Normal tongue coating: The normal tongue coating is thin and white with clear grains, evenly scattered and rooted to the tongue. It cannot be wiped off, and is neither wet nor dry, sticky nor greasy.

Tongue coating formation: Generated by stomach qi, it is created by the upward tide of the Spleen and Stomach yang qi evaporating and transforming damp turbidity.

In *Thorough Understanding of Cold Damage* (傷寒指掌, 1892), Wu Kun-An wrote that "The tongue has a coating just like the earth has moss. Moisture arising from the earth gives rise to the growth of moss. The Stomach vaporizes the Spleen's dampness, which rises upward to appear on the tongue coating."

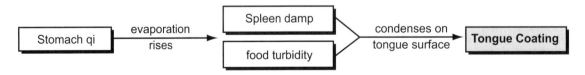

Chart 1.5.17 Physiology of Tongue Coating Formation

Biomedical perspective: the tongue coat is a layer of material on the surface of the tongue. Important elements in its creation include a combination of keratinized squamous epithelium and scaling epithelium of the filiform papillae, dregs of food, saliva fluids, bacteria and oozing matter from white blood cells. The major changes of the tongue coating are changes in the filiform papillae.

Clinical Significance of Tongue Coating Inspection: Inspecting the tongue coating allows one to:

- determine the depth of the disease

- identify pathogenic factors and the thermal nature of the disease (heat/cold)

- assess the condition of the Stomach

Scope of tongue coating inspection

Inspection of the tongue coating includes two major categories: the color of the coating and the qualities of the coating, which includes such parameters as thickness, viscosity, distribution, etc.

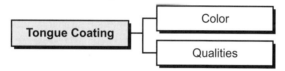

Chart 1.5.18 Scope of Tongue Coating Inspection

Caution: The color of the tongue coating is readily affected by food, drink, and medications. In particular, bismuth-based antacids can produce a false black coating. Coffee, tea, or recent meals can generate a yellow coating that does not necessarily indicate the presence of heat. Candies or other artificially-colored products can also produce abnormal tongue coating colors that do not indicate pathology.

Some people will brush off their tongue coating in the morning as part of their daily oral hygiene. This too can affect the quality of the tongue coating.

(1) Tongue Coating Color

Tongue coatings can be white, yellow, gray, or black. Since colors are associated with pathogenic factors, the color of the tongue coating can reflect certain aspects of a disease.

— A. White coating

Indications:

- exterior pattern

- cold pattern

Location: Lung and Large Intestine

The white coating can be found in exterior, interior, excessive, and deficient patterns.

White Coating Variations		Indications
Thin		normal, mild, or early stage disease
		exterior pattern: wind cold, wind damp, cold damp
Thick and Greasy		Spleen/Stomach yang deficiency causes an accumulation of food or dampness
		turbid dampness or phlegm accumulation
Thick, Greasy and Glossy		Spleen yang deficiency with retention of cold damp phlegm
		interior cold with phlegm and dampness
Dry	thin	wind heat invades or dryness attacks the Lungs, yang deficiency prevents water from being transformed into body fluids and so fails to nourish the tongue
	thick	early stage of febrile disease, body fluid is injured by excess heat
Powdery		toxic heat in the interior, seen in contagious epidemic diseases

Table 1.5.26 White Tongue Coating and its Indications

— *B. Yellow coating*

Indications:

- interior pattern
- heat pattern

The different hues of yellow reflect the increasing severity of pathogenic heat.

Location: Spleen and Stomach

Yellow Hue	pale yellow	dark yellow	brown yellow
Indications	mild heat	severe heat	heat accumulation

Table 1.5.27 Yellow Tongue Coating Hues and their Indications

The yellow coating can be seen in exterior, interior, hot, excessive, and deficient patterns.

Yellow Coating Variations		Indications
Thin and Slightly Yellow		exterior wind heat
		wind cold transforming into wind heat
Thick and Slightly Yellow		damp heat accumulation with qi stagnation
Yellow and Greasy		damp heat or phlegm heat
		food stagnation with heat
Greasy and Sticky	pale yellow	more damp than heat
	dark yellow	more heat than damp
Glossy with Pale Tongue Body		yang deficiency loses its function of transforming the water leading to an accumulation of water which generates heat.
Yellow Partially Covers Tongue Body	tip white root yellow	exopathogen penetrating deeper, more interior than exterior
	tip yellow root white	heat in the upper burner
	double yellow strips	exopathogen penetrating the interior
		heat in the Spleen / Stomach
	dark yellow	heat in the Liver / Gallbladder

Table 1.5.28 Yellow Tongue Coating and its Indications

— *C. Gray coating*

The gray coating is the same as a slightly black coating. It represents a development of the white or yellow coating.

Indications:

- interior pattern
- heat pattern
- cold dampness

The gray coating can only be seen with interior and excess heat patterns, never with exterior or deficiency cold patterns.

Gray Coating Variations		Indications	
Glossy		Cold pattern	damp
			damp phlegm
Dry		Heat pattern	yin deficiency with heat

Table 1.5.29 Gray Tongue Coating and its Indications

— D. Black coating

The black coating usually evolves from a gray or yellow coating.

Indications:

- interior pattern
- extreme heat
- extreme cold

The black coating reflects a disease of long duration and a critical condition. The black coating can also arise after the use of bismuth-based antacids (e.g., Pepto-Bismol®), in which case it does not indicate a pathology.

The black coating can be seen only with interior patterns, never with exterior patterns.

Black Coating Variations	Indications	
Glossy and Greasy	Cold pattern	excess cold damp
		yang deficiency
Dry and Cracked	Heat pattern	Kidney exhaustion

Table 1.5.30 Black Tongue Coating and its Indications

Eight Principles	White	Yellow	Gray	Black
Exterior	+	+		
Interior	+	+	+	+
Heat	+	+	+	+
Cold	+	+	+	+
Excess	+	+	+	+
Deficiency	+	+	no deficiency cold	+
Yang		+		+
Yin	+		+	+

Table 1.5.31 Eight Principles Applied to Tongue Coating Color

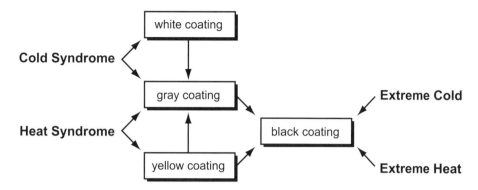

Chart 1.5.19 Summary of Tongue Coating Color

(2) Tongue Coating Qualities

The qualities of the tongue coating include its thickness, moisture, distribution, and other aspects listed below. The tongue coating reflects the condition of the antipathogenic qi and the state of the *zàng fǔ* organs, especially the Stomach.

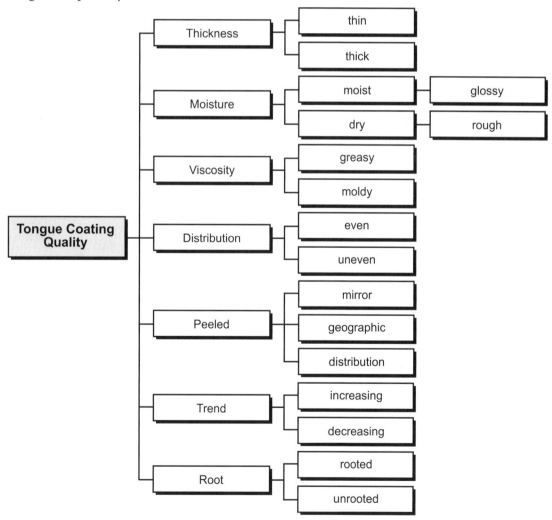

Chart 1.5.20 Scope of Tongue Coating Inspection

— A. Thickness

DEFINITION: The tongue coating is considered thin if the underlying tongue body shows through faintly, whereas a thick coating is one that completely blocks the tongue surface.

CLINICAL SIGNIFICANCE: Differentiating the thickness of the tongue coating can help distinguish the condition of the antipathogenic qi as well as the depth of the disease.

PATHOPHYSIOLOGY OF THE TONGUE COATING THICKNESS: The tongue coating is generated by the Stomach qi. It is created by the upward tide of the Spleen and Stomach yang qi evaporating and transforming damp turbidity. If the Spleen or Stomach functions are impaired, there is not enough power to evaporate and transform damp turbidity. Alternatively, if the Kidney and Stomach yin is insufficient, there will not be enough body fluids or damp turbidity to steam upward, resulting in a thin tongue coating.

When the Spleen and Stomach's transportive and transformative functions are compromised by food stagnation or by phlegm dampness, accumulation will result. These problems will increase the turbidity in the Stomach and thus more steam will rise, causing the tongue coating to grow thicker.

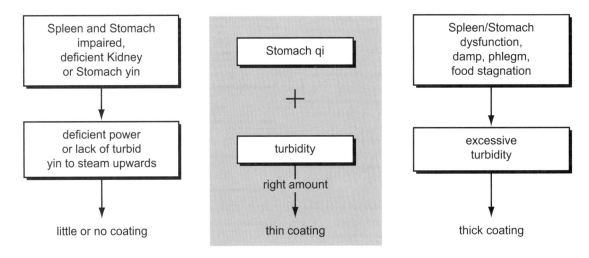

Chart 1.5.21 Pathophysiology of Tongue Coating Thickness

	Thin Coating	**Thick Coating**
Description	tongue body is clearly seen through the coating	tongue body is not clearly seen through the coating
Indications	normal, exterior syndrome, mild, or early stage disease	retention or stagnation of damp, phlegm, food, or water
Pathogenesis	Stomach qi generates the tongue coating	retention of phlegm, damp, or food causes Stomach qi to combine with turbidity which rises upward and accumulates on the surface of the tongue
Pathogen Strength	weak	strong
Location	exterior	interior
Severity	mild	severe
Stage	early stage	later stage
Prognosis	thin to thick: worse	thick to thin: better

Table 1.5.32 Thickness of Tongue Coating and its Indications

— B. Moisture

DEFINITION: A healthy tongue is kept moist naturally by saliva. A normal tongue coating is moist and lustrous.

CLINICAL SIGNIFICANCE: Examining the moisture of the tongue coating can help one assess the condition of the body fluids.

PATHOPHYSIOLOGY OF THE TONGUE COATING MOISTURE: Saliva keeps the tongue coating moist. Saliva is a body fluid, and thus the condition of the body fluids affects the moisture on the tongue. If excessive pathogenic heat injures the body fluids, or if dysfunction in the internal organs gives rise to yin deficiency, a dry tongue coating may result. If body fluids are severely impaired, a rough tongue coating can be seen.

When dampness or water attacks the body, an excessive amount of dampness and saliva may cause the tongue coating to appear glossy (slippery). In the case of Spleen or Kidney yang deficiency, this dampness can arrive from the exterior or the interior; when this occurs, consumed liquids cannot be transformed into body fluids, which gives rise to the accumulation of dampness.

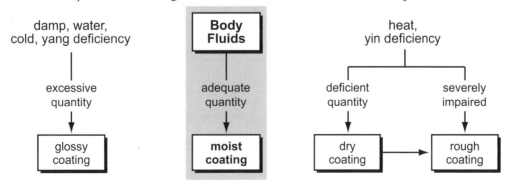

Chart 1.5.22 Pathophysiology of Tongue Coating Moisture

	Moist Coating	Dry Coating
Description	normal condition, neither glossy nor dry	dry without adequate fluid on the coating
Indications	healthy person, or body fluids have not been injured even during illness	external dryness invades Lung
		excess heat
		yin deficiency
		yang deficiency
Pathogenesis	body fluids from Stomach and Kidney rise up to nourish the tongue	dryness or heat cause injury to the body fluids; Stomach, Kidney yin deficiency; yang qi deficiency unable to transform water into body fluids
Body Fluids	sufficient	injured or deficient
Prognosis	from dry to moist: better	from moist to dry: worse

Table 1.5.33 Moisture of the Tongue Coating and its Indications

	Glossy Coating	Rough Coating
Description	tongue is covered with a transparent or semitransparent film of fluid, even to the point of dripping off the tongue when extended	tongue coating granules are very rough like sandpaper which is rough when touched by the fingers
Indications	cold syndrome	severe injury to the body fluids
	damp, phlegm, water accumulation	
	yang deficiency	
Pathogenesis	yang qi deficiency fails to transform water into body fluids which becomes dampness and water accumulation that rises to the tongue surface	severe damage to the body fluids leads to a lack of nourishment for the tongue surface
Body Fluids	sufficient	severe injury

Table 1.5.34 Comparison of Glossy and Rough Tongue Coatings

	Dry Coating	Rough Coating
Dryness	++	+++
Granules	±	+++
Body Fluid Injury	++	+++

± = may or may not be evident

Table 1.5.35 Comparison of Dry and Rough Tongue Coatings

— *C. Viscosity*

DEFINITION: This refers to the "stickiness" and turbidity of the tongue coating.

A normal healthy tongue has a fine coating with a grainy appearance, described as a "clean coating."

CLINICAL SIGNIFICANCE: Examining the viscosity of the tongue coating can help one identify which pathogenic factors are causing turbidity as well as assess the condition of the fluid metabolism.

PATHOPHYSIOLOGY OF TONGUE COATING VISCOSITY: The tongue coating is engendered by the upward flow of the Stomach's steaming of Spleen dampness (turbidity). The viscosity of the tongue coating reflects the amount of turbidity. When there is dampness, phlegm, water, or food stagnation and accumulation, the Stomach qi will produce excessive amounts of turbidity that steam upward and result in a greasy or moldy tongue coating.

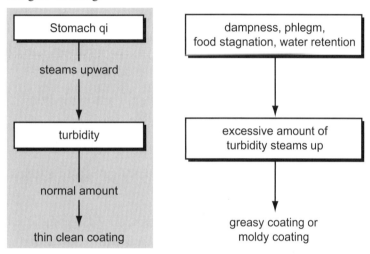

Chart 1.5.23 Pathophysiology of Tongue Coating Viscosity

	Moldy Coating	**Greasy Coating**
Description	The coating is thick and patchy, with coarse granules. Some texts describe this coating as "bean curd", "tofu" or "cottage cheese."	The greasy coating is sticky and made of fine particles that are thicker in the middle and thinner on the margins, like greasy fat or peanut butter
Indications	food stagnation	damp
	phlegm	phlegm
	internal abscess	food stagnation
Adherence	easily wiped or scraped off	difficult to wipe or scrape off
Pathogenesis	excessive yang heat steams the turbid, then putrid qi rises to the tongue's surface	excess pathogenic factors obstruct the yang qi followed by stagnation of dampness on the tongue
Remark	The moldy and greasy coatings can appear simultaneously.	

Table 1.5.36 Comparison of the Moldy and Greasy Tongue Coatings and their Indications

	Moist	Glossy	Greasy
Wetness	+	+++	++
Viscosity	-	+	++
Turbidity	-	+	+++
Thick	±	+	-
Indications	sufficient body fluids	dampness, cold	phlegm, food stagnation

± = may or may not be present, + = likely, - = unlikely

Table 1.5.37 Comparison of the Moist, Glossy, and Greasy Tongue Coatings

— D. Distribution

DEFINITION: Under normal circumstances, there is a thin white coating distributed evenly over the tongue surface, with the center and rear portions being slightly thicker.

- *Even coating*: a tongue coating that completely covers the tongue body.

- *Uneven coating*: also called a partial coating, it covers only certain localized areas of the tongue surface such as the anterior, posterior, left, right, central, or peripheral areas.

CLINICAL SIGNIFICANCE: Examination of the distribution of the tongue coating helps one identify the location and depth of a disease.

PATHOPHYSIOLOGY OF TONGUE COATING DISTRIBUTION: Different parts of the tongue reflect the health of different organs. When pathogens are widespread, or when dampness obstructs the middle burner, the tongue coating will be distributed evenly and will completely cover the tongue surface. When pathogens attack only certain parts of the body, or when only certain organs undergo pathological change, there may be an uneven distribution of tongue coating which appears only on those areas of the tongue associated with the affected organs.

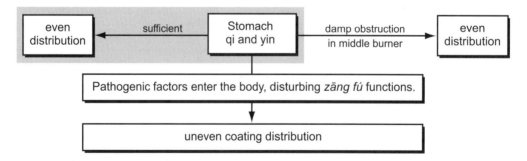

Chart 1.5.24 Pathophysiology of Coating Distribution

Uneven Distribution of Coating			
front half	rear half	one side	absent in center
Description	coating is found on parts of the tongue and absent elsewhere		
Indications	pathogenic factor entering the interior but not yet deep, or Stomach qi deficiency	mild exopathogenic factor invading with Stomach dysfunction	pathogenic factor in the *shào yáng*, or Liver and Gallbladder	Stomach qi or Kidney yin deficiency; or deficiency of yin, essence, qi, and blood
Pathogensis	Different portions of the tongue reflect the functions of different organs. When damp turbidity arises from the Spleen and Stomach, the distribution of the coating will reflect the location of any pathogenic factors or processes.		

Table 1.5.38 Tongue Coating Distribution and its Indications

— E. Peeling

DEFINITION: In a healthy person, a thin white coating will tightly cover the entire tongue surface. However, under certain conditions, the tongue coating will peel off, completely or in part, exposing the tongue body underneath. Different terms are used based upon the location, thickness, and size of the exfoliated area.

CLINICAL SIGNIFICANCE: Examining the tongue for peeling of the coating allows one to assess the condition of the Stomach qi and yin.

PATHOPHYSIOLOGY OF PEELED TONGUE COATING: The tongue coating is engendered by the steaming of the Spleen's turbidity by the Stomach yang. When the Stomach qi and/or yin are insufficient, the tongue coating can partially peel off. If the Stomach yin is exhausted and/or the Stomach qi fails to steam the Spleen's turbidity, there will be no coating on the tongue surface.

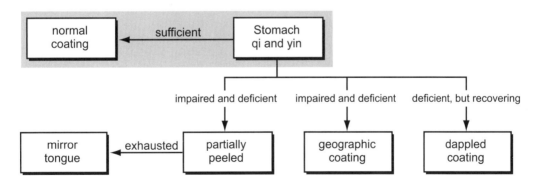

Chart 1.5.25 Pathophysiology of Peeled Tongue Coatings

	Peeled Coating			
Name	partially peeled	geographic coating	mirror tongue	dappled coating
Description	portions of coating are missing, where coating is peeled, tongue's surface is shiny	scattered areas of peeled tissue, with borders that rise above the surface	tongue completely lacks coating, looks as smooth and shiny as a mirror	portions of coating are missing, however tongue's surface is not shiny due to new coating growth
Indications	Stomach yin and qi deficiency			
Remarks		mostly seen in children	exhausted Stomach yin	chronic illness though Stomach yin still exists
Pathogenesis	When Stomach yin is exhausted or Stomach qi fails to produce a tongue coating, the peeled tongue arises.			

Table 1.5.39 Peeled Tongue Coatings and their Indications

— F. Trend in thickness of coating

DEFINITION: This refers to changes in the thickness of the tongue coating. The presence and the thickness of the tongue coating reflect the strength of pathogenic factors as well as the health of the Stomach qi and antipathogenic qi. If the coating thickens, it is increasing, and if it thins, it is decreasing.

CLINICAL SIGNIFICANCE: Noting the trend in the thinning or thickening of the tongue coating provides insight into the health of the Stomach qi and the state of the antipathogenic qi, as well as the prognosis of the disease, since the prognosis is most often based on the condition of the Stomach qi.

PATHOPHYSIOLOGY OF THE INCREASE AND DECREASE IN THE TONGUE COATING: The tongue coating reflects the health of the Stomach qi and severity of the pathogens. In most cases, when pathogens grow in strength or penetrate deeper into the body, the tongue coating will thicken. As the antipathogenic qi overcomes the pathogens, the tongue coating will grow thinner.

In the critical phase of a disease, if a thick or thin tongue coating should disappear it indicates the failure of the Stomach qi and/or yin. If the tongue coating was absent, but then returns, it indicates that the Stomach qi and/or yin has recovered.

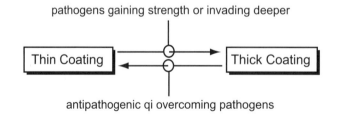

Chart 1.5.26 Trend in Appearance of Thin and Thick Coatings

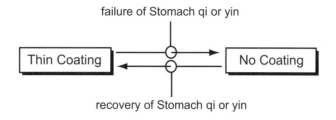

failure of Stomach qi or yin

Thin Coating ← → No Coating

recovery of Stomach qi or yin

Chart 1.5.27 Trend in Appearance of Thin and No Coating

	Decreasing Coating		Increasing Coating	
Description	tongue coating gradually thinning or decreasing		tongue coating gradually thickening or reappearing	
Indications	thick to thin	thin to none	none to thin	thin to thick
	antipathogenic qi recovering	Spleen or Stomach qi failure	Spleen Stomach qi recovery	disease worsening
Prognosis	better	worse	better	worse
Remarks	Sudden disappearance of coating indicates exhaustion of Stomach qi.		Sudden appearance of a thick coating indicates a rapid decline of antipathogenic qi and a quick invasion of the pathogenic factor.	

Table 1.5.40 Trend in Tongue Coating Thickness and its Indications

— *G. Rooted and unrooted tongue coatings*

DEFINITION: Under normal circumstances, the tongue coating should attach to the tongue surface tightly and be relatively difficult to scrape or wipe off. It grows out of the tongue body much like grass grows from the soil.

CLINICAL SIGNIFICANCE: Examining whether the coating is rooted is important in assessing the severity of the pathogens, as well as the condition of antipathogenic qi and Stomach qi.

PATHOPHYSIOLOGY OF THE TONGUE COATING ROOT: The Stomach's yang steams the Spleen's turbidity and gives rise to the tongue coating. Stomach yang (qi) is the power that engenders the coating and Stomach yin supplies material for the creation of the coating; thus the Stomach and Kidney (as source of the body's yin) are the basis for the tongue coating. When the Stomach qi is sufficient, the tongue coating will be rooted. Should the Stomach qi fail, there will be an absence of tongue coating or it will be unrooted.

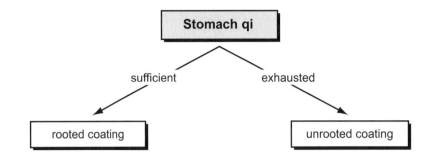

Chart 1.5.28 Pathophysiology of Rooted and Unrooted Tongue Coatings

	Rooted Coating	**Unrooted Coating**
Description	This coating is closely adhered to the tongue body and is difficult to scrape off. It appears to be growing out from the tongue body.	This coating has a clear boundary and is easily scraped off. It appears to have been applied to the tongue body. The surface of the tongue body looks very smooth after coating has been scraped off.
Indications	sufficient antipathogenic and Stomach qi	failure of antipathogenic and Stomach qi
Pathogenesis	Stomach qi and antipathogenic qi are strong enough to rise up to the surface of the tongue.	Stomach qi and antipathogenic qi are exhausted leading to an inability to rise up and generate new coating, so the old coating separates from the tongue body.
Remarks	can be seen in early, middle, or late stage disease	only seen in chronic or critical conditions

Table 1.5.41 Rooted and Unrooted Tongue Coatings and their Indications

In the clinic, it is important to differentiate the unrooted coating from the so-called "false coating," which is a thicker coating that one may encounter in a patient with a moldy coating or one who has recently awakened from sleep. In both cases, we see a thick coating that is easily removed; however, the "false coating" does have a root and should be differentiated from the unrooted coating.

	False Coating	Unrooted Coating
Definition	coating can be easily scraped or wiped off, but retains a root	patchy tongue coating without root
Description	This thick coating without clear boundary is usually distributed evenly and is easily scraped off. The tongue's surface doesn't look very smooth after scraping off the coating, or the coating reappears very quickly after the coating is scraped off.	This tongue coating has a clear boundary and is easily scraped off. It looks like it has been applied to the tongue body. The surface of the tongue body looks more smooth after having the coating scraped off.
Indications	Stomach qi still exists	failure of antipathogenic qi
Prognosis	good	poor
Remarks	The moldy coating is a form of false coating	Dappled is a form of unrooted coating.
	The false coating and the unrooted coating can appear simultaneously, however the false coating doesn't always lack root. A false coating can be seen in the healthy individual. For instance, a thick coating may cover the entire tongue on waking, but end up thinner after eating breakfast.	

Table 1.5.42 Comparison of False and Unrooted Coatings

IV. COMBINING THE CONSIDERATION OF TONGUE BODY AND TONGUE COATING

Generally, the manifestations of the tongue body and tongue coating will be consistent with each other. However, pathological changes are intricate and variable, and sometimes the manifestations of the tongue body, coating, and hypoglossal veins will be inconsistent. Thus, in order to make an accurate diagnosis, both the tongue body and coating should be examined meticulously and assessed together by taking all factors into consideration.

In TCM, there are many ways to interpret signs and symptoms. What follows are three common methods to organize the diagnostic information provided by the appearance of the tongue that are used in modern China.

• EXAMINING THE TONGUE BODY: Helps to assess the state (excess and deficiency) of antipathogenic qi and the condition of the *zàng fǔ* organs, and to differentiate the thermal nature of the pathogenic factors.

• EXAMINING THE TONGUE COATING: Helps to differentiate the thermal nature and location of the pathogenic factors.

• EXAMINING THE TONGUE BODY: Provides insight into pathogens at the blood level.

• EXAMINING THE TONGUE COATING: Provides insight into pathogens at the qi level.

• EXAMINING THE TONGUE BODY: Provides insight into yin, yang, excess, and deficiency.

• EXAMINING THE TONGUE COATING: Provides insight into the thermal nature of the pathogen as well as its location.

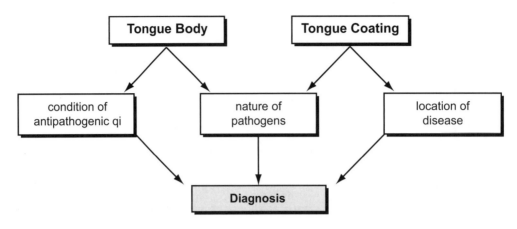

Chart 1.5.29 Combining the Inspection of the Tongue Coating and Body

Section 6

Questions and Answers for Deeper Insight into Inspection

1. How is it that inspecting the outside of the body can help us understand and predict internal pathological changes?

Inspection is one of the four diagnostic methods. In order to understand and predict pathological changes of the *zàng fǔ* organs, the practitioner observes abnormal changes in the patient's spirit, complexion, tongue, secretions, and excreta.

Over the course of thousands of years of clinical practice, traditional Chinese medicine practitioners correlated manifestations on the outside of the body with the condition of the *zàng fǔ* organs, the state of the qi and blood, and pathological changes in the channels and collaterals. The human body is a holistic entity, with the five *zàng* organs in the center and the six *fǔ* organs in an exterior/interior relationship. Through the channels and collaterals, the *zàng fǔ* organs connect with the five orifices, the surface of the body, and the four extremities. They all mutually impact each other physiologically and pathologically. Hence, external manifestations—especially changes in the spirit, complexion, and tongue—are closely related to the excess or deficiency of the *zàng fǔ* organs and to the flourishing or decline in the state of the qi and blood.

Pathological changes in the *zàng fǔ* organs, qi and blood, channels and collaterals, or yin and *yang* will manifest externally. This is why observation of the outside of the body can help one to understand internal pathological changes.

2. Why is inspection of a patient's eye movement so important to the assessment of her spirit?

Spirit is the general manifestation of the vital activities of the human body and the outward sign of the relative strength of the qi and blood in the *zàng fǔ* organs. Spirit includes mental activities such as consciousness, thinking, and emotions, as well as vital activities. It is based on yin essence, which is formed by congenital essences, and nourished and supported by acquired essences. Spirit can be observed in various manifestations, such as facial expression, eye movement, mental state, physical activity and reactivity, voice, tongue, and pulse.

Inspecting the spirit means observing whether the patient's mental state is normal, whether her consciousness is clear, movements are harmonious, and whether or not her reactions are timid. These observations allow the practitioner to determine the state of excess or deficiency of the yin, yang, qi, blood, and *zàng fǔ* organs as well as to make a prognosis about a disease.

Observing eye movement is one of the most important components in inspection of the spirit. This is because the eye is regarded as the window of the Liver and the messenger of the Heart. All the essences and qi of the five *zàng* organs flow up to the eyes.

As we know, the Heart stores the spirit and is related to mental activities. It governs the blood and controls the blood vessels. Heart qi is the power behind blood circulation. The essence and qi of the five *zàng* organs flow through the blood up to the eyes. When Heart function is normal, the eyes will receive sufficient nourishment from the qi and blood and therefore appear bright, move freely, and be able to identify and distinguish things. *The Divine Pivot*, Chapter 80 (靈樞。大惑论) states that "The eyes are the messengers of the Heart, and the Heart houses the spirit." *Basic Questions*, Chapter 81 (素問。解精微論) teaches that "The Heart concentrates the essence from the five *zàng*, and the eyes are its nest."

The Liver stores the blood and opens to the eyes. If Liver blood is abundant, the eyes will be appropriately moist and the vision will be clear. *Basic Questions* states that "When the Liver receives blood, the eyes can see." *The Divine Pivot* states that "Liver qi extends to the eyes; when the Liver is healthy the eyes can distinguish the five colors."

Therefore, when inspecting the spirit, one should pay special attention to the movement of the patient's eyes.

3. What is the relationship among the essence, qi, and spirit?

Essence is the original substance of human life. It makes up the human body. Essence is composed of congenital essence, which is inherited from the parents, and acquired essence, which is derived by the Stomach and Spleen from food. Qi is the essential substance in the human body that maintains its vital activities as well as the functional activities of the *zàng fǔ* organs and tissues. Spirit is the sum total of all external manifestations of life and thus reflects *zàng fǔ* organ functions. The spirit also includes mental activities such as consciousness and thinking.

Essence, qi, and spirit are also called the "three treasures." Essence is the source of life, qi is the force of life, and spirit is the controller and manifestation of life. They work together as one, physically and functionally. The three treasures are inseparable. The coitus of the parental essences produces life, and then the mental and physical activities (spirit) appear. Spirit is the manifestation of the vital activities of life. After spirit is formed, it is enriched and nourished by the qi and blood, which is generated and supplied by acquired essence. When the qi, blood, and essence are sufficient, one will have spirit. If they are insufficient, one will manifest fatigued spirit, or the more severe loss or lack of spirit.

4. What is the difference between spirit disturbance (神亂 *shén luàn*) and loss of spirit (失神 *shī shén*)?

Both spirit disturbance and loss of spirit have mental symptoms, however a spirit disturbance and loss of spirit are fundamentally different in their etiology and pathogenesis.

Spirit disturbance refers to mental disorder. Clinical manifestations include agitation, irritability, restlessness, mental depression, manic behavior, possible hallucinations, disorientation, or a sudden loss of consciousness. Spirit disturbance is commonly seen in a patient who has been diagnosed with a psychological or neurological disorder such as depression, manic psychosis, hysteria, or epilepsy. Symptoms may be recurrent, but during the remission stage, one's mental status may remain normal. The specific symptoms and their frequency arise from their unique etiology and pathogenesis. Spirit disturbances are mostly caused by pathogenic factors that disturb the Heart spirit, such as manic disorder, vexation, or agitation due to phlegm-fire disturbing the Heart spirit. Apathy or dementia might arise from turbid phlegm obstructing the Heart spirit. Sudden syncope can arise from wind-phlegm disturbing the Heart spirit. These are mostly patterns of excess and usually occur toward the onset or during the course of an illness, rather than at its end. Spirit disturbances do not indicate critical conditions. Although the illness may be of long duration, the antipathogenic qi may not be severely impaired.

Loss of spirit manifests as mental disorders such as confusion, agitation, sudden loss of consciousness, delirium, or hallucinations. However, in the case of loss of spirit, these mental disorders are manifestations of *zàng fǔ* organ failures. The antipathogenic qi has been exhausted and the essence has declined. It is a pattern of deficiency. Loss of spirit usually occurs in the later stage of an illness. It indicates a critical condition and the prognosis is usually unfavorable.

Therefore, in general, it can be said that spirit disturbance is a pattern of excess while loss of spirit is a pattern of deficiency.

5. Why do TCM practitioners examine the vein of the index finger instead of taking the pulse in children under the age of three?

Young children have very short radial arteries which are difficult to palpate with adult fingers. They easily cry and become distressed by unfamiliar surroundings. It is therefore difficult to keep them calm and in a stable position for a regular pulse examination.

Based on thousands of years of clinical practice, Chinese medicine practitioners have obtained diagnostic information through finger examination in children under the age of three before the natural thickening of the skin prevents the finger veins from being seen. This information is particularly useful in judging the severity of a disease.

The Divine Pivot, Chapter 10 (靈樞。經脈篇) says of the hand *tài yīn* channel of Lung: "Then it runs along the inner side of the forearm and the lower end of the radius to reach the radial artery pulse location, and then, runs along the thenar eminence to reach the tip of the thumb; its branch starts from the rear of the wrist and runs to the tip of the inner side of the forefinger." In other words, since the vein of the palmar side of the index finger lies on a branch that separates from the main channel at a point proximal to the wrist, and since it provides diagnostic information that accords with that of the radial pulse, we can see changes on this vein that would normally be palpated at the radial artery.

6. Both the greenish complexion and the blackish (dark) complexion indicate blood stagnation. What is the difference between their pathogenesis?

Cold is a yin pathogen that causes contraction and stagnation. When pathogenic cold attacks the body, it will lead to qi and blood stagnation as well as contraction and spasms in the vessels and channels. Since the vessels themselves have a green to purple-green hue and cold causes them to contract, their color deepens and concentrates such that it shows through to the skin of the face. Hence, the pathogenesis of the green or purple-green colors on the face signifies pathogenic cold invading the blood vessels. This is a condition of excess.

The other cause is deficiency cold. Kidney yang deficiency results in internal cold. Cold impedes the flow of blood because it causes the blood to stagnate. When the deep purple color of blood stagnation combines with the greenish hue of the blood vessels, a dark or blackish color will appear on the complexion.

The greenish or purple-green complexion arises from excess cold attacking the channels, while the dark or blackish complexion arises from Kidney yang deficiency.

7. In regard to the facial complexion, it is written that "if there is qi (luster), then one should not worry too much about color, but if there is color, there can be no life without qi (luster)" (有氣不患無色，有色不可無氣). What is the meaning of this classic statement?

This passage was written by Wang Hong (汪宏) (Qing dynasty, 1875) in his book *Classic on the Principles of Observation* (望診遵經). Qi in this context means *zàng fǔ* organ essence qi (精氣　 *jīng qì*). When the essence qi of the *zàng fǔ* organs is sufficient, it rises upward to flourish on the face; the facial complexion will then have sheen, luster, and appropriate moisture. This is what Wang Hong means by saying that "there is qi." If the *zàng fǔ* organ essence qi is insufficient or in a state of failure, the qi cannot rise upward to flourish on the face, in which case the facial complexion will appear withered and dim. Wang Hong refers to this as "without qi."

Color means facial color, which is a combination of yin, blood, and skin color. Different facial colors signify different characteristics of an illness, which are the manifestations of pathology in the five *zàng* organs.

When a patient's facial complexion has sheen, the skin color looks moist and lustrous. It indicates that the essence qi is not severely impaired and the *zàng fǔ* organs are still functional. Even when facial color lacks redness, it may only be a deficiency of blood; because qi can transform into blood, with proper treatment the patient can recover, and the prognosis is therefore favorable. Thus, "if qi shows up on the face, but color does not, the patient can survive" and "if qi exists, then one should not worry too much about color."

When the patient's facial complexion is withered and dim, it indicates *zàng fǔ* organ essence qi failure. In this case, the functions of the *zàng fǔ* organs are severely impaired. Regardless of the color on the face, this is always a critical condition that is difficult to treat and the prognosis is therefore unfavorable. Thus, the complexion that "has color, but is without qi," or a complexion in which "color shows on the face, but not qi, then the patient will die." Because the condition of the *zàng fǔ* organ essence qi is reflected in the facial sheen, observing the facial sheen, luster, and moisture can help predict the prognosis of the illness.

8. What is the difference between a macule and a papule?

Both the macule and the papule are skin rashes that appear during a disease process. Generally speaking, macules erupt from the muscle layer while papules erupt from the skin layer and collaterals. Macules are also called plaques. They are characterized by red patches, spots, or a net-like crisscross pattern (usually secondary to scratching). Macules are flat, non-swollen, and have a clear edge on the skin. The red color of the macule will not disappear by pressing. Macules are usually caused by exogenous heat invading the nutritive and blood levels. The heat compels the blood to overflow from the muscles to form macules.

Papules are also called rashes. Papules are seed-sized eruptions with a red color and distinct borders. Papules arise from the level of the skin and can be felt with palpation. They can arise as scattered eruptions or accumulate in patches. Their red color fades with pressure. Papules are usually caused by an invasion of exogenous factors stagnated in the Lung that enter the nutritive level which then erupt on the skin through the collaterals.

		Macule	**Papule**
similarities		red skin rash caused by exopathogenic heat	
differences	rash shape	bigger spots, patches, or net-like shape, flat, clear edge without swelling on the skin	smaller size, like millet seeds, distinct border, raised from skin, palpable with touch
	color	red or deep red, color does not disappear when pressing	light red to red, color fades with pressure
	severity	severe, heat invading the nutritive and blood levels, rash erupting from muscle layer	mild, heat invading nutritive level, rash erupts from skin and collateral layer

Table 1.6.10 Comparison of Macules and Papules

9. What are the distinguishing characteristics that differentiate measles from German measles?

Both will manifest with seed-sized red skin rashes caused by attack of exogenous wind-heat. Before the skin rash appears there will be symptoms of fever, runny nose, red eyes, etc. However, the way in which the rash appears, its shape, and accompanying symptoms are different.

	Measles (Rubeola)	German Measles (Rubella)
similarities	millet-sized skin rashes, caused by exopathogenic wind heat attack	
fever	high fever for three or four days	mild fever for one to two days
distribution	rash first appears on forehead, then spreads downward over face, neck, body, and down to the feet; rash disappears in the same order	rash begins on face and spreads downward; as it spreads, it clears up on the face
shape	red or reddish brown blotchy appearance, raised from the skin with distinct borders	either pink or light red spots which may merge to form evenly colored patches; the rash can itch and last up to three days; as the rash clears, the affected skin occasionally sheds very fine flakes
accompanying symptoms	hacking cough, sneezing, runny nose, red watery eyes, cold ears, red lines on posterior aspect of auricle, Koplik's spots which are small red spots with light blue centers that appear in the mouth	swollen and tender lymph nodes, usually on the back of the neck or behind the ears
occurrence	mostly seen in children	can arise in both children and adults, when rubella occurs in a pregnant woman, it may cause congenital rubella syndrome with potentially devastating consequences for the developing fetus

Table 1.6.11 Comparison of Measles and German Measles

10. Why is yellow urine *not always* indicative of heat?

Yellow urine is a common clinical sign and can appear in any pattern. Even when it is not a major symptom, it can provide additional information for differentiation.

Generally speaking, yellow urine indicates the presence of heat. Excess heat, damp-heat, and deficient heat can all consume body fluids and thereby lead to concentrated urine. For example, excess Heart fire can pour downward into the Small Intestine where the heat disturbs its function of separating the clear from the turbid, leading to burning, painful, yellow urine. Overconsumption of greasy and spicy food or an invasion of damp-heat can lead to an accumulation of damp-heat in the Bladder. This compromises the Bladder's qi transformation function leading to symptoms of urgent, painful, and burning yellow urine. Yin deficiency can be constitutional, due to chronic illness, or to excessive sexual activity. Yin deficiency leads to deficiency heat which consumes more body fluids and causes scanty yellow urine, with a mild burning sensation during urination.

However, in clinical practice, we can also see some patients with cold-damp accumulation who present with yellow urine. Cold-damp can accumulate in the middle burner where it obstructs and contracts the Gallbladder, leading to the leaking of bile that causes yellow urine. It usually appears in chronic processes. This yellow urine is unique in that its quantity will not be scanty, as is the case when heat is consuming body fluids. Other signs and symptoms include a dim yellow complexion, dim yellow sclera, poor appetite, abdominal bloating, cold extremities, loose stools, a pale tongue with a white greasy coating, and a soft pulse. This is known as yin jaundice.

There are also many non-pathological presentations of yellow urine. Because of higher temperatures and more physical activity in the summer, profuse sweating can lead to urine that is scanty and yellow. Medication, certain foods, and some herbs and vitamins can also cause yellow urine in the absence of pathology.

Children can present with yellow urine because they are full of vitality, are rapidly developing and growing, and have a high level of metabolic activity. This too is a normal physiological phenomenon which is not associated with heat. If one uses cool or cold herbs to clear heat based solely on the color of the urine, the treatment may impair the child's Spleen and Stomach functions and affect their development.

11. How is the tongue coating formed according to TCM theory?

The tongue coating is a layer of material on the surface of the tongue. According to TCM theory, the tongue coating is created from the rising and evaporation of Stomach qi. Spleen and Stomach qi evaporate and steam the food turbidity from the Stomach upward, where it condenses on the surface of the tongue. Wu Kun-An noted that "The tongue has a coating just like the earth has moss. Moisture arising from the earth gives rise to the growth of moss. The Stomach vaporizes the Spleen's dampness, which rises upward to appear on the tongue coating."

The normal tongue coating is thin, white, moist, and evenly distributed. It may be slightly thicker in the middle and rear areas. When Stomach qi is sufficient, there is a coating on the tongue like a layer of grass growing on fertile earth. When there is a failure of the Stomach qi, there will be no coating on the tongue.

12. What is the relationship between the tongue and qi, blood, and body fluids?

The tongue is a muscle with abundant blood vessels. It depends on qi, blood, and body fluids for its nourishment. The tongue body shape and color is dependent on the quantity and circulation of qi and blood. When the qi and blood is sufficient, the tongue body shape is normal with a pink color. If the qi or blood is insufficient, the tongue body will shrink in size or become pale. When the circulation of qi and blood is smooth, the color of the tongue body will be normal and maintain its proper shape. But if the circulation is impaired, it will appear purple, or develop purple spots on the lateral margins. If the qi and blood overfills the tongue body, it will become swollen and red or crimson.

The moisture of the tongue body and coating depends on the status of the body fluids. Acupoints M-HN-20 (*jīn jīn* 金津 and *yù yè* 玉液) are two holes beneath the tongue through which saliva is secreted. According to TCM theory, spittle is the fluid of the Kidney and drool is the fluid of the Spleen. Both are considered body fluids. The generation and distribution of fluids depends on the functioning of the *zàng fǔ* organs, especially the Kidney, Spleen, and Stomach. By observing the moisture on the tongue body and coating, we can assess the status of the body fluids and any pathogenic heat that may be consuming them.

13. Why examine the tongue body first and the tongue coating second?

In the clinic, when we examine the tongue we should first pay attention to the tongue body, and then the tongue coating. The tongue body is anatomically deeper. It is both a muscle and a sensory organ with abundant blood vessels. When it protrudes outside the mouth for too long, the blood vessels will overfill and the tongue color will take on a light purple hue. The tongue coating, however, lies superficially on the tongue and is easily observed. Unlike the body of the tongue, the coating does not change after a long period of exposure outside the mouth. So it is best to first observe the tongue body and then the coating.

To obtain the most clinically relevant information from tongue examination, do not let the patient protrude his tongue for over 30 seconds. Allow the tongue to remain inside the mouth for three to five minutes between periods of protruding and observation.

14. How do you define the "normal" tongue?

The normal tongue means the appearance of the tongue in a healthy person or one with a mild illness. The normal tongue is neither too large nor too small, has a texture that is neither tough nor tender, is soft and moves freely and smoothly, and is a vivid pink in color. It is covered by a thin and even white coating with moderate moisture. The coating cannot be easily scraped off because it is well rooted to the tongue body. A shorter description of the normal tongue used in TCM is simply a pink tongue with a thin white coating. A normal tongue indicates that the *zàng fǔ* organs are functioning normally, that there is sufficient qi, blood, and body fluids, and that the Stomach qi is exuberant.

15. What does "spirit" of the tongue mean? What are its clinical manifestations and significance?

Spirit means vitality manifested on the tongue. The tongue vitality is observed as the flourishing or withering of the tongue texture. It reflects the conditions of the *zàng fǔ* organs as well as the state of the qi, blood, and body fluids.

When the tongue has spirit, the texture is flourishing. This refers to the brightness of the tongue body with appropriate moisture and energetic movement. It indicates that the Stomach qi is normal and hence the prognosis is favorable. If the tongue body is withering, dark, dry, and sluggish in movement, it lacks vitality or spirit. This indicates failure of the Stomach qi, and a poor prognosis.

16. What are the physiological mechanisms that allow us to infer diagnostic information from the appearance of the tongue?

Every part of the human body is connected by the flow of qi, blood, and body fluids through the channels and collaterals. Every illness will affect the normal movement of qi and blood and cause local pathological changes. All *zàng fǔ* organs are directly or indirectly connected with the tongue, and the tongue has abundant blood vessels. As a sensory organ, it has a lot of qi and blood. Thus, the tongue is sensitive to changes and serves to expose the state of the internal organs. Any changes in the qi, blood, or body fluids will be transmitted through the channels and collaterals and reflected in the appearance of the tongue.

The tongue is the "sprout" of the Heart, which governs the blood vessels and stores the spirit. The movement of the tongue regulates the voice and sound to form speech. Thus the tongue primarily reflects the condition of the Heart. The Heart serves as the king who controls all other organ functions and governs the qi and blood of the entire body. Thus every pathological change in any of the *zàng fǔ* organs or in the qi or blood will have some affect on the Heart, which in turn will be reflected on the tongue.

The sensation of taste can affect the appetite. Saliva, which is secreted beneath the tongue, not only moisturizes the tongue, but also helps in digestion and the transport of food into the Stomach and Spleen. The Spleen and Stomach are the acquired root of the human body. They are the source of the qi, blood, and body fluids. Thus the tongue not only reflects the functions of the Spleen and Stomach, but also the health of the entire body's qi, blood, and body fluids.

The Kidney channel connects with the root of the tongue and the fluid of the Kidney secretes from beneath the tongue, where it is called spittle (涎 *xián*). The Kidney is also the congenital root of the human body and stores the essence. Thus the tongue not only reflects the functioning of the Kidney, but also the condition of the essence in all the *zàng* organs.

Based on the relationship between the tongue and the *zàng fǔ* organs, as well as the qi, blood, and body fluids, the appearance of the tongue can provide accurate information for diagnosis.

17. How does the diagnostic information gleaned from examination of the tongue body differ from the information derived from examination of the tongue coating?

The most common opinion says that the tongue body reflects the condition of antipathogenic qi and the thermal character of the pathogens, while the tongue coating reflects the location and thermal character of the pathogens and the condition of the Stomach qi.

A second opinion suggests that changes in the tongue body can help identify the pathological change at the blood level and five *zàng* organs, while the tongue coating is more a reflection of the qi level and pathological changes in the six *fǔ* organs.

A third opinion says that the tongue body enables one to assess whether the disease is one of yin or yang, excess or deficiency, while the coating reflects the location of a disease and whether it is hot or cold in nature.

In order to make a correct diagnosis, we must combine information from inspection of both the tongue body and coating. Generally speaking, the tongue body and coating will agree. For instance, if the tongue reflects a pathogenic change such as interior heat, wc should see a red tongue body with a dry yellow tongue coating; for interior cold, we should see a pale tongue with a white moist coating. However, sometimes changes in the tongue body and coating do not match. In these cases, we should combine our observations with symptoms derived from the other diagnostic methods to make a more comprehensive analysis. For example, a black tongue coating can be found in both a cold as well as a hot pattern, however one is moist and the other is dry; a deep red tongue body with a dry white coating indicates dry heat injuring the body fluids. Because dryness can quickly transform into heat, the color of the tongue body may change—indicating that pathogenic heat has entered the nutritive level—before the color of the tongue coating has had a chance to change.

18. What are the differences between a purple tongue body that arises from extreme heat and one that arises from extreme cold?

The pathogenesis of the purple tongue body color is qi and blood stagnation, or contraction of the blood vessels. In the extreme cold pattern, excessive cold causes contraction and stagnation, and thus qi and blood stagnation. When the vessel is contracted, the blood cannot flow and thus turns purple, or it cannot enter the tongue, in which case a pale purple hue may arise. If the vessel is heavily contracted, there will be little blood color there; instead, the color of the vessels themselves will appear, which is thought of as blue-green in TCM. In that case, the tongue is purple and pale, or green purple, and moist.

In a pattern of extreme heat, the heat will consume the body fluids. This causes the blood to become more concentrated, and its increased viscosity will slow and stagnate the circulation of blood. The tongue body will manifest with a deep-red purplish color with a dry coating.

So, a purple tongue body can indicate either extreme heat or extreme cold. However the purple color indicating heat will have some red in its hue, while the purple color indicating cold will also be somewhat pale, blue, or green-purple.

19. How can one differentiate the physiological (congenital) cracks on the tongue from pathological cracks?

Cracks in the tongue body do not always accompany pathological change. One-half percent of the general population has congenital cracks on the tongue. Congenital tongue cracks are usually coated inside, and there are no concurrent symptoms or complaints. Pathological cracks on the other hand are usually accompanied by other complaints as well as a lack of coating inside the cracks.

20. What is the pathogenesis of the pale tongue with a yellow greasy coating?

When the appearance of the tongue body and coating do not agree, we should analyze the etiology and pathogenesis of each to determine the diagnosis. When a patient has a pale tongue with a yellow greasy coating, the pale tongue mostly indicates deficiency and cold, however the yellow greasy coating indicates damp heat. Although the tongue body and coating indicate cold with heat, the tongue body mostly reflects the condition of the antipathogenic qi, and the tongue coating reflects the pathogenic factors. Thus this tongue would suggest deficiency cold of the Spleen and Stomach with accumulation of damp heat. The root (*běn*) is deficiency and the branch (*biāo*) is excess. This is therefore a complex pattern of heat and cold. Damp heat may arise from either the accumulation of dampness transforming into heat, or from a direct exopathogenic attack of damp heat.

21.   What is the pathogenesis of a deep red tongue with a greasy white coating?

A deep red tongue usually indicates the presence of internal heat, while a moist greasy white coating may be caused by an accumulation of cold dampness. Thus a deep red tongue body and a greasy white tongue coating reflect two opposing pathological changes: heat and cold.

There are two situations that may create this unusual pathological phenomenon. The first is exopathogenic heat invading the nutritive level while there is an accumulation of cold dampness remaining at the qi level. When exopathogenic heat invades the nutritive level, the heat consumes the blood and body fluids. This causes the blood to become more concentrated. As the concentrated blood fills up the blood vessels of the tongue, the tongue body will become deep red in color. Meanwhile, there is an accumulation of cold dampness in the qi level. This pathogen may preexist or attack the body and combine with the exopathogenic heat. Turbid cold dampness is steamed upward by the Stomach qi and condenses on the surface of the tongue to form a greasy white tongue coating.

The second possible explanation for this presentation is when a person with constitutional yin deficiency with empty fire is attacked by cold dampness or food stagnation. Because blood is a part of the yin and body fluids, when the yin is deficient or exhausted, the blood will concentrate and manifest on the tongue with a deep red color. Because the deficient yin fails to nourish and moisten, the tongue may also appear small and dry. On top of this yin deficiency, cold dampness can attack, or the patient may have an improper diet that leads to food stagnation. The turbidity thus formed is steamed upward by the Stomach qi and deposited on the tongue surface where it forms a greasy tongue coating. Since deficiency heat is not strong enough to transform the color of the tongue coating from white to yellow, it remains white.

When changes in the tongue body and coating do not agree, this usually indicates that there are two or more pathological changes occurring simultaneously in the body. In such cases, the circumstances are relatively complicated. The appearance of the tongue can summarize these changes.

Chapter Two

Listening (Auscultation) and Smelling (Olfaction) 聞診

■ CONTENTS

LISTENING (AUSCULTATION) AND SMELLING (OLFACTION) 聞診

Both sounds and smells are produced by the physiological and pathological activities of the zàng fǔ organs. They are an external manifestation of life activities, and reflect the condition of the zàng fǔ organs and state of the qi and blood. Thus, listening and smelling for abnormal changes can provide diagnsostic insight into the condition of the zàng fǔ organs and the nature of disease.

Section 1

Listening (Auscultation)

I. INTRODUCTION

(1) Definition of Listening

Listening is also called "auscultation": it means listening to the patient's voice, breathing, coughing, vomiting, belching, sneezing, and language. Listening is a method through which pathological changes of the *zàng fǔ* organs can be assessed. The thermal nature of a disease, as well as its excessive or deficient nature, can be assessed as well.

(2) Clinical Significance

Listening to the sounds and changes in the voice and breathing can help identify the thermal nature of the pathogens, and the excessive or deficient state of the antipathogenic qi.

Sound	Indications
loud volume, strong force	heat, excess
soft volume, weak force	cold, deficiency

Table 2.1.1 Sounds and their Indications

(3) Scope of Listening

The scope of listening include two aspects. The first is listening to changes in speech and breathing. This means listening to the volume (loud or soft), strength (strong or weak), clarity (clear or turbid), and rate (rapid or slow). The second aspect means listening to the abnormal sounds such as coughing or vomiting which are caused by pathological changes in the *zàng fǔ* organs.

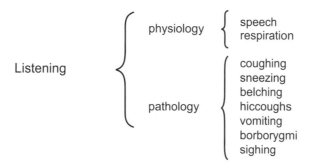

Chart 2.1.1 Scope of Listening

II. LISTENING TO VOCAL SOUNDS

Vocalization mainly depends on the function of qi and forms the basis of speech. It is associated not only with the phonic organs, but also with the functional activities of the Lung, Heart, Kidney, and other *zàng fǔ* organs. The normal voice reflects the harmony of the *zàng fǔ* organs and sufficiency of the qi and blood. Thus, listening to the voice provides insight into changes in the phonic organs and pathological changes in the *zàng fǔ* organs, as well as the state of the pathogen.

(1) The Vocal Sounds and *Zàng Fǔ* Organ Relationships

According to TCM theory, vocalization is produced by the coordinated actions of the Lung, throat, epiglottis, lips, tongue, teeth, and nose. Since yang qi is the power underlying the production of vocal sounds, the Lung and Kidney are the two organs most closely related to the production of vocal sounds.

Lung: movements of qi create sound. Abnormal changes in the qi result in changes of the voice. Since the Lung governs the qi, and the larynx and vocal cords are part of the Lung system, the Lung is directly involved in the production of sound. The Lung is thus the gateway of the voice.

Kidney: the root of source qi (原氣 *yuán qì*) controls the reception of qi. The Kidney channel enters the Lung, runs along the throat, and terminates at the root of the tongue. Since the original qi is the dynamic motive force that arouses and moves the functional activity of all the organs, the volume of the voice is directly related to the function of the Kidney. The Kidney is thus the root of the voice.

Stomach and Spleen: the acquired root of the qi. The Stomach channel also passes through the throat and influences vocalization. The transformation and transportation functions of the Spleen and Stomach send food qi (穀氣 *gǔ qì*) up to the Lung where it combines with air (清氣 *qīng qì*) and transforms into gathering qi (宗氣 *zōng qì*). The gathering qi controls speech and the strength of the voice. Thus, the Spleen and Stomach are also related to the strength of the voice.

(2) Normal Vocal Sounds

Normal vocal sounds are natural, clear, and smooth. Though the structures of the body are the same, individual differences exist. As such, normal vocal sounds differ in volume, tone, and clarity. Normal vocalization also changes in accordance with differences in constitution, age, gender, and emotional status.

(3) Pathological Vocal Sounds

— A. *Definition:* the voice loses its clarity and smoothness, leading to acute or chronic hoarseness, raspiness, or a complete loss of voice.

— B. *Etiology and pathogenesis:* abnormal vocalization is caused by a disorder of the larynx and vocal cords. This disorder can be divided into three aspects.

- Loss of moisture in the larynx and vocal cords may be due to an attack of exogenous dryness or a deficiency of Lung and Kidney yin. Yin deficiency can arise from chronic illness, aging, smoking, profuse sweating, bleeding, or improper treatment.

- Loss of force and power to produce sound is caused by qi stagnation or qi and yang deficiency, which may result from emotional stress or chronic illness.

- Pathogens obstructing or lodged in the larynx and vocal cords, such as phlegm or blood stasis, which result from dysfunctions of the *zàng fǔ* organs; or exogenous pathogens such as wind-heat or wind-cold.

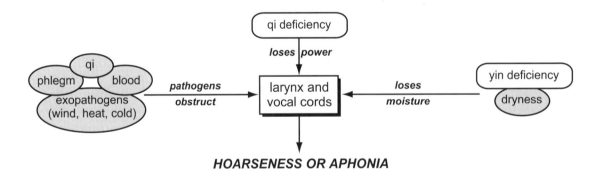

Chart 2.1.2 Etiology and Pathomechanisms of Abnormal Sounds

— C. *Clinical Significance:* listening to the voice can help identify the thermal nature of the pathogens and state of the antipathogenic qi.

Voice Sounds	Indications
loud volume	heat, excess
low volume, vague	exterior wind cold, dampness invasion
low volume	cold, deficiency

Table 2.1.2 Pathological Voices Sounds and Indications

— *D. Pathological vocalizations:* abnormal vocal sounds can be further divided into two categories: hoarseness, which is a partial loss of vocal sounds, and aphonia, which is a total loss of vocal sounds.

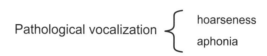

Pathological vocalization { hoarseness / aphonia }

Chart 2.1.3 Abnormal Vocalizations

··· a) Hoarseness

DEFINITION: voice and cough lose their clear and smooth qualities.

Hoarseness	Accompanying Symptoms	Indications
sudden onset, voice is low in pitch and raspy	chills and fever, sore or itchy throat, cough, floating pulse	exterior syndrome
chronic with gradually increasing intensity	dry and sore throat, mass or nodule on neck, dry mouth without desire to drink, purple tongue	blood stagnation
hoarseness with plum-pit sensation, coughing	cough with thick yellow phlegm, severe sore throat or plum pit sensation, fever, red tongue with slippery rapid pulse	phlegm heat
chronic onset, gradually increasing intensity, worse in evening	dry itchy throat with slight soreness, night sweats, dry cough without phlegm, thready pulse	Lung and Kidney yin deficiency

Table 2.1.3 Hoarseness and its Indications

··· b) Aphonia

DEFINITION: also called "loss of voice," this is a condition in which one is unable to produce vocal sounds.

Classification		Indications	Prognosis
Tongue disorder: aphonia due to lack of free tongue movement. The voice is normal and can produce sound. This is not true aphonia.			
wind stroke		exogenous or endogenous pathogen	
Throat disorder: tongue movement is normal, but vocal sounds cannot be produced			
acute	wind cold invading epiglottis	exopathogenic factor	curable
	damp phlegm stagnating in Lung collateral		
	follows violent cough or loud shouting		
chronic	Lung / Kidney yin deficiency	endopathogenic factor	difficult to cure
	Lung / Spleen qi deficiency		
	qi and blood stagnation		
remark	pregnancy aphonia: a temporary condition		

Table 2.1.4 Aphonia and its Indications

III. LISTENING TO SPEECH

Speech is the most important communication tool for humans. It expresses and conveys thinking and consciousness. Because speech follows thought, it is considered a manifestation of mental activities.

(1) Speech and Relationships to *Zàng Fǔ* Organs

According to TCM theory, normal speech is the result of the coordination of all the *zàng fǔ* organs. It reflects harmony of the *zàng fǔ* organs, sufficient qi and blood, and good health of the spirit (*shén*).

Speech is a manifestation of consciousness and mental activity. Qi, essence, and blood are the fundamental materials that form the basis of the spirit; thus, all *zàng fǔ* organs that are related to the formation and transportation of the qi, blood, and essence are implicated in the creation of speech. As such, the Lung, Kidney, Liver, Heart, Spleen, and Stomach are all related to speech. Among these, the Heart is the organ most directly related to speech.

The Heart houses the spirit, and the condition of the Heart affects one's mental activities and consciousness. Since speech is a manifestation of mental activity and consciousness, it is said to be the "voice of the Heart." The Heart controls not only the color, form, and appearance of the tongue, but also the sense of taste and movements of the tongue. Hence, the Heart controls speech.

(2) Normal Speech

Normal speech is the product of thought and consciousness. It should sound natural, clear and fluent, and be able to express and convey one's thoughts and feelings.

(3) Pathological speech

— *A. Definition:*

- dysarthria: difficult, poorly articulated speech, e.g., slurring
- aphasia: impaired expression or comprehension of written or spoken language

— *B. Etiology and pathogenesis:* abnormal speech can be caused by either a disorder of the tongue, or pathological changes of the spirit.

Disorders of the tongue usually cause *indistinct speech* related to inflexible movement in the tongue body. There are two major pathogeneses. The first is phlegm or blood stasis obstructing the channels and collaterals, which blocks qi and blood from nourishing the tongue. The second is yin deficiency that again causes a lack of nourishment in the tongue. This may be the result of pathogenic heat that consumes the yin, chronic illness, or aging.

Spirit disorders usually cause *incoherent speech*. The Heart houses the spirit and is nourished by the Heart qi and blood. When pathogenic factors (heat, phlegm, blood stasis, etc.) attack the Heart, or the qi and blood is insufficient, the spirit may be disturbed, leading to incoherent speech.

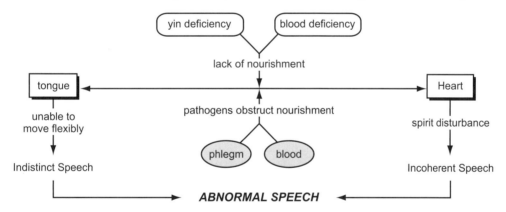

Chart 2.1.4 Etiology and Pathomechanisms of Abnormal Speech

— *C. Clinical Significance:* variations in the patient's speech are associated with the state of the spirit and Heart functions. The excessive or deficient qualities of disease can be known by listening to the speech

Speech	Indications
taciturn (silent or dislike of speaking)	cold, deficiency
persistent talking	heat, excess

Table 2.1.5 Variations in Speech and their Indications

— *D. Abnormal speech:* abnormal speech can be classified into two categories. The first is *indistinct speech,* which is related to inflexible movements of the tongue body; the other category is *incoherent speech,* which is due to a lack of spirit or to a disturbance of the spirit.

Abnormal speech { indistinct speech
incoherent speech

Chart 2.1.5 Abnormal Speech

··· a) Indistinct Speech

DEFINITION: broken speech, a hard, inflexible tongue, or slurred speech with unclear words and a soft voice which makes it difficult to be understood by others.

PATHOGENESIS: either the tongue body lacks nourishment due to wind-phlegm or blood stasis obstructing the channels and collaterals of the tongue, or there is an insufficiency of body fluids.

INDICATIONS:

- wind-phlegm or blood stasis obstructing the channels and collaterals
- yin impairment due to febrile disease

··· b) Incoherent Speech

DEFINITION: speech that is unable to express or convey thought. It is spoken without thinking and cannot be controlled. It is often found in a patient who also displays abnormal mental behavior (spirit disturbance), unclear consciousness, or loss of consciousness.

PATHOGENESIS: failure of the Heart to store the spirit.

INDICATIONS:

i. Raving (狂言 *kuáng yán*) and muttering (癲語 *diān yǔ*)

	Raving	**Muttering**
common	incoherent speech with dementia or disturbance in thought patterns	
description	rude and incoherent speech with cursing and shouting in a loud voice	incoherent speech, talking to one's self silently or quietly
accompanying symptoms	irregular movements, singing loudly in high places, exposure of one's naked body	disorientation, irregular and inappropriate crying and laughter, avoids people
pathogenesis	1. phlegm fire disturbing the Heart 2. Liver / Gallbladder heat accumulation	1. phlegm obstructing Heart orifices 2. Spleen / Heart deficiency
eight principles	yang, excess, heat	yin
remarks	mostly associated with mania	mostly associated with depression

Table 2.1.6 Raving and Muttering and their Indications

ii. Soliloquies (獨語 *dú yǔ*) and wrong speech (錯語 *cuò yǔ*)

	Soliloquy	Wrong Speech
common	abnormal speech with clear consciousness, though reactions are slow, mostly seen in older patients or those with chronic illness.	
description	murmuring to one's self with repetition and interuptions, the content is incoherent and stops when in the presence of other people	words or sentences express the wrong meaning when spoken aloud, however the patient recognizes and corrects immediately
accompanying symptoms	poor memory, fatigue, slow reactions, pale face, thin pulse	dizziness, fatigue, palpitations, frequent sighing, depression, irritability
pathogenesis	phlegm obstructing the Heart, or Heart qi and blood deficiency which fails to support the spirit	
indications	Heart qi and blood deficiency, or turbid phlegm obstructing the Heart orifices	Heart and Spleen deficiency, Liver qi stagnation, or turbid phlegm accumulation

Table 2.1.7 Soliloquy and Wrong Speech and their Indications

iii. Delirium (譫語 *zhān yǔ*) and faint murmuring (鄭聲 *zhèng shēng*)

	Delirium	Faint Murmuring
common	Abnormal speech even while patient is unconscious, it is a sign of a severe or critical condition, and a symptom of loss of spirit.	
description	speech is incoherent, forceful and loud, and cannot be understood	speech arrives in broken sentences, repeated words, vague and feeble voice
accompanying symptoms	high fever, irritability	low energy, feeble pulse
pathogenesis	heat disturbs the Heart or Pericardium	Heart qi impaired
illness	febrile disease	later stage of illness
eight principles	yang, excess, heat	yin, deficiency
remark	Delirium can also be seen during the stage in which yin and yang are separating.	

Table 2.1.8 Raving and Faint Murmuring and their Indications

IV. Listening to Respiration

Respiration is the process by which the human body exchanges turbid qi (濁氣 *zhuó qì*) for clear qi (清氣 *qīng qì*) through the act of exhalation and inhalation. Respiration exchanges and renews qi to ensure the proper functioning of all the body's physiological processes, which require qi. When respiration is normal, it indicates that the qi is normal, even when there are other pathological changes in the body. When respiration is abnormal, it indicates that the qi as well as the body is in a pathological state.

(1) Respiration and Relationship to the *Zàng Fǔ* Organs

Respiration is the physiological process of inhaling and exhaling air. These physiological activities are performed by the joint efforts of various *zàng fǔ* organs, primarily the Lung and Kidney, but also the Liver, Spleen, Stomach, and Heart.

Lung: governs the qi and controls respiration by controlling the inhalation of clear qi and exhalation of turbid qi. The constant exchange and renewal of qi performed by the Lung ensures the proper functioning of all the body's physiological processes which utilize qi as their basis.

Kidney: receives qi, is the root of qi, and grasps clear qi that is made to descend by the Lung. Thus, when the Lung and Kidney cooperate and respond to each other, deep and smooth breathing can be achieved.

Liver: ensures the free flow of qi. When Liver qi stagnates, it can obstruct the flow of Lung qi, impairing its descending function and causing abnormal respiration.

Stomach and Spleen: the root of the acquired qi. When there is Spleen and Stomach qi deficiency, the transformation of food essence may be insufficient, leading to a systemic qi deficiency, particularly Lung qi deficiency, causing abnormal respiration.

Heart: governs the blood while the Lung governs the qi. The qi and blood are mutually dependent, with qi governing the blood and the blood nourishing the qi. Thus, dysfunction of the Heart will affect the Lung.

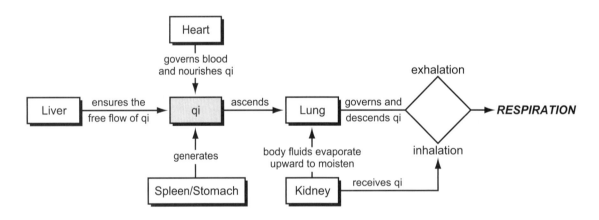

Chart 2.1.6 Respiration and the *Zàng Fǔ* Organs

(2) Normal Respiration

Normal respiration is described as a rate of breathing that is neither too rapid nor too slow (about 12-15 times per minute), with a regular rhythm, smooth and even flow, and without audible sounds.

(3) Pathological Respiration

— A. *Definition:* respiration changes in rate, rhythm, smoothness, strength, and sound quality (clear or turbid). Abnormal respiration is the external manifestation of pathological changes in the Lung.

— B. *Pathomechanism:* the Lung is the organ most directly involved with respiration. There are two major causes of abnormal respiration.

The first cause is excessive in nature. Pathogens obstruct the Lung qi. Pathogens such as wind, heat, cold, damp, or dryness may attack the Lung from the exterior. Other excessive pathogenic factors include those created by dysfunctions of the *zàng fǔ* organs such as phlegm, blood stasis, qi stagnation, or dampness. These pathogenic factors result from improper diet, emotional stress, chronic illness, or a weak constitution. When the Lung qi is obstructed, its descending function is impaired and causes rebellious Lung qi, which manifests as wheezing, asthma, upper stifling breath, shortness of breath, or shortage of qi.

The second cause of abnormal respiration is deficient in nature, especially of the Lung and Kidney qi. When the Lung qi is too weak to descend under its own power, or when the Kidney qi is unable to aid the Lung by grasping the qi, the qi may accumulate in the chest or it may ascend, leading to an abnormal state of respiration.

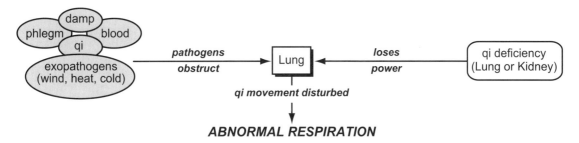

Chart 2.1.7 Etiology and Pathomechanisms of Abnormal Respiration

— C. *Clinical Significance:* listening to the sound of respiration can help identify the thermal nature (hot or cold) of the pathogens and the excessive or deficient nature of the antipathogenic qi.

Respiration Sound	Indications
loud, harsh, rapid	heat, excess
weak, deep, slow	cold, deficiency
deep breathing	excess qi in the Heart and Lung
weak breathing	deficiency of both the Liver and Kidney
rough respiration with rapid exhalation and slow inhalation	heat, excess, exogenous disease
faint respiration with slow inhalation and exhalation	deficiency, chronic endogenous disease

Table 2.1.9 Respiration Sounds and their Indications

— D. Abnormal respiration

Asthma, wheezing, upper stifling breath, shortness of breath, and shortage of qi are the types of abnormal respiration that are commonly seen in the clinic. Asthma and wheezing are two different diseases. Depending on the sound of the breathing, phlegm, and other signs and symptoms, these can be classified as hot, cold, excessive, and deficient conditions. Upper stifling breath, shortness of breath, and shortage of qi are all symptoms that can appear in a variety of diseases.

Abnormal respiration
{
asthma
wheezing
upper stifling breath
shortness of breath
shortage of qi
}

Chart 2.1.8 Abnormal Respiration

··· a) Asthma (喘 *chuǎn*)

DEFINITION: also called "panting," respiration is difficult, short, and rapid. There is a sense of tightness, congestion, breathlessness, or constriction in the chest with difficulty inhaling. In severe cases, the patient gasps for breath with his mouth open, lifting his shoulders and flaring his nostrils to assist in respiration. During an attack, the patient is unable to lie flat.

PATHOGENESIS: Lung qi failure to descend

SYMPTOMS AND INDICATIONS:

Asthma Sounds	Accompanying Symptoms	Indications
Excess type: acute onset; deep and long breathing, relieved by exhalation; harsh and loud sound of breath. Patient prefers supine position when laying down, protruding eyes, accompanied with cough and phlegm, strong body movements and breathing, forceful pulse		
asthma with harsh and loud sounds, breathlessness, cough with thin sputum	chills and fever, headache, floating and tight pulse	wind cold attack in the Lung
asthma, cough with yellow sputum, labored breathing, hot sensation in the chest	fever, aversion to cold, thirst, red tongue with yellow coating, floating and rapid pulse	wind heat attack in the Lung
asthma, difficulty in exhaling, a sensation of fullness in the chest, cough with profuse thick phlegm	nausea or vomiting, thick white tongue coating, slippery pulse	turbid phlegm in the Lung
asthma that is induced or aggravated by emotional stress, plum-pit sensation in the throat	irritability, hypochondriac pain and distention, stifling sensation in the chest, wiry pulse	Liver attacking the Lung
Deficiency type: chronic and gradual onset; short, shallow, and difficult breathing, relieved by inhalation; soft and weak voice, induced or aggravated by exertion		
chronic asthma, shortness of breath, shallow breathing	spontaneous sweating, aversion to wind, frequent colds and flus, weak pulse	Lung qi deficiency
shallow or difficult breathing, shortness of breath, exhalation larger than inhalation	edema, weak lower extremities, dark complexion, pale tongue, deep and weak pulse	Kidney deficiency
shortness of breath with a relatively labored inhalation but smooth exhalation, cough + watery copious sputum	stifling sensation in the chest, low back and knee weakness, a deep and weak pulse	Kidney qi deficiency with phlegm
difficulty in breathing, especially when lying down, worse at night and in the winter, copious and bubbly sputum	palpitations, edema, chest oppression, cold limbs, weak and slow pulse	Kidney yang deficiency with water accumulation

Table 2.1.10 Symptoms and Indications of Asthma

··· b) Wheezing (哮 *xiào*)

DEFINITION: respiration is rapid and makes a whistling sound. Recurrent attacks are likely. This condition is difficult to cure.

PATHOGENESIS: Lung qi fails to descend, with phlegm obstruction.

SYMPTOMS AND INDICATIONS:

Wheezing	Accompanying Symptoms	Indications
Heat wheezing: occurs during summer or fall, and is induced by hot and dry weather.		
wheezing with rapid respiration, loud, heavy and rough sound	thick yellow phlegm, red face, thirst, slippery and rapid pulse	phlegm heat accumulation in the Lung
dry wheezing with little or no phlegm, rapid respiration, soft voice	night sweats, dry mouth and throat, thin and rapid pulse	yin deficiency with phlegm
Cold wheezing: occurs during winter or spring, and is induced by cold and damp weather.		
wheezing with heavy and stifling sensation in the chest	profuse white or foamy phlegm, green and dim complexion, tight pulse	cold phlegm accumulation in the Lung
wheezing with short inconsistent respiration, aggravated by exertion	cold limbs, pale face, spontaneous sweating, pale tongue, submerged pulse	yang deficiency with phlegm

Table 2.1.11 Symptoms and Indications of Wheezing

··· c) Upper Stifling Breath (上氣 *shàng qì*)

DEFINITION: respiration is rapid, exhalation more evident than inhalation, and may be accompanied by shortness of breath and edema of the face and eyes.

PATHOGENESIS: Lung qi rises upward to the throat and obstructs the air tract.

SYMPTOMS AND INDICATIONS:

Breath Sounds	Accompanying Symptoms		Indications
rapid respiration, difficult breathing with rattling sound in throat	stifling sensation in chest, relieved with exhalation or sitting, worse when lying down	E X C E S S	phlegm accumulation in Lung
harsh and rapid respiration, cough with phlegm	chills and fever, possibly with facial edema		exopathogenic attack on the Lung
short and rapid respiration, dry cough or phlegm that is difficult to expectorate	night sweats, five center heat	D E F I C I E N C Y	yin deficiency with heat

Table 2.1.12 Symptoms and Indications of Upper Stifling Breath

··· d) Shortness of Breath (短氣 *duǎn qì*)

DEFINITION: respiration is inconstant, shallow, and rapid without sounds. It is like asthma, but without lifting the shoulders to breathe.

PATHOGENESIS: Lung qi deficiency.

SYMPTOMS AND INDICATIONS:

Main Symptoms	Accompanying Symptoms	Indications	
inconsistent shallow and rapid respiration without sounds	coughing with watery white sputum, stifling sensation in the chest	water retention in the chest	excess
	low energy, spontaneous sweating, frequent colds and flus, tongue with teeth marks	Lung qi deficiency	deficiency

Table 2.1.13 Symptoms and Indications of Shortness of Breath

··· e) Shortage of Qi (少氣 *shǎo qì*)

DEFINITION: respiration is feeble and short. It is difficult to produce the sound required for speech, but otherwise the breathing sounds normal.

PATHOGENESIS: antipathogenic qi insufficiency is a systemic deficiency in which all of the zang fu organs are in a state of hypofunction.

SYMPTOMS AND INDICATIONS: antipathogenic qi insufficiency.

COMPARISON OF UPPER STIFLING BREATH, SHORTNESS OF BREATH, AND SHORTAGE OF QI

Name	Symptoms	Pathogenesis
upper stifling breath	rapid breathing, exhales more than inhales	Lung qi obstruction
shortness of breath	short, rapid, and interrupted breathing without anguish or lifting of the shoulders	Lung qi deficiency
shortage of qi	breathing is feeble, short, and with low volume, difficult to produce speech, otherwise no other symptoms	antipathogenic qi insufficiency

Table 2.1.14 Comparison of Upper Stifling Breath, Shortness of Breath, and Shortage of Qi

V. COUGH

(1) Definition: cough is a common symptom arising from pathological changes of the Lung. Expelling air from the Lung suddenly and noisily keeps the respiratory passages free of irritating material (phlegm or other). Therefore, cough not only suggests pathological changes, but is also a response for self-protection.

(2) Pathomechanism: spasmodic contraction of the thoracic cavity causes the Lung qi to ascend, leading to a sudden closing of the glottis which produces the sound of coughing.

The Lung governs the qi and controls respiration. It is connected to the throat, opens to the nose, and governs the hair and skin. It is located on top of all the organs, and is regarded as the "delicate" organ because it is easily affected by environmental conditions. When exogenous pathogens attack the body, the Lung is often the first organ to be affected. Exogenous pathogens disturb the movement of the Lung qi and cause it to become rebellious, leading to cough. Additionally, cough is the body's natural attempt to expel the pathogens.

Zàng fǔ organ dysfunctions are also a major cause of cough. There are two endopathological changes that can cause cough: excess and deficiency.

Excess-type cough is due to pathogenic factors such as phlegm obstructing the Lung qi. This phlegm may arise from a dysfunction of the Spleen, Kidney, or Lung and can be caused by improper diet or chronic illness. Another cause of excess-type endopathogenic cough is Liver fire attacking the Lung, which may result from emotional stress.

Deficiency-type cough can appear in a patient with chronic illness, or a weak constitution. Deficiency-type cough includes Spleen and Lung qi deficiency, both of which can lead to a condition in which the Lung qi is too weak to descend. Another deficiency condition that causes cough is when the Kidney and Lung yin are deficient. The Lung loses nourishment and is unable to perform its descending function.

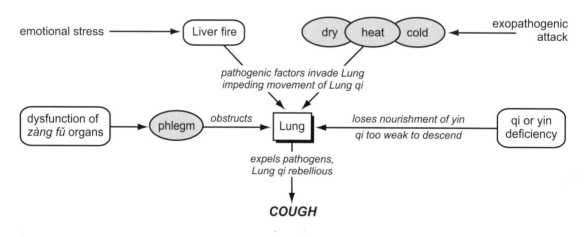

Chart 2.1.9 Etiologies and Pathomechanisms of Cough

(3) Clinical significance: the sound of the cough can help one determine the cause (etiology) and thermal nature of the disease.

(4) Symptoms and Indications

Cough				Indications
acute onset, harsh and loud cough, daytime worse than nighttime	harsh coarse and loud sound	**E X T E R I O R**		wind cold attack in Lung
	hacking, choking cough with coarse sound			wind heat attack in Lung
	dry hacking cough with clear, crisp sound			dryness attack in Lung
chronic recurrent onset, cough with loud coarse sound	paroxysmal, severe cough, the cough comes in bursts	**I N T E R I O R**	**E X C E S S**	Liver fire attacking Lung
	cough with rattling loose sound, worse in the morning and after meals			phlegm accumulation in the Lung
chronic cough with feeble and weak sound	feeble sound, low volume, worse in the afternoon and evening		**D E F I C I E N C Y**	Lung qi deficiency
	protracted dry and feeble cough with hoarse sound, worse in the evening			Lung yin deficiency
	low feeble volume, discontinuous cough			Kidney / Spleen yang deficiency
paroxysmal cough characterized by uninterrupted cough, even leading to vomiting, and making a sound like the call of the whooping crane, followed by recurrences.				whooping cough
spasmodic cough that sounds like the bark of a dog				diphtheria cough

Table 2.1.15 Symptoms and Indications of Cough

VI. Sneezing

(1) Definition: a sneeze is an autonomic, convulsive expulsion of air from the nose and mouth. In TCM theory, sneezing is the sound caused by Lung qi suddenly flowing upward through the throat and nose. It is a clinical manifestation of yang qi that is stimulated to brace up to pathogens. Sneezing is not only a pathological change, but a response for self-protection. *The Divine Pivot*, Chapter 28 (靈樞。口問) points out that "when yang qi is harmonious and sufficient, [it] fills the chest; [when] it arises from the nose, this is sneezing."

(2) Pathomechanism: there are two causes of sneezing, one being due to exogenous pathogens attacking the Lung and the other due to insufficient Lung qi. When exogenous pathogens attack the Lung, yang qi stirs upward to push the pathogens out. When the Lung qi suddenly flows upward through the nose and throat, this causes sneezing. When the Lung qi is insufficient, the nose loses nourishment, and this causes obstruction or abnormal sensations. The yang qi is then stimulated to flow upward and brace against the pathogenic factor, if it exists, resulting in sneezing.

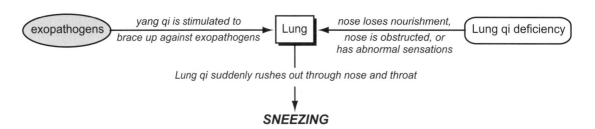

Chart 2.1.10 Etiology and Pathomechanism of Sneezing

(3) Clinical Significance: the sound of the sneezing can help one assess the thermal nature of the pathogenic factor as well as the state of the antipathogenic qi. It also helps in forming a prognosis for the disease.

(4) Symptoms and Indications

Sneezing	Indications
acute onset, constant loud sound	heat, excess
chronic frequent attack, soft volume	Lung qi deficiency
sudden sneezing in critical stage of chronic illness	yang qi recovery, improvement in disease state
sneezing due to external stimulation	normal

Table 2.1.16 Symptoms and Indications of Sneezing

VII. Vomiting

(1) Definition: vomiting (or emesis) is the forceful expulsion of the contents of the stomach through the mouth.

- vomiting: emesis with sound and vomitus
- silent vomiting: emesis without sound but with vomitus
- retching: emesis with sound but no vomitus or scanty fluid

(2) Pathomechanism: rebellious Stomach qi forces the Stomach contents out through the mouth. The Stomach is a *fǔ* organ, which has an abundance of qi and blood. It prefers moisture and dislikes dryness. It is responsible for receiving, decomposing (rotting and ripening), and causing the food to descend. There are three pathogeneses for rebellious Stomach qi: Stomach qi obstruction (stagnation), exopathogenic attack, and a loss of nourishment in the Stomach.

Improper diet, emotional distress, or *zàng fǔ* organ dysfunction may produce phlegm, qi stagnation, or food stagnation, any of which can obstruct the Stomach qi. When the Stomach qi is obstructed, the descending function becomes impaired, and instead of descending, the Stomach qi rises upward to cause vomiting.

Invasion by external pathogens into the Stomach is another common cause of vomiting. The external pathogen is usually dampness combined with a seasonal pathogen or the ingestion of spoiled food. External pathogens impair the descending of the Stomach qi, which causes the Stomach qi to rise up, resulting in vomiting.

Chronic illness or a weak constitution may lead to Spleen and Stomach qi deficiency or Stomach yin deficiency. When there is Spleen and Stomach qi or Stomach yin deficiency, there isn't enough power or nourishment to make the food descend, and vomiting results.

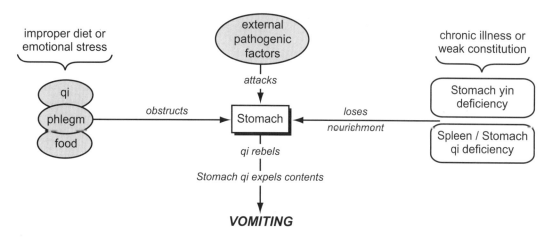

Chart 2.1.11 Etiology and Pathomechanism of Vomiting

(3) Clinical Significance: the sounds accompanying the vomiting can help one determine the thermal nature of the pathogen or disease, and whether it is excessive or deficient.

(4) Symptoms and Indications

Vomiting Sound		Indications
vomiting with deep sound, vomitus is made up first of clear fluids, followed by food, severe abdominal pain that is relieved by vomiting, usually occurs after overconsumption of raw or cold foods	E X C E S S	cold damp attacks Stomach
vomiting with loud and forceful sound, turbid vomitus has acidic taste and foul odor, usually occurs after over consumption of food		food stagnation
vomiting with deep loud sound, or retching without vomiting, intermittent attacks of nausea and sighing, usually occurs with emotional stress		Liver / Stomach disharmony
vomiting comes slowly with a weak sound, usually after a meal, and little quantity of vomitus	D E F I C I E N C Y	Spleen / Stomach yang deficiency
violent vomiting with sharp and crisp sound, vomitus is made up first of food, then clear fluids or green mucus, occurs immediately after eating, usually in the wake of febrile disease or over consumption of hot spicy food		Stomach yin deficiency

Table 2.1.17 Vomiting Sounds and their Indications

VIII. BELCHING

(1) Definition: also known as eructation, burping, or ructus. It is a normal process to relieve distention from the air that accumulates in the Stomach.

(2) Pathomechanism: rebellious Stomach qi makes a sound when flowing through the throat. Rebellious Stomach qi can be caused by conditions of either excess or deficiency. Excessive pathogens such as food, qi, or phlegm may accumulate in the Stomach and obstruct the descent of Stomach qi. Or, deficiency of the Spleen and Stomach qi may be unable to cause the Stomach qi to descend on its own. Thus, qi begins to accumulate in the Stomach and later rebels upwards as belching.

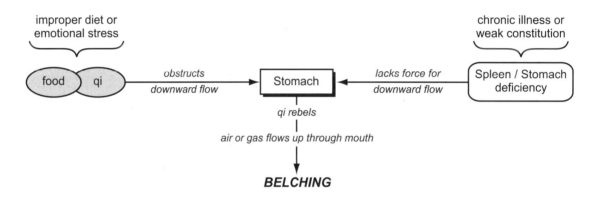

Chart 2.1.12 Etiology and Pathomechanism of Belching

(3) Clinical Significance: the sound of the belching can help one distinguish whether the pattern is excessive or deficient in nature.

(4) Symptoms and Indications

Belching Sounds	Accompanying Symptoms	Indications
Excess type: long, loud, and tight sound		
heavy and unclear sound with strong foul odor, induced or aggravated by overeating	abdominal pain aggravated by pressure, aversion to food	food stagnation
frequent attacks with loud and clear sound, induced or aggravated by emotional stress	hypochondriac pain and distention, easily angered, frequent sighing	Liver qi stagnation
Deficiency type: low volume, feeble, short sound		
belching with low, feeble, inconstant sound without odor	poor appetite, abdominal distention, fatigue, weak pulse	Spleen / Stomach deficiency

Table 2.1.18 Belching Sounds and their Indications

IX. HICCOUGHS

(1) Definition: reflexive spasms of the diaphragm accompanied by a rapid closure of the glottis produce an audible sound. Hiccoughs can occur alone or as part of some other condition.

(2) Pathomechanism: Stomach qi rebellion causes an involuntary spasm of the diaphragm and glottis. Many factors can contribute to this condition. Hiccoughs can be classified as excessive or deficient. Excessive conditions are due to external or internal pathogens which accumulate in the Stomach and obstruct the descent of Stomach qi. Deficiency of qi or yin causes the Stomach qi to lose its power to descend, which causes an accumulation of qi that rises in the form of hiccoughs.

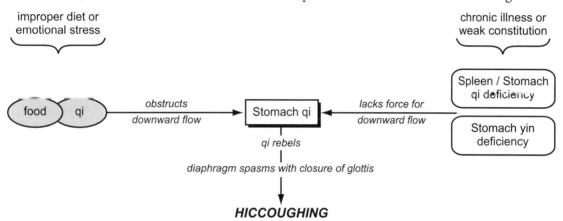

Chart 2.1.13 Etiology and Pathomechanism of Hiccoughs

(3) Clinical Significance: the sound of the hiccoughs enables one to distinguish whether it is a symptom of heat or cold, excess or deficiency.

(4) Symptoms and Indications

Hiccough Sounds			Indications
acute onset with loud, high-pitched, forceful, and consistent sound	deep, slow and forceful sound which may be relieved by heat and aggravated by cold	E X C E S S	pathogenic cold attacks the Spleen and Stomach
	frequent attacks that are induced by emotional stress; loud, sonorous, and clear sound		Liver fire attacks Stomach
	loud and clear sound, rushes out from the throat with a strong foul odor		Stomach fire
chronic onset, with low, weak, and intermittent sound	short and intermittent hiccough sounds with recurrent attacks	D E F I C I E N C Y	Stomach yin deficiency
	weak sound, low volume, intermittent, chronic		Spleen / Kidney yang deficiency
critical patient suddenly hiccoughs which is weak and interrupted and recurs after a long break			exhausted Stomach qi

Table 2.1.19 Hiccoughs and its Indications

Comparison of Vomiting, Belching, and Hiccoughs:

Symptoms	Common	Differences
vomiting	rebellious Stomach qi	food, fluid, or sputum flows up from the Stomach and out of the mouth, with sound
belching		air or gas flows up from the Stomach and makes sound when passing through the throat
hiccoughing		Stomach channel's qi rebellion causes involuntary spasms of the diaphragm and makes a short sound

Table 2.1.20 Comparison of Vomiting, Belching, and Hiccoughs

X. BORBORYGMI

(1) Definition: also called "bowel sounds" or "abdominal rumbling," this refers to the sounds associated with intestinal movement.

(2) Pathomechanism: Large Intestine qi disorder is the pathomechanism for borborygmi and is related to the function of the Spleen, Stomach, Liver, and Kidney. Qi obstruction, or qi and dampness lodged in the Large Intestine, are the two causes of pathological change affecting the qi of the Large Intestine.

An attack of external pathogens can lead to internal dampness. Improper diet can lead to an accumulation of food or phlegm in the middle burner. Dampness, food, and phlegm all block the circulation of qi . When qi and dampness strike and attack each other, intestinal sounds ensue. When the qi is stronger than the dampness, the sound is loud.

Both emotional stress and chronic illness can lead to qi obstruction. Following the Large Intestine's movement, qi stagnation can suddenly abate, giving rise to sudden borborygmi.

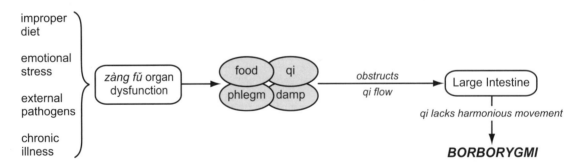

Chart 2.1.14 Etiology and Pathomechanism of Borborygmi

(3) Clinical Significance: the sound of borborygmi can help one distinguish whether the nature of the disease is one of excess or deficiency, hot or cold.

(4) Symptoms and Indications

Borborygmi Sounds	Accompanying Symptoms	Indications
Excess type: loud volume, acute attack, usually accompanied by diarrhea or dysentery		
thunder-like sound, frequent attacks	cold abdominal pain, loose stools, vomiting of clear fluids, cold limbs	cold damp in the middle burner
sounds like water sloshing in a bottle, if patient stands up or abdomen is pressed, the location of the sound descends	dizziness, retching, nausea, slippery pulse and greasy tongue coating	phlegm damp in the middle burner
borborygmi induced or aggravated by emotional stress and relieved by happiness, associated with slight abdominal pain	hypochondriac pain and distention, frequent sighing, irritability, wiry pulse	Liver / Spleen disharmony
loud volume, acute attack, usually occurs in the summer or late summer, can be induced by impropor diot, roliovod by paccagc of diarrhea	diarrhea or dysentery with burning sensation in anus, bitter taste in thc mouth	damp heat in the Stomach and Large Intestine
Deficiency type: weak volume, chronic condition, inconsistent sounds, recurrent attacks		
restless sounds as if due to hunger, chronic abdominal pain, relieved by warmth and aggravated by cold	loose stools in the morning, weakness or aching in the lower back or knees	Spleen / Kidney yang deficiency
weak volume, relieved by food and aggravated by hunger	fatigue, bloating, loose stools, or rectal prolapse	middle burner qi deficiency

Table 2.1.21 Symptoms and Indications of Borborygmi

XI. Sighing

(1) Definition: patient feels chest distress and makes a deep expiration with a short sound, which relieves the sensation of distress in the chest.

(2) Pathomechanism: sighing is an involuntary process to relieve chest distress. The chest distress is caused by qi obstruction, due to either emotional stress which causes qi stagnation in the chest, or to chronic illness which leads to qi deficiency and the loss of power to circulate qi in the chest.

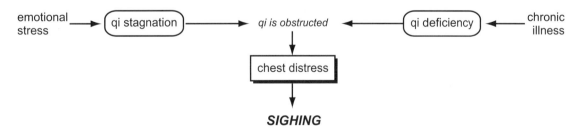

Chart 2.1.15 Etiology and Pathomechanism of Sighing

(3) Clinical Significance: the sound of the sighing can help one understand the condition of the qi.

(4) Symptoms and Indications

Symptoms	Accompanying Symptoms	Indications
sighing due to chest distress which is aggravated by emotional stress	hypochondriac pain and distention, irritability, anger, bitter taste, wiry pulse	Liver qi stagnation
sighing with a low and feeble sound, shortness of breath, chest distress, aggravated by exertion	voice with weak volume, pale tongue, frail pulse	yang qi deficiency

Table 2.1.22 Symptoms and Indications of Sighing

Section 2

Smelling (Olfaction)

I. Introduction

(1) Definition of Smelling

Smelling, also called "olfaction," means assessing the patient's odors, which include body odors, the odors of excreted materials, and the odors in a patient's room. The sense of smell is used to distinguish abnormal odors in the excreta and secretions, and to determine the cold or hot, excessive or deficient nature of a disease. It includes smelling the odor of sputum, nasal discharge, sweat, stool, urine, menstrual blood, vaginal discharge, etc.

When something is stale, there are changes in its odor. In a healthy body, the qi and blood circulate smoothly, the *zàng fǔ* organs and channels and collaterals function well, and there is accordingly no abnormal odor.

(2) Clinical Significance

The perception of an abnormal odor through the sense of smell can help one identify the thermal nature of the pathogens (hot or cold) and the state of the antipathogenic qi (excess or deficiency).

Odor	Indications
foul, rotten, fetid, stinking	heat, excess
fishy or odorless	cold, deficiency

Table 2.2.1 Abnormal Odors and their Indications

(3) The Scope of Smelling

Smelling for abnormal odors includes the odors of the body; odors of the orifices including the mouth (breath), nose, ears, and eyes; odors of the excreta and secretions including sweat, urine and stools, menstrual blood and vaginal discharge, vomit, ructus (belching), and flatulence; and finally the odor of the ward (or patient's room) are taken into consideration for purposes of diagnosis.

Abnormal odors {
  odor of the body
  odor of the orifices
  odor of excreta and secretions
  odor of ward (patient's room)
}

Chart 2.2.1 Abnormal Odors

II. Smelling

(1) Body Odor

Body odor is usually caused by pathological changes to the sweat. Sweating is a metabolic product of the body's physiological activities. It is body fluid which is evaporated and sent to the skin through the pores of the body by the yang qi. When there are pathological changes in the human body, sweating is one physiological method to expel the pathogens. Different pathogens cause different odors in the sweat.

Odor	Indications
goatish odor	wind damp heat accumulation
foul stinking odor	epidemic infection disease, or summer heat toxic syndrome
foul sweat odor in the armpit ("fox-like" smell)	damp heat accumulation

Table 2.2.2 Abnormal Odors of the Body and their Indications

(2) Odors of the Orifices

— A. Mouth Odor

Mouth odor can be caused by tissues in the oral cavity, or dysfunction of the internal organs. The most common cause is Stomach heat, however other causes include heat-phlegm in the Lungs, and Kidney yin deficiency with heat. Mouth odors can also be related to diet, drink, and medications.

Symptoms		Indications
fetid odor that is stinking and foul	**M O U T H**	gingivitis
sour and foul		tooth decay
foul odor that disappears after brushing teeth		bad mouth hygiene
foul odor with hot, swollen gums; or ulcers in the mouth and on the tongue; thirst with desire to drink cold fluids, red tongue with yellow coating	**S T O M A C H H E A T**	Stomach fire flaring upward
sour and stinking odor like rotten eggs, belching with foul smell, acid regurgitation, abdominal distention and pain that refuses pressure, red tongue, thick yellow greasy coating that looks like cottage cheese		food stagnation
foul odor with yellow eyes and skin, heavy sensation in the body, fatigue, poor appetite, nausea, bitter taste in the mouth, yellow greasy tongue coating		damp heat in the Liver and Gallbladder
foul fishy odor; cough with turbid sputum, or pus and blood; chest pain and distress, dry mouth and throat, no desire to drink, fever		phlegm heat accumulation in the Lung
foul odor, frequently recurring canker sores, chronic gum ulcers, hot flashes, night sweats		Kidney yin deficiency with fire

Table 2.2.3 Abnormal Odors of the Mouth and their Indications

— B. Odor of the Nose

Odor of the nose can arise from nasal discharge or internal organ disorders, such as *xiāo kě* (wasting and thirsting disorder) and yin-water pattern.

Symptoms			Indications
nasal discharge	yellow sticky discharge with foul odor	coughing with phlegm	excess heat in Lung
		poor appetite, distention and bloating	damp heat in the Spleen and Stomach
nasal ulcer	foul stinking odor with ulcer in the nose		syphilis, leprosy, rhinocarcinoma
internal organ disorder	rotten apple odor		late stage or severe *xiāo kě* syndrome
	smell of urine		late stage of yin-water syndrome (uremia)

Table 2.2.4 Abnormal Odors of the Nose and their Indications

— C. Odor of the Ears

SYMPTOMS: foul, fishy odor emanating from the ears with turbid pus and discharge

INDICATION: damp-heat accumulation in the ear

— D. Odor of the Eyes

SYMPTOMS: red and swollen eyes with turbid tears accompanied by a foul, fishy odor, or ulcerations around eyes

INDICATION: damp-heat in the Liver channel

(3) Odor of the Excreta and Secretions

— A. Vomiting and belching

Symptoms	Indications
sour and foul vomiting or belching with thirst for cold fluids	Stomach heat
putrid odor belching or vomiting with undigested food	food stagnation
vomit with pus and blood, and a **fishy foul odor**	Stomach abscess
vomit without odor or **slight fishy odor**, prefers warm fluids	cold in the Stomach / Spleen
odorless belching, abdominal cold pain, nausea	Liver attacking Stomach, or Stomach cold

Table 2.2.5 Vomiting and Belching Odors and their Indications

— B. Urination

Symptoms	Indications
frequent, urgent, painful, burning urination; turbid yellow urine with a **foul odor**	damp heat in the Bladder
heavy **smell of urea**, scanty yellow urine	Heart fire pouring downward into Bladder
clear frequent odorless urination or with a slight **fishy odor**	Kidney deficiency
odorless urinary incontinence	exhaustion of Kidney fire

Table 2.2.6 Urination Odors and their Indications

— C. Stool and Flatulence

Symptoms	Indications
fetid, stinking, foul odor, diarrhea with pus or blood, flatulence, tenesmus	damp heat in the Large Intestine
sour and foul odor with indigestion in pediatric cases	food stagnation
fishy odor with loose stools	cold in the Spleen / Stomach
slight odor or **odorless** flatulence, aggravated by emotional stress	Liver qi stagnation
abnormal stool color, but **without odor**, or frequent flatulence without strong odor	Stomach / Large Intestine qi deficiency

Table 2.2.7 Odors of Stool and Flatulence and their Indications

— D. Menstrual Blood and Vaginal Discharge

Symptoms	Indications
foul fishy odor with profuse yellow sticky vaginal discharge	damp heat in Liver channel
strong foul odor with yellow, green, and/or red color discharge	uterus ulceration
mild fishy odor with profuse white sticky discharge	damp cold in Liver channel

Table 2.2.8 Odors from Menstrual Blood and Vaginal Discharge and their Indications

(4) Ward Odor

An offensive odor in the patient's room or ward indicates a serious condition.

Symptoms	Indications
offensive odor	pestilent disease
bloody and fishy odor	profuse bleeding
smell of **rotten apples**	late stage of *xiāo kě* disease (diabetes mellitus)
urine odor	late stage of yin-water pattern (uremia)

Table 2.2.9 Ward Odors and their Indications

Section 3

Questions and Answers for Deeper Insight into Smelling and Listening

1. What are the differences between shortness of breath and shortage of qi?

Shortness of breath is short, rapid, and interrupted breathing. It is similar to asthma, but without the lifting of the shoulders. Shortage of qi is more difficult to see as it is very close to one's natural breathing; however, it is feeble, shallow, and light. Additionally, it limits one's ability to produce sounds, as the expiration is weak.

The pathomechanism of both shortness of breath and shortage of qi is insufficient Lung qi, however the pathogenesis of these two conditions is different.

Shortness of breath can arise from either excess or deficiency. Excess-type shortness of breath is caused by water retention in the chest, which limits the space available to inhale the clear qi. With a lack of qi entering, the Lung responds with rapid and shallow breathing in order to overcome the insufficiency of qi, resulting in "shortness of breath." This condition can also arise from chronic illness which consumes the Lung qi, or some other *zàng fǔ* organ dysfunction whereby the production of qi is compromised, leading to Lung qi deficiency.

By contrast, shortage of qi can only arise from deficiency. It is most commonly due to a deficiency of antipathogenic qi associated with chronic illness, weak constitution, malnutrition, or aging. Insufficient antipathogenic qi leads to a deficiency of Lung qi, which also gives rise to symptoms of fatigue and weak respiration, aggravated by slight exertion.

2. How is it that listening to a patient's vocal sounds can help predict pathological changes in the *zàng fǔ* organs?

Vocal sounds are produced by the coordinated functions of the Lung, throat, epiglottis, lips, tongue, teeth, and nose. The Lung governs the qi. While the Lung is by definition a *zàng* (solid) organ, it is unique in that it is also considered to be hollow, with many holes (中空有竅 zhōng kōng yǒu qiào). Because it is hollow, it can fill with clear qi, and the holes can reverberate when air is pushed upward through the throat. This produces sound.

While sound originates in the throat, it is the numerous movements of other structures that modify that sound into speech and other vocalizations. These include the opening and closing of the epiglottis, movement of the tongue, shape of the lips, and position of the teeth. Hence, listening to the changes in the sounds and vocalizations of the patient can help one identify pathological changes in the phonic organs.

According to five-phase theory, the sounds, *zàng* organs, and phonic organs all cooperate in a balanced manner to produce sound and vocalizations.

Phase	Wood	Fire	Earth	Metal	Water
pitch	mi (角 *jiǎo*)	so (徵 *zhǐ*)	do (宮 *gōng*)	re (商 *shāng*)	la (羽 *yǔ*)
vocalization	shouting	laughing	singing	crying	groaning
záng organ	Liver	Heart	Spleen	Lung	Kidney
phonic structure	tongue	teeth	throat	mouth	root of tongue

Table 2.3.1 The Five Phases and their Phonic Structures

Under normal circumstances, sound is produced harmoniously. It may deviate up or down by a few levels of pitch in accordance with one's constitution, age, sex, and emotional status, but the deviations are generally very small. However, when pathogens attack and cause pathological change in the *zàng fǔ* organs, an imbalance of the qi and blood can ensue. Thus, sound will lose its harmonious, smooth, and fluid qualities. Depending on the location of the pathology, the sound and voice will undergo a corresponding change. Therefore, listening to the changes in the sound and vocalizations can help one identify pathological changes in the phonic organs and, by extension, the *zàng fǔ* organs.

Phase	Wood	Fire	Earth	Metal	Water
normal sound characteristics	gentle and smooth; not too long nor short, pitch not too high nor low, sound not too tight nor loud	slightly short and high, clear with appropriate pitch and volume dynamics	long, thick deep, and free-flowing	slightly long, sharp, with a clang and jingle	short, high, thin
key characteristics	long	clear	deep	sharp	thin
abnormal characteristics	urgent, hurried	robust, strong	slow	sad, sorrowful	low volume, feeble

Table 2.3.2 Normal and Abnormal Sound Characteristics of the Five Phases

3. How can one differentiate asthma due to Lung qi deficiency from that due to Kidney qi deficiency?

In asthma, respiration is difficult, short, and rapid. There is a sense of tightness, constriction, and congestion in the chest. In severe cases, the patient gasps for breath with the mouth wide open. The shoulders may also lift and the nostrils may flare to assist with breathing. The patient cannot lie supine.

Asthma usually results from pathological changes to the Lung or Kidney, and is classified into excess and deficient types.

Excess-type asthma is commonly caused by wind-cold attack, heat-phlegm, or water retention in the Lung. All of these causes result in the Lung qi becoming constricted and unable to disperse.

Deficiency-type asthma can arise from either deficiency of Lung qi or Kidney qi. When the Lung's qi is deficient, it loses its ability to control and cause the qi to descend. When Kidney qi is deficient, it loses its ability to grasp the qi. Asthma due to both Lung qi deficiency and Kidney qi deficiency both share symptoms of short and difficult breathing. However, asthma due to Lung qi deficiency manifests with difficulty during the exhalation phase of respiration, with short and shallow inhalations. By contrast, asthma caused by Kidney qi deficiency presents with difficulty during inhalation, while exhalation is deep and long.

4. In which patterns can hiccoughs arise?

Hiccoughs is a spasm of the diaphragm accompanied by a rapid closure of the glottis, producing an audible sound. It can occur alone or as part of some other condition. In every case, the pathomechanism of hiccoughs is rebellious Stomach qi. Clinically, we can differentiate based on the volume of the sound (loud or weak volume), its pitch (high or low), and frequency (length of time between hiccoughs) to predict the thermal nature (heat or cold) and excess or deficient cause of the disease.

An acute onset, loud and forceful sound with high pitch, and frequent attacks all indicate an excess pattern due to an attack of pathogenic heat or cold in the Stomach. Chronic, low and weak volume with a deep pitch, and a long period of time between hiccoughs all suggest an association with Spleen and Stomach deficiency with cold. If the patient is in critical condition, but suddenly starts to hiccough frequently, but with a low, weak sound, it indicates Stomach qi failure.

5. What are the indications of pathological yawning?

Yawning due to normal fatigue or desire to sleep, such as just before bedtime or upon awakening, is considered normal. If one suffers from frequent yawning attacks or yawning in the absence of fatigue, these are considered pathological.

Yawning Description	Accompanying Symptoms	Indications
frequent yawning with loud sound, need is relieved after yawn, induced by emotional changes	depression, stifling sensation or discomfort in the chest and hypochondriac areas, belching, moodiness, wiry pulse	Liver qi stagnation
yawning accompanied with chest pain, may occur after injury or chronic illness	tight and stifling sensation in the chest, or with sharp pain; shortness of breath, dizziness, poor memory, purple tongue, choppy pulse	qi and blood stagnation
infrequent attack, weak or no sound	physical or mental fatigue, cold limbs, pale face, poor appetite, loose stools, pale tongue, deep and thin pulse	Spleen and Kidney yang deficiency

Table 2.3.3 Yawning and its Indications

Chapter Three

INQUIRY 問診

■ CONTENTS

Inquiry 問診

Section 1

Introduction

Inquiry allows the practitioner to obtain information about the patient's experience of pain or other non-observable phenomena, making it a very important component of the patient-practitioner interaction. Inquiry is one of the four key diagnostic methods in TCM. Practitioners inquire of the patient or her representative about the disease process' onset, development, treatment, present symptoms, and other information.

I. Definition

Inquiry examination is verbal interaction with the patient or her representative to obtain information used to develop an accurate diagnosis

II. Purpose of the Method of Inquiry

Inquiry can assist in collecting information where the other three methods (observation, listening and smelling, and palpation) were insufficient. Aspects of the patient need to be understood in order to determime the etiology, thermal nature, and history of the disease. These aspects include her pastimes, living environment (both climate and social environment) and customs, as well as the onset, development, and prior treatment of the illness. This additional information will assist in making a diagnosis and developing an appropriate treatment strategy.

III. Method

In order to obtain the most accurate information from the patient, the following items should be considered:

- The practitioner should be amiable and sympathetic to the patient's feelings.

- The practitioner should focus on the patient's chief symptoms or complaints.

- The practitioner should give the patient necessary prompts if the patient fails to talk about his or her disease clearly or comprehensively.

- A patient in critical condition should be given immediate emergency treatment after a brief inquiry and examination.

- During an inquiry, the practitioner should use simple language, rather than relying on medical terms.

• The practitioner is expected to accept the patient's answers with the utmost concentration and natural expression on her face, and without surprise, frustration, or a pessimistic reaction to the patient's responses.

Section 2

Scope of Inquiry

Inquiry is one of the most important examination techniques in TCM diagnosis. There are two main areas of questioning. First, there is the standard biographical information provided during a patient's first encounter with the practitioner, such as name, contact information, previous medical history, personal life history, and the family's medical history. Second, there are questions unique to the changeable nature of a health condition such as the chief complaint and present medical history.

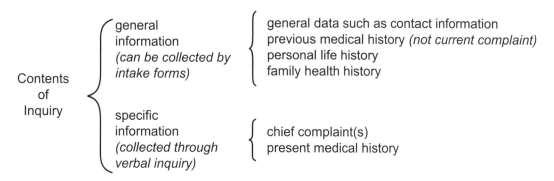

Chart 3.2.1 Scope of Inquiry

I. General Data

General data can help the practitioner get to know the patient, contact and follow-up with her, as well as provide basic reference information to help manage the case. General data includes the following:

• name

• gender

• age

• marital status

• occupation

• race

• birth place and nationality

• address

• phone number, email address, etc.

II. CHIEF COMPLAINT

The chief complaint are the symptoms the patient feels with the most severity, and are usually the main cause for visiting a practitioner. They include the following:

- major symptoms (chief symptoms)
- duration and frequency
- severity
- character

Chief complaint example #1: Dull lower back pain *(chief symptom)* over three years *(duration)* which has become severe *(severity)* with intermittent *(frequency)* and sharp pains *(character)* over the past two days *(duration)*.

Chief complaint example #2: Cough and constant *(frequency)* high fever with dull chest pain *(chief symptom, severity, and character)* for two days *(duration)*.

III. PRESENT MEDICAL HISTORY

Present medical history comprises the primary content of inquiry. It refers to the entire developing course of a condition, from its onset up to the present, and includes the following aspects:

(1) Onset of the Disease

This will help the practitioner assess the deficient or excessive condition of the antipathogenic qi, and the thermal nature of a disease. This includes:

- time and duration (date of onset and period since)
- cause or inducing etiological factors
- mode of onset (sudden or gradual)

(2) The Characteristics of the Chief Symptoms

These will help the practitioner identify the location and the thermal nature of pathological changes.

- location
- thermal nature (heat or cold)

(3) Accompanying Symptoms

These are other symptoms that accompany the chief complaint or symptoms.

(4) The Development of the Disease

Inquiring about the development of a disease chronologically, from its onset to its present state. These questions include the following:

- when and why the symptom is aggravated or alleviated
- whether its existence is temporary or persistent
- when and why it changes

(5) The Course of Diagnosis and Prior Treatment by Other Practitioners

- practitioner or other physician
- examination and results
- diagnosis
- treatment
- medication: dosage, method of application, duration, result and side effects

IV. PREVIOUS MEDICAL HISTORY

The patient's past health condition and diseases. This serves as a reference for the present disease, and includes the following:

- past health condition (both health or illness)
- past diseases

V. PERSONAL LIFE HISTORY

This includes the history of the patient's life style, such as:

- life experience (personal and work history)
- pastimes, recreation, addictions
- emotional status
- diet
- lifestyle
- working condition

VI. FAMILY MEDICAL HISTORY

Learning about the state of health and diseases that the patient's relatives had may be helpful to making a diagnosis about certain infectious or hereditary diseases.

Section 3

Present Symptoms and the Ten Questions

Inquiring about present symptoms means asking the patient about her suffering or discomfort, and the condition of the whole body as it may relate to her illness.

Symptoms reflect pathological changes and provide the basis for diagnosis and differentiation. In the clinic, many symptoms are subjective, e.g., stifling sensation, bloating, heavy sensations, pain, numbness, etc. There are no objective indications for these kinds of patient experiences. They can only be obtained through the method of inquiry.

TEN QUESTIONS

Present symptoms include the patient's daily experience with diet, elimination, discomfort, or unusual symptoms. This information will reflect the body's physiological and pathological condition.

The "Ten Question Song" (十問歌 *shí wèn gē*) was originally written in the Ming dynasty by Zhang Jing-Yue (張景岳). It provides the practitioner with a template whereby important clinical information can be obtained in a manner that is easy to remember.

First, ask about hot and cold (chills and fever)

Second, ask about sweat (sweating)

Third, ask about head and body (head and limbs)

Fourth, ask about stools and urine (urination and defecation)

Fifth, ask about food and drink (diet)

Sixth, ask about chest

Seventh, ask about hearing (deafness)

Eighth, ask about thirst

Ninth, ask women's questions (gynecology)

Tenth, ask children's questions (pediatrics).

In the clinic, these ten questions are a good guide to follow, however questions not included above should also be considered such as asking about emotional disturbances, the patient's pain, and sleeping. For this reason, the remainder of this chapter will not always correspond exactly with the ten question song as listed above.

Question One: Chills and Fever

I. INTRODUCTION AND DEFINITION

In Chinese medicine, chills and fever are two opposing phenomena which are objective or subjective symptoms of physiological or pathological processes. They are common symptoms over the course of a disease, and reflect the status of yin and yang, as well as the thermal nature of the pathogenic factor(s).

Chills: the cold sensation felt by a patient. Depending on the character and degree of cold, chills are classified into three levels: aversion to wind, aversion to cold, and intolerance of cold.

Fever: the sensation of heat or warmth in a patient. Depending on whether the fever is manifest in the body's temperature or is just the subjective sensation of the patient, fever can be divided into two levels: feverish sensation, and fever or higher body temperature.

II. ETIOLOGY AND PATHOMECHANISMS OF CHILLS AND FEVER

Chills and fever are usually associated with the thermal nature of the pathogenic factor and with the state of the yin and yang of the body.

Thermal Nature of the Pathogenic Factor:
Generally speaking, when exopathogenic factors cause disease, pathogenic cold mostly causes an aversion to cold, but the cold can also transform into heat. Pathogenic heat mostly causes fever, but can also lead to false cold.

Condition of Yin and Yang:
When the disharmony between yin and yang leads to pathological changes in the body, the following can occur: if yang predominates, the result will be external heat; if yin predominates, the result will be internal cold; if yang declines, the result will be external cold; if yin declines, the result will be internal heat.

Fever / Chills	Pathogenesis	
	exopathogenic factor	yin / yang disharmony
Heat (fever)	pathogenic heat	yin deficiency or yang excess
Cold (chills)	pathogenic cold	yin excess or yang deficiency

Table 3.3.1 Pathogenesis of Chills and Fever

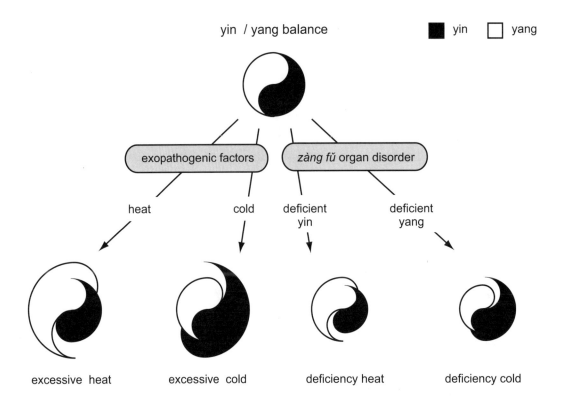

Chart 3.3.1 Pathogenesis of Chills and Fever

III. CLINICAL SIGNIFICANCE:

Inquiry into the details of chills and fever can help one to:

- infer the disease etiology
- distinguish the disease location
- determine the thermal nature of the pathogenic factor
- know the condition of yin and yang in the body
- provide a reliable treatment principle

IV. SCOPE OF INQUIRY INTO CHILLS AND FEVER

When asking about chills and fever, the following five areas are the most important:

1) Existence of chills and fever
2) Relationship of chills and fever. If fever and chills are present, their relationship should be determined:
   - simultaneous chills and fever
   - chills only or fever only
   - alternating chills and fever

3) Severity: if chills and fever are simultaneous, which is more severe?

- mild aversion to cold and high fever

- severe aversion to cold and slight fever

- severe aversion to cold and high fever

- mild aversion to cold and slight fever

4) Onset and duration

- do the chills or fever get worse in the morning, noon or evening?

- chills first and then fever, or fever first and then chills?

- duration: chronic or acute?

5) Concomitant symptoms

Are there other symptoms that accompany the chills and fever such as cough, headache, anorexia, etc.?

V. Pathological Chills and Fever

Pathological chills and fever can be classified into four categories: chills without fever, fever without chills, simultaneous chills and fever, and alternating chills and fever.

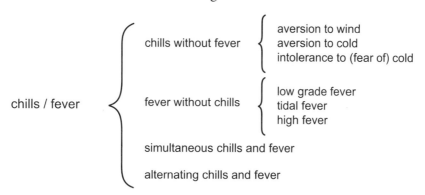

Chart 3.3.2 Chills and Fever

(1) Chills without Fever

— A. Definition

The condition in which the patient feels cold but there is no fever or feverish sensation. Chills may appear in the early stage of an exterior pattern before the fever appears; or it may be due to pathogenic cold directly attacking the *zàng fǔ* organs and/or channels, or to deficiency of the internal organs. The severity and character of the chills can be classified according to three levels of severity: aversion to wind, aversion to cold, and intolerance of cold.

Aversion to wind (惡風 *wù fēng*): a slight aversion to cold, feeling chills when exposed to even a slight draft.

Aversion to cold (惡寒 *wù hán*): feeling chills that are not relieved by putting on more clothes or warming oneself from a heat source.

Intolerance of cold (fear of cold) (畏寒 *wèi hán*): chills that are relieved by putting on more clothes or warming oneself from a heat source.

— B. Etiology and pathomechanisms of chills

Yin excess is the pathomechanism of cold or chills. There are two causes of yin excess. The first is due to exopathogenic cold attack, and the second to a disorder of the *zàng fǔ* organs.

When exopathogenic cold attacks the body surface, defensive qi will rise up against the pathogen. This process may weaken or even impair the defensive qi's warming function. Therefore, the patient feels aversion to wind or to cold. Pathogenic cold can also attack the *zàng fǔ* organs, which damages the yang and obstructs circulation, thereby causing sensations of cold and pain.

A *zàng fǔ* organ disorder can cause yang deficiency, especially Kidney yang deficiency, which makes yin relatively excessive. When deficient Kidney yang can no longer maintain its warming function, the patient feels an intolerance of cold.

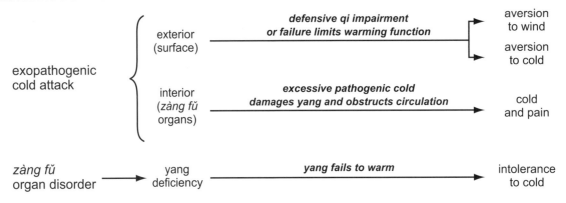

Chart 3.3.3 Etiology and Pathogenesis of Chills

— C. Symptoms and indications

Chills	Description	Indications	Pathogenesis
aversion to wind	feels cold when exposed to wind	nutritive/defensive qi disharmony, *tài yáng* deficiency type syndrome	defensive qi impairment or failure leads to compromised warming function
aversion to cold	chills and cold sensations not relieved by more clothes or heat source	exterior cold	defensive qi fights with exopathogens, cannot maintain warming function
shivers	severe aversion to cold with shivering		
intolerance (or "fear") of cold	cannot tolerate cold, sensation relieved by more clothes or external heat source	interior cold due to yang deficiency	yang qi deficiency fails to warm the surface

Table 3.3.2 Symptoms and Indications of Chills

Be aware that aversion to wind, aversion to cold, and shivering last for only a short time in an exterior condition before the body temperature rises.

(2) Fever without Chills

— A. Definition

The condition in which the patient's body temperature rises or the patient reports feeling warm. Depending on the severity of the heat, its time of occurrence and duration, and its characteristics, it can be classified as one of three types: low-grade fever, tidal fever, and high fever.

Low-grade fever (低燒 *dī shāo*): the body temperature is consistently between 98.6° and 100.4° F (37° - 38° C) over a period of at least two weeks. In TCM, low-grade fever also includes a patient's subjective sensation of heat, even in the absence of a measurable rise in body temperature.

Tidal fever (潮熱 *cháo rè*): occurs or worsens at a fixed hour of the day, just like the regular rise and fall of the tides. Tidal fever can also include a patient's subjective sensation of heat, without any measurable increase in body temperature.

High fever (高燒 *gāo shāo*): a body temperature above 102° F (38.8° C), which persists without aversion to cold.

— B. Etiology and Pathomechanisms of Fever

Fever is a symptom of antipathogenic qi resisting pathogens. The fever's severity depends on the strength of both the antipathogenic qi as well as the strength of the pathogenic factor.

Fever is essentially an excess state of yang arising from either exposure to pathogenic factors or a *zàng fǔ* organ disorder.

Pathogenic factors can enter from the exterior, such as heat, cold, dryness, or damp-heat, or they can arise from a *zàng fǔ* organ disorder, such as blood stasis, phlegm, or food stagnation. Generally speaking, pathogenic factors from the exterior lead to acute high fevers, while pathogenic factors associated with internal disorders cause chronic lower-grade fevers.

Zàng fǔ organ disorders usually cause a deficiency of yin, blood, qi, or yang, any of which can cause a relative excess of yang, giving rise to either a chronic low-grade fever or to feverish sensations.

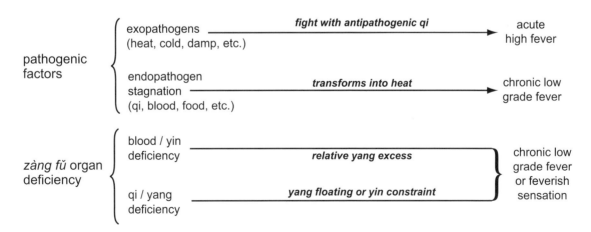

Chart 3.3.4 Pathogenesis of Fever

— C. Symptoms and Indications

Fever	Description	Indications	Pathogenesis
high fever	temperature above 102° F (38.8° C), may be accompanied by thirst, sweating, and flooding pulse	excess type interior heat syndromes	transmission of the pathogenic factors from the exterior to the interior with excessive heat in the interior
tidal fever	high grade tidal fever, occurs and is aggravated between 3-5 pm	*yáng míng fǔ* syndrome	*yáng míng* qi reaches its peak between 3-5 pm. It creates a stronger battle between antipathogenic qi and the pathogen at this time of day.
tidal fever	Upon initial touch, skin feels normal, however upon prolonged touch, skin feels hot. Fever gets worse in afternoon, decreases a little after sweating, but fever soon returns.	hidden-fever due to damp heat	Damp heat in the middle burner - dampness prevents heat from radiating outward, the fever is then hidden. The dampness is sticky and difficult to clear, so it becomes prolonged and stubborn.
low-grade fever or feverish sensation	low-grade fever or feverish sensation occurs in the late afternoon or night	yin deficiency	yin deficiency leads to a relative yang excess which results in endogenous heat
low-grade fever or feverish sensation	afternoon or nighttime low-grade fever, or localized sensations of heat, fixed and sharp pain, follows traumatic injury	blood stagnation	stagnation transforms into heat
low-grade fever or feverish sensation	intermittent low-grade fever, usually occurring in the morning or afternoon, induced or worse after exertion	qi deficiency	middle burner qi deficiency with empty fire - qi deficiency leads to stagnation which causes heat

Table 3.3.3 Symptoms and Indications of Fever

(3) Simultaneous Chills and Fever

— A. Definition

The condition in which the patient has a sensation of chills accompanied by a higher body temperature (measured). It is seen in the initial stage of an exterior pattern caused by exogenous pathogens. Because the exopathogens have different thermal natures, simultaneous chills and fever can be divided into three types:

- Severe chills and slight fever
- Slight chills with high fever
- Fever with aversion to wind

— B. Etiology and Pathomechanisms of Chills and Fever

Chills and fever reflect the struggle between defensive qi and the pathogenic factor. When exogenous pathogens attack the body, defensive qi will rise up against the pathogen. This process may weaken or impair the defensive qi's warming function. Therefore, the patient feels aversion to wind or aversion to cold. Meanwhile, the struggle between the defensive qi and the exopathogens will create heat and lead to an increase in body temperature.

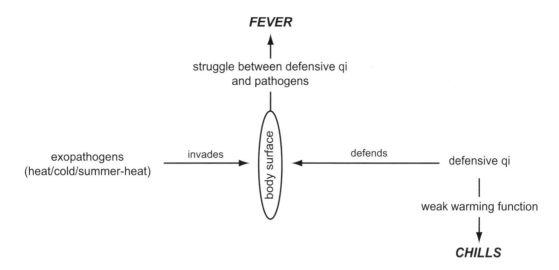

Chart 3.3.5 Pathology of Simultaneous Chills and Fever

The severity of the chills and fever helps one judge the thermal nature of the exopathogens. Generally speaking, if the fever is high with mild chills, this indicates an exterior attack of wind-heat; if there are severe chills with mild fever, this indicates exterior wind-cold.

The severity of the chills and fever can also help one understand the condition of the antipathogenic qi and the pathogens. Generally speaking, if the pathogen is weak and the antipathogenic qi is strong, the fever and chills are both mild. When there are strong pathogens and weak antipathogenic qi, the chills are severe and the fever is mild; if the pathogens and antipathogenic qi are both strong, the chills and fever are both severe.

— *C. Symptoms and Indications*

Symptoms	Additional Symptoms	Season	Indications	
severe chills and slight fever	bodyaches and wheezing, no sweating	winter	wind cold attack	excess type
chills and fever, aversion to wind	spontaneous sweating, sneezing	winter and spring		deficiency type
slight chills, severe fever	sore throat, cough, thirst headache	spring	wind heat attack	
high fever with slight chills	distending headache, stifling sensation in chest, nausea, sweating, thirst, greasy tongue coating	summer or late summer	summer heat	

Table 3.3.4 Symptoms and Indications of Fever and Chills

(4) Alternating chills and fever

— *A. Definition*

The condition usually seen in the middle stage of an exopathogenic factor's attack (*shào yáng* stage or malaria). The chills and fever occur one after the other.

— B. Etiology and Pathomechanisms of Alternating Chills and Fever

When the pathogen invades deeper into the body and struggles with antipathogenic qi between the exterior and interior, the antipathogenic qi and pathogens become locked. When antipathogenic qi is stronger than the pathogens, or the pathogens decline, yang will dominate and the body temperature will rise; when the pathogens predominate, or antipathogenic qi is weaker, yin will dominate and there will be chills.

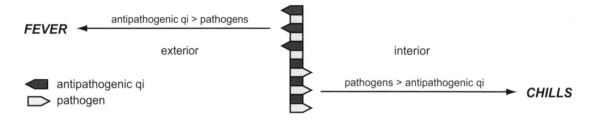

Chart 3.3.6 Pathogenesis of Alternating Chills and Fever

— C. Symptoms and Indications

	Symptoms		Indications	Pathogenesis
alternating chills and fever	irregular occurance	bitter taste in mouth, fullness and pain in chest and flanks, wiry pulse	*shào yáng* pattern	pathogen can't completely enter the interior while antipathogenic qi is unable to expel the evil
	regular occurance	severe headache, profuse sweating, and thirst	malaria	exopathogen hides in the *mò yuán**, located between interior and exterior

Table 3.3.5 Alternating Chills and Fever in Shào yáng Pattern and in Malaria

---

*Mò yuán (膜原) is also known as the "membrane source", an anatomical location unique to the warm-febrile disease school which describes the diaphragm.

■ Question Two: Sweating

I. INTRODUCTION

Sweating is both a physiological and pathological clinical phenomenon. When we eat spicy or pungent foods, do physical work, undergo sudden emotional changes, or wear too many clothes, there will be sweating. This is a normal physiological process. Sweating is generated by the body fluids. *The Divine Pivot*, Chapter 30 (靈樞。決氣) states that "when the interstitial (腠理 *zòu lǐ*) spaces open, the body fluids come out to form sweat." This means that body fluids and sweat are the same substance. When it is inside the body we call it body fluids, and when it is outside the body, escaping through the skin pores, we call it sweat.

(1) Physiology of Sweat Formation

Sweat is body fluids which have been steamed and sent to the skin through the pores by the yang qi. To form sweat, three things are required: material substance, power, and open skin pores. Body fluids transform from food essence, which depends on the function of the Spleen and Stomach. Yang qi provides the power to push the body fluids out of the body in the form of sweat. *Basic Question*, Chapter 7 (素問。陰陽別論) points out: "When yang is more abundant than yin, the yang energy will force the yin fluids to discharge and cause sweating."

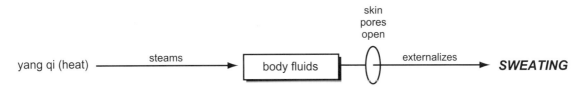

Chart 3.3.7 Physiology of the Formation of Sweat

(2) Sweat and *Zàng Fǔ* Organ Relationships

Since sweat is the body fluids that have been pushed out by yang qi, any organ related to the formation of body fluids, such as the Lung, Spleen, Stomach, or Kidney, plays an important part in the formation of sweat. Among these organs, the Heart plays the most important part in sweat formation.

Heart: sweat is also called the fluid of the Heart. Sweat is a body fluid. Body fluids and blood are mutually interchangeable. The Heart governs the blood. Therefore, the Heart has an intimate relationship with sweat.

Spleen and Stomach: body fluids originate from food and drink, which are transported and transformed by the Spleen and Stomach. The Spleen and Stomach are therefore the source of sweat.

Kidney: a water organ, the Kidney supplies the power to the Spleen to perform the function of transformation, and assists the Small Intestine in its function of separation of body fluids into pure and impure parts. The Kidney is also in charge of the excretion of fluids. The Kidney is the root of sweat.

Lung: said to regulate the "water passages" because it controls the dispersion of the body fluids, the Lung also controls the opening and closing of the skin pores.

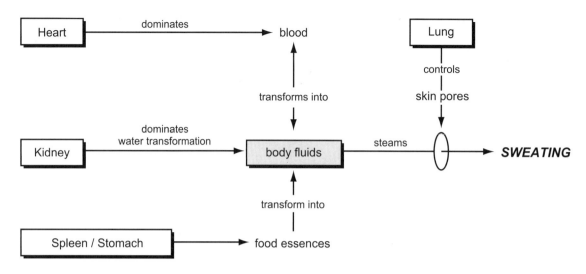

Chart 3.3.8 Sweating and the *Zàng Fǔ* Organs

(3) Functions of Physiological Sweating

Sweat is an important physiological product that performs the following functions:

- regulates body temperature
- maintains balance between yang qi and yin fluid
- expels metabolic waste
- expels pathogenic factors
- harmonizes the nutritive and defensive qi
- moistens the skin

II. ETIOLOGY AND PATHOMECHANISM OF SWEAT:

There are two major causes for abnormal sweating. One is pathogenic heat that originates either from the exterior or the interior due to yang excess or yin deficiency. In either case, the pathogenic heat steams and pushes the body fluids outward. The other cause is qi deficiency, especially Lung qi deficiency, in which the Lungs lose control over the opening and closing of the skin pores, leading to the leakage of body fluids.

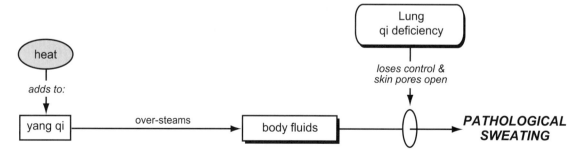

Chart 3.3.9 Pathogenesis of Pathological Sweating

III. CLINICAL SIGNIFICANCE:

Inquiry into the details about sweating can help one to:

- assess the condition of the antipathogenic qi, which helps determine the treatment principle
- determine the disease location and its thermal nature
- assess the state of the body fluids

IV. SCOPE OF INQUIRING OF SWEATING

When asking about sweating, one should focus on the following:

- whether or not there is sweating
- time of occurrence: when is the sweating most pronounced? (daytime, nighttime, after exercise, eating, etc.)
- location: where on the body is it sweating (head, back, hands)?
- severity: quantity of sweat (slight or profuse)
- character of sweat: thin, thick, sticky, or oily
- symptoms accompanying sweating
- any signs or symptoms that change after sweating

V. PATHOLOGICAL SWEATING

Pathological sweating can present as either anhidrosis (no sweating) or morbid sweating. Depending on the amount, time, and location, morbid sweating may be further subdivided into profuse sweating, spontaneous sweating, night sweats, partial sweating, and improper sweats.

abnormal sweating {
    no sweating
    morbid sweating {
        profuse sweating
        spontaneous sweating
        night sweats
        partial sweating
        improper sweats (gold or yellow sweating)
    }
}

Chart 3.3.10 Pathological Sweating

(1) Anhidrosis (no sweating)

— A. Definition

A condition in which there is a lack of physiological sweating.

— B. Etiology and Pathomechanisms

Sufficient body fluids, abundant yang qi, and open skin pores are the three conditions required for the body to sweat. When exopathogenic cold attacks the body surface, it constricts and blocks the skin pores, preventing body fluids from escaping. In chronic conditions, *zàng fǔ* organ disorders result in a deficiency of yin or yang. When there is yin deficiency, there is not enough body fluids to dispatch to the body surface; when there is yang deficiency, the yang qi will not be strong enough to steam the body fluids, and therefore no sweat is produced.

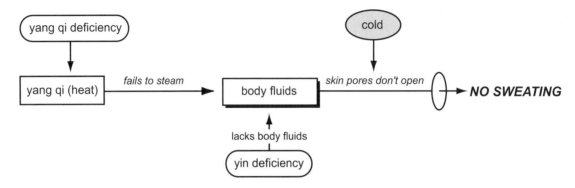

Chart 3.3.11 Pathogenesis of Anhidrosis

— C. Symptoms and Indications

Description	Indications		Pathogenesis
acute onset, severe chills with mild fever, no sweating, headache, nasal obstruction	**exterior** wind cold		pathogenic cold causes constriction and blockage of skin pores
chronic illness, dry skin and dry hair, five center heat, irritability	**interior**	yin deficiency	shortage of body fluids cannot product sweat
intolerance to (fear of) cold, desire for warm drinks, pale face and tongue, deep, weak, and slow pulse		yang deficiency	declining yang can no longer evaporate body fluids

Table 3.3.6 Symptoms and Indications of Anhidrosis

MORBID SWEATING

(2) Profuse sweating

— A. Definition

Excessive perspiration on the skin; overevaporation of body fluids.

— B. Etiology and Pathomechanisms of Profuse Sweating

There are two causes of profuse sweating. The first is body fluids being steamed by excessive pathogenic heat. This pathogenic heat can come from either an external invasion, such as an attack of wind-heat or summer heat, or excessive interior heat. The second cause of profuse sweating is loose interstitial spaces and open skin pores due to the failure of yang qi. The yang fails to consolidate the body surface, allowing the body fluids to escape from the body.

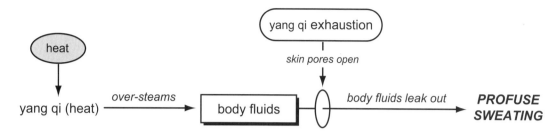

Chart 3.3.12 Pathogenesis of Profuse Sweating

— C. Symptoms and Indications

Description	Indications	Pathogenesis
profuse warm (hot) sweating with red face, high fever, thirst and big pulse	excessive heat	excessive heat steams and pushes body fluids out
cold and clear sweat, or oily sweat with pale face and cold limbs	yang exhaustion	yang fails and skin pores open, fluids leak out
sticky, warm, and yellowish sweat with warm limbs, thirst, sunken eyes, thin or faint pulse	yin exhaustion	yang fails following yin failure, deficient heat pushes out remaining body fluids

Table 3.3.7 Symptoms and Indications of Profuse Sweating

(3) Spontaneous Sweating

— A. Definition

Frequent sweating during the daytime in the absence of any sweat-inducing activity. Spontaneous sweating is aggravated by slight exertion.

— B. Etiology and Pathomechanisms of spontaneous sweating

Because of yang qi deficiency, or the failure of defensive yang to consolidate the body surface or to regulate the opening and closing of the skin pores, the interstitial spaces loosen and there is a leakage of body fluids. Physical exertion consumes more qi, and thus the sweating is aggravated by slight exertion.

Another reason for spontaneous sweating is disharmony between the nutritive and defensive qi. Under normal circumstances, the nutritive and defensive qi mutually control each other. Defensive qi circulates on the surface of the body and consolidates the nutritive qi so as to keep it inside. Meanwhile, the nutritive qi supplies nutrition for the defensive qi. When exopathogenic factors attack the body, the defensive qi rises up against the pathogens, and this action may disrupt the balance between the nutritive and defensive qi. Defensive qi then fails to consolidate the nutritive qi and the body fluids leak out.

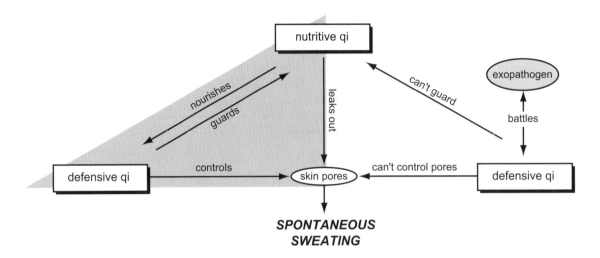

Chart 3.3.13 Pathogenesis of Spontaneous Sweating

— C. Symptoms and Indications

Description		Indications	Pathogenesis
spontaneous sweating, aversion to wind, body aches, possible fever and chills, sneezing, thin white coating, moderate pulse		nutritive / defensive qi disharmony	defensive qi fails to consolidate the surface, interstitial space is loose and skin pores open, body fluids escape
spontaneous sweating worse after exertion	frequent colds, aversion to cold, shortness of breath	qi deficiency	Heart / Lung qi deficiency, not consolidating the surface, allows body fluids to escape
	cold limbs, poor appetite, weak low back	yang deficiency	Kidney / Spleen yang deficiency - yang cannot control yin, yin escapes

Table 3.3.8 Symptoms and Indications of Spontaneous Sweating

(4) Night Sweats

— A. Definition

Sweating that occurs while asleep and stops upon awakening.

— B. Etiology and Pathomechanisms of Night Sweats

As a physiological function, the defensive qi circulates on the skin's surface during the daytime and then enters the interior and moves into the yin phase with the nutritive qi during sleep. Since the defensive qi is not on the surface, the interstitial spaces are slightly loose and the skin pores open easily. At this time, a very mild heat, such as deficiency heat or heat generated by stagnation, may be able to steam the body fluids outward.

If yin essence is insufficient it will be unable to control the yang. This will lead to a relative predominance of yang qi, which will give rise to endogenous deficiency heat during sleep when the defensive qi is completely interior. The defensive qi is also yang, so when it enters the interior at night and combines with deficiency heat, it will produce a stronger heat that pushes out the body fluids.

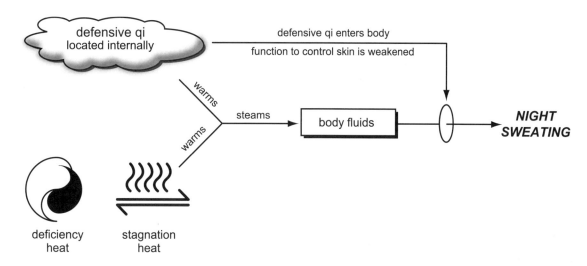

Chart 3.3.14 Pathogenesis of Night Sweats

— C. Symptoms and Indications

Description	Indications		Pathogenesis
frequent night sweating, dull and heavy headache, poor appetite	excess	dampness accumulation	During the sleeping period, yang retreats to the interior, so defensive qi is weaker in the skin. Deficiency or stagnation heat alone is then strong enough heat to push outward the body fluids that would not otherwise be expressed when yang is controlling the exterior.
night sweats with short term illness, alternating chills and fever		*shào yáng* pattern	
palpitations, pale face, dizziness, insomnia, shortness of breath, poor memory	deficiency	Heart blood deficiency	
hot flashes, five center heat, thirst, low grade fever, emaciation		Kidney yin deficiency	

Table 3.3.9 Symptoms and Indications of Night Sweats

(5) Pathological Sweating at Different Locations

— A. Definition

Sweating is present only in certain parts of the body, or is profuse or excessive only in those areas.

— B. Etiology and Pathomechanisms of Pathological Sweating at Different Locations

In TCM, we view the body as a whole. Local areas are governed by the internal organs. Connections occur via the channels and collaterals. Thus, sweating in a particular part of the body will reflect the condition of a specific organ. Inquiry about the location of abnormal sweating helps us identify the location of the disease in a channel, collateral, or *zàng fŭ* organ. Generally speaking, abnormal sweating at different locations is caused by an imbalance in the distribution of body fluids due to either stagnation or excess heat in certain parts of the body; or it is caused by disorders of the *zàng fǔ* organs.

— C. *Symptoms and Indications*

Location	Differentiations and Symptoms	
half of the body (left / right)	***wind dampness or cold dampness stagnation in the channels and collaterals:*** sweating with hemiplegia, or stiff joints and muscle aches	
	nutritive and defensive qi disharmonies: spontaneous sweating with aversion to wind	
	qi and blood deficiency: spontaneous sweating, night sweats that are induced or aggravated by exertion	
upper body	***damp heat accumulation:*** fever, irritability, insomnia, carbuncles and deep-rooted boils	
lower body	***damp heat in the lower burner:*** sweating in external genital area, may be swollen, UTI	
head	excess type	***dampness with heat:*** sticky, warm, sweat has a foul odor
	deficiency type	***yang collapse:*** cold sweat beads up like pearls
	zhēng lóng tóu	***normal:*** baby's head sweats while sleeping without other symptoms
chest	***Heart and Spleen qi deficiency:*** palpitations, fatigue, pale face, aversion to cold	
	Heart and Kidney yin deficiency: night sweats, restlessness, insomnia, and palpitations	
hands & feet	excess type	***excess heat in the yáng míng fǔ:*** severe constipation, fever possible
		damp heat in the middle burner: stifling sensation in chest, loose stools
	deficiency type	***Spleen and Stomach qi deficiency:*** cold limbs, fatigue, pale tongue
		Liver and Kidney yin deficiency: night sweats, five center heat
armpit	***damp heat in the Liver and Gallbladder channel:*** sweating with strong odor	
	Liver yin deficiency with deficiency heat: sweating without odor	

Table 3.3.10 Pathological Sweating at Different Locations and their Indications

■ Question Three: Pain

I. INTRODUCTION AND DEFINITION

Pain is one of the most common pathological clinical phenomena. It refers to an unpleasant or uncomfortable feeling in the body, which may be accompanied by aching or sore sensations. Pain is a subjective feeling and, based on its severity, can be divided into three levels of intensity:

- mild pain: patient can ignore the sensation
- moderate pain: interferes with tasks or concentration
- severe pain: interferes with basic needs or requires bedrest

II. Etiology and Pathomechanisms of Pain

When tissues and organs lack nourishment, the body will generate an unpleasant feeling: pain. There are two pathomechanisms whereby tissues or organs may lack nourishment. The first is stagnation, which prevents qi, blood, body fluids, or other nutrients from nourishing local tissues; this causes pain. The stagnation may arise from a dysfunction of the *zàng fǔ* organs, local trauma, or from invasion of pathogenic cold. In the case of stagnation, the pain is often sharp and severe. The second cause is deficiency of qi, blood, body fluids, or essence, which results in a lack of nourishment to the tissues and organs. This too causes pain, which in this case is usually dull, aching, and mild.

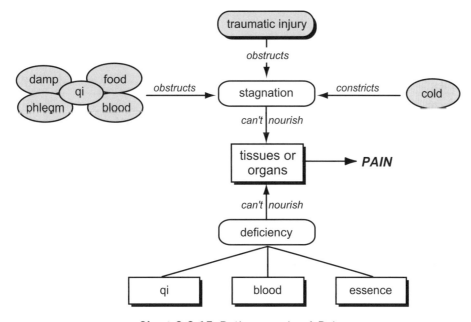

Chart 3.3.15 Pathogenesis of Pain

III. Clinical Significance

Inquiring into the condition of the patient's pain will provide insight into its etiology, thermal nature, location, and the excessive or deficient nature of the antipathogenic qi.

IV. Scope of Inquiring about Pain

The main subjects of inquiry about pain are its character and location, however we should also ask about its history and accompanying symptoms.

(1) Characteristics of Pain Include

- quality of the pain: sharp, dull, distending, etc.

- severity of pain: excruciating or mild

- factors affecting the pain: anything that can trigger or relieve, aggravate, or ameliorate the pain, such as heat or cold, activity or rest, or changes in the weather

- frequency and duration: better or worse at a specific time of the day, consistent or intermittent, chronic or acute

(2) Location of Pain

Head, shoulder, back, lower back, channel trajectory, etc.

(3) Etiology or Cause of Pain or How the Pain Started

History of trauma or surgery, gradual or sudden onset, etc.

(4) Accompanying Symptoms

V. INDICATIONS OF PAIN

(1) Characteristics of Pain

Different etiologies will give rise to different body responses and sensations. Inquiring into the character of the pain can help to distinguish the etiological agent.

Pain	Definition	Characteristics	Indications
distending pain	pain with distention in the same location	sudden onset, comes and goes, or pain relieved by passing gas	qi stagnation
stabbing pain	pain with sensation of being needled or stabbed	fixed in location, sharp in character, small area	blood stagnation
colicky pain	severe pain as if the body is being twisted	larger area, a violent cut or twisted pain	obstruction of excessive pathogenic factor
unfixed pain	migrating pain that moves without definite location	migrates without stable location	pathogenic wind attacking the body
retraction pain	pain with pulling sensation	radiating pain, with starting point and pulling feeling	malnutrition of tendons
scorching pain	pain feels as if one is being burning	heat and burning sensation at location with a preference for cold	pathogenic heat injuring the channels
cold pain	pain feels as if one is being frozen	cold sensation at location of pain, relieved by warmth	pathogenic cold constricting channels
heavy pain	pain with a sensation of heaviness	heaviness of the limbs with achy sensation	pathogenic dampness in the channels
hollow pain	pain with sensation of emptiness	empty and light feeling with a preference for pressure and warming	deficiency of blood, essence, yin, or yang
dull pain	pain lingering and mild	tolerable pain that lingers for a long period of time	deficiency of qi, blood, yin, or yang
aching pain	pain that aches, accompanied by weariness	mild, may be accompanied by other pain such as heavy or dull	exterior dampness or Kidney deficiency

Table 3.3.11 Characteristics of Pain and their Indications

(2) Location of Pain

Inquiry into the location of pain can help determine the location of pathogenic changes, including *zàng fǔ* organs and related channels.

— A. Headache

The head is the meeting place of all the yang channels and houses the brain, which is the sea of marrow. Qi and blood of the five *zàng* and six *fǔ* organs all rise to the head. If pathogenic factors invade the head and block the clear yang, or if stagnation of qi and blood in endogenous disease blocks the channels and deprives the brain of nourishment, headache will ensue.

Signs and Symptoms		Indications		Pathogenesis
headache that is persistent and severe	chills and fever, cough, seasonal, acute and short course	excess	exterior	phlegm, cold, or blood stasis obstructs the channels or pathogenic heat disturbs the head
	longer duration with excess type pulse image		interior	
chronic headache, pain is intermittent and mild		deficiency		qi, blood, essence, or body fluids deficiency fails to nourish the brain and head

Table 3.3.12 Headache and its Indications

Headache Location	Channels
occipital, radiating to nape	*tài yáng*
forehead and periocular region	*yáng míng*
lateral aspect of head	*shào yáng*
vertex of head	*jué yīn*
side of head which radiates to the teeth and throat	*shào yīn*
headache with heavy sensations and diarrhea	*tài yīn*

Table 3.3.13 Channel Differentiation of Headache

— B. Chest Pain

The chest belongs to the upper burner. It is the house of the Heart and Lung and the place of gathering qi (宗氣 *zōng qì*). Hence, chest pain is mostly seen in diseases of the Heart and Lung.

Chest yang can be suppressed by pathogenic cold, blood stasis, or phlegm. Pathogenic heat can damage the channels and collaterals in the chest. All of these factors can lead to inadequate circulation of qi and blood in the chest, causing pain.

Signs and Symptoms		Indications	
severe pain, sudden onset, pain may radiate to left arm and shoulder	severe stabbing chest pain with fixed location, worse at night	excess	blood stagnation
	distending pain, may occur suddenly, can be induced by emotional stress, frequent sighing		qi stagnation
	dull chest pain, stifling sensation in the chest, cough with profuse sputum		phlegm obstruction
	expectoration of yellow thick phlegm or pus, with blood and foul odor		lung abscess
vague, chronic, mild pain	chest pain induced or aggravated by exertion, intermittent attacks, palpitations, shortness of breath, and oppression in the chest	deficiency	qi deficiency
	continual vague chest pain, intermittent palpitations, dream disturbed sleep, feverish sensation in the chest		qi and yin deficiency

Table 3.3.14 Chest Pain and its Indications

— C. *Hypochondriac pain*

Hypochondriac pain refers to pain under the ribcage margin on one or both sides, or beneath the ribs in the back. This is the house of the Liver and Gallbladder. The hypochondriac region is traversed by the Liver and Gallbladder channels. Obstruction or undernourishment of these channels and organs may produce hypochondriac pain.

Signs and Symptoms		Indications	
severe and incessant pain	mild pain or discomfort in hypochondriac region, fixed in location, alternating chills and fever	excess	*shào yáng* pattern
	unilateral pain with distension which makes it painful to twist the body, pain aggravated by breathing		fluid retention
	distending pain without fixed location, induced or aggravated by emotional stress		liver qi stagnation
	stabbing pain which is fixed in location and worse at night, or with fixed masses in hypochondrium that are resistant to pressure		blood stagnation
	severe hypochondriac pain that may be accompanied by burning and stifling sensation, bitter taste in the mouth		damp heat in the Liver and Gallbladder
vague, chronic, mild pain	chronic, persistent, dull and vague hypochondriac pain	deficiency	Liver yin deficiency

Table 3.3.15 Hypochondriac Pain and its Indications

— D. Epigastric Pain

The epigastric region is the upper half of the upper abdomen and is related to the Stomach. The physiological function of the Stomach is to govern reception, decomposition, and descending.

Because the Stomach is a *fǔ* organ which continuously receives, moves, and transports, any stagnation will interfere with Stomach function and lead to pain. Stagnation may be caused by pathogenic factors such as cold, heat, food, blood stasis, or phlegm. It may also be caused by Stomach yin or Spleen qi deficiency, which inhibits the descending function of the Stomach and and thereby leads to stagnation.

Signs and Symptoms			Indications
acute onset, short duration, severe pain with distention, worse after eating, resistant to pressure	excruciating pain with strong sensation of cold, pain relieved by warmth	excess	excess cold in the middle burner
	severe epigastric burning pain		excess heat in the middle burner
	epigastric and abdominal pain, distention that is relieved after bowel movement		food stagnation
	distending pain that comes and goes, no fixed location, pain can radiate to the hypochondrium or lower abdomen, can be induced by emotional stress or menstrual period		qi stagnation
	sharp and fixed in location, may be accompanied by hematemesis, hematochezia, or masses in the epigastric region		blood stagnation
chronic onset, long duration, vague pain, induced or aggravated by hunger, relieved by eating, relieved with pressure	pain with burning sensation, epigastric discomfort, hunger without desire to eat, dry heaves, hiccups	deficiency	Stomach yin deficiency
	persistent vague pain with empty feeling, consumption of cold food will induce or aggravate the pain, there is a desire for warm food		Spleen and Stomach qi deficiency with cold

Table 3.3.16 Epigastric Pain and its Indications

— E. Abdominal pain

The abdomen is divided into the upper abdomen, which refers to the region between the xiphoid process and umbilicus, and the lower abdomen, which refers to the area below the umbilicus.

The upper half of the upper abdomen is called the epigastrium and pertains to the Stomach, while the lower half of the upper abdomen is called the "big abdomen" and pertains to the Spleen channel. The medial part of lower abdomen is called the "little abdomen" and is the region where the Kidney, Bladder, Large and Small Intestines, uterus, and the channels of the Spleen and Stomach are located. The bilateral sides of lower abdomen are referred to as the "junior abdomen"; this is the region through which the channels of the Liver and Gallbladder pass. By localizing the pain, the diseased *zàng fǔ* organs and channels can be identified. See Illustration 4.2.1 on page 336.

Signs and Symptoms		Indications	
severe pain that is resistant to pressure, aggravated by food intake	excruciating cold pain, patient cannot tolerate being touched, severe vomiting, unable to eat	excess	excess cold accumulation
	burning pain, severe constipation and flatulence, tense and firm abdomen, focal distention and abdominal fullness		*yáng míng fǔ* pattern
	pain that comes and goes, no fixed location, pain may radiate to the hypochondrium and lower abdomen, induced by emotional stress		qi stagnation
	abdominal pain that is fixed in location, worse in the evening, or with masses in the abdomen		blood stagnation
	sudden onset, increasing over time, or paroxymal attack, aggravated by pressure, bloating and distention		damp heat in the middle burner
	cold pain with pulling sensation in the "junior abdomen" and radiating to the genital region		cold in the Liver channel
dull and vague pain in "big abdomen" that comes and goes, relieved by warmth or pressure, aggravated by hunger and exertion		deficiency	middle burner deficiency cold

Table 3.3.17 Abdominal Pain and its Indications

— *F. Back Pain*

The lower back houses the Kidney. Lower back pain may result from obstruction of the local channels, or it may be due to deficiency of the Kidney, which fails to nourish the lumbar region.

Signs and Symptoms		Indications	
shorter duration, more severe, more common among younger patients	patient has no history of back pain, acute onset, pain has tight sensation, pain in neck, shoulders or joints, aggravated by cold weather	excess	exterior wind cold attack in the *tài yáng* channel
	chronic or intermittent attack which is aggravated by cold or damp weather, relieved by warmth; dull or vague pain with sensation of stiffness, but range of motion is normal		obstruction of wind damp cold
	back pain with burning sensation that is relieved with cold, aversion to heat		damp heat accumulation
	acute onset, history of injury, extremely sharp pain with fixed location, resistant to pressure, pain is aggravated by movement, back's range of motion is limited		blood stagnation
longer duration, aching pain, more common among older patients	chronic and persistent low back pain that is vague, relieved by rest and aggravated by overwork or cold weather	deficiency	Kidney yang deficiency
	chronic back pain that is accompanied by soreness in the lower back and knees, sensation of heat in the palms and soles		Kidney yin deficiency
	low back ache that is relieved by slight movement, induced or aggravated by the body remaining in one position for extended periods of time		injury due to extended periods of standing in one place (勞損 *láo sǔn*) or repetitive stress

Table 3.3.18 Back Pain and its Indications

— *G. Limb Pain*

Pain in the four limbs may involve the joints, muscles, or channels. This pain is caused by retardation of qi and blood circulation due to invasion of exogenous pathogenic factors.

Signs and Symptoms		Indications
shorter duration, more severe, more common among younger patients	migrating joint pain that involves the upper extremities	**excess**	wind attack to the channels and collaterals
	severe joint pain that increases with cold and diminishes with warmth, no redness or swelling		attack of pathogenic cold
	pain and heaviness sensation in the joints, usually attacks the lower back or lower extremities, muscle numbness or stiffness, joint deformities		obstruction of dampness in channels
	pain and burning sensations in the joints, visible redness and swelling		pathogenic heat blocks the channels
	sharp pain with fixed location, resistant to pressure, worse at night, joint stiff or deformed		blood stagnation in the channels
longer duration, aching pain, more common among older patients	chronic joint ache, worse after exertion, muscle weakness or atrophy	**deficiency**	qi and blood deficiency
	chronic fixed ache in the lower back and lower extremities, weakness and stiffness, worse in the evening		Kidney and Liver yin deficiency

Table 3.3.19 Limb Pain and its Indications

■ Question Four: Symptoms of the Head and Body

Besides pain, there may be other pathological signs, symptoms, or discomfort in the head and body, such as dizziness, stifling sensation in the chest, bloating and distention, palpitations, numbness, heavy sensations, etc.

I. Dizziness

Dizziness is a visual distortion with a whirling sensation in the head. In mild cases, the patient will feel better after they close their eyes. In severe cases, the patient may feel as if she is riding in a vehicle or boat. The dizziness may even upset one's sense of balance or be accompanied by nausea, vomiting, sweating, or fainting.

Many diseases in biomedicine, such as aural dizziness, cerebral dizziness, hypertension, hypotension, anemia and neurosis, with dizziness as their main symptom, can be diagnosed and treated as dizziness.

(1) Definition: the general name for dizziness and vertigo.

Dizziness (眩 *xuàn*): refers to dim eyesight or blackened and blurred vision or spots in the visual field. This may only occur upon moving and last just a few seconds.

Vertigo (暈 *yùn*): an inability to stand firmly because one's surroundings seem to be revolving.

Vertigo and dizziness often appear simultaneously, in which case we simply call it dizziness (眩暈 *xuàn yùn*).

(2) Etiology and Pathomechanisms of Dizziness

The two major causes of dizziness are a disturbance of the clear orifices (清竅 *qīng qiào*) brought on by pathogenic factors, or a lack of nourishment to the clear orifices. Dizziness is closely related to wind, fire, phlegm, blood stasis, and deficiency. The "clear orifices" refers to the sensory orifices of the head and includes all seven orifices as well as the brain.

Pathogenic wind and fire tend to rise upward. When they attack the head, they disturb the clear orifices, which can lead to dizziness. Wind and heat can arise from either an exterior invasion or from a dysfunction of the *zàng fǔ* organs, especially the Liver, because it is the organ related to wind. Ancient medical books say that "all wind, shaking, and dizziness pertain to the Liver."

The Divine Pivot, Chapter 33 (靈樞。海論) says that "deficiency of the brain leads to dizziness." Deficiency of the brain can be caused by a lack of nourishment due to qi, blood, or essence deficiency; or it may be due to pathogenic factors such as blood stasis or phlegm obstructing the channels and collaterals. In either case, the qi and blood cannot adequately circulate, leading to a lack of nourishment in the head. Ancient medical books say that "without phlegm, there is no dizziness," thus phlegm is another major cause of dizziness.

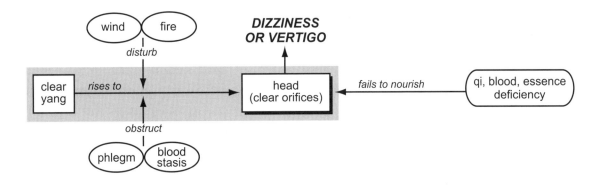

Chart 3.3.16 Pathogenesis of Dizziness or Vertigo

(3) Symptoms and Indications

Signs and Symptoms		Indications	
dizziness with distending pain in the head	paroxysmal dizziness and rotary vertigo, heaviness of the head, aggravated by motion; difficulty in thinking or concentration, especially in the morning; stifling sensation in the chest, nausea, profuse sputum	excess	wind phlegm or phlegm heat
	dizziness and vertigo that feels like motion sickness, tinnitus, red face, irritability, distending headache, symptoms aggravated by emotional stress		Liver yang rising or Liver fire blazing upward
	dizziness after head injury, accompanied by sharp pain		blood stasis
chronic, hollow and heavy sensations in the head	dizziness with desire to lie down, worse in standing position, induced by exertion	deficiency	qi deficiency
	dizziness which is worse when standing up from a sitting or laying position, blurred vision		Heart and Spleen blood deficiency
	persistent dizziness and vertigo with empty feeling in head, worse in afternoon and evening, aggravated by overwork or overthinking		Kidney essence deficiency

Table 3.3.20 Symptoms and Indications of Dizziness

II. STIFLING SENSATION IN THE CHEST

(1) Definition

Also called "chest oppression," the patient feels a stifling or tight sensation in the chest. It is an uncomfortable and unpleasant feeling.

(2) Etiology and Pathomechanisms of Stifling Sensation in the Chest

Usually caused by qi obstruction in the chest area related to a dysfunction of the Lung or Heart. Qi obstruction may be due to excess or deficiency. The excess could be stagnation of pathogens which may include qi, blood, or phlegm. Stagnant pathogens may by due to either an exopathogenic attack, which causes an accumulation of Lung qi, or to a *zàng fǔ* organ dysfunction that produces phlegm, blood stasis, or qi stagnation. The deficiency could arise from dysfunction of the *zàng fǔ* organs. When qi is deficient, there isn't enough power to circulate the qi and blood, and stagnation results.

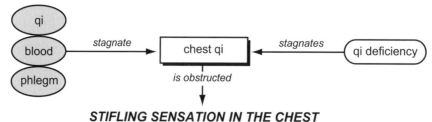

Chart 3.3.17 Pathogenesis of Stifling Sensation in the Chest

(3) Symptoms and Indications

Signs and Symptoms	Indications		
acute onset, stifling sensation in the chest, cough, chills and fever, floating pulse	excess	Lung qi accumulation	wind cold attacking the Lung
stifling or tight sensation in the chest, rapid and shallow respiration, cough or asthma			pathogenic heat lodged in the Lung
stifling sensation with dull pain in the chest; expectoration of thick yellow phlegm, pus, or blood with foul odor			Lung abscess
stifling sensation in the chest, aggravated when lying horizontally, cough with profuse sputum		phlegm accumulation in the Lung	
stifling sensation in the chest which is worse at night, accompanied by chest pain, or pain that radiates to the shoulder		Heart blood stagnation	
stifling sensation in the chest, accompanied by hypochondriac pain, frequent sighing		Liver qi stagnation	
stifling sensation in the chest, shortness of breath, wheezing	deficiency	qi and blood deficiency	

Table 3.3.21 Symptoms and Indications of Stifling Sensation in the Chest

III. Palpitations

(1) Definition

The sensation of the heart beating felt in the chest by the patient. It is caused by either an increase in heart rate, an increase in heart contraction, or by irregular heart beats. It is often present in various kinds of coronary heart disease, cardioneurosis, anemia, and hyperthyroidism. Palpitations can also arise in a healthy person during periods of exercise or emotional excitement. Depending on its severity, palpitations can be divided into the following categories:

Fright palpitations (驚悸 *jīng jì*): refers to heart palpitations that occur when there is a fright. It is usually due to some external cause. They come and go quickly, and are of short duration. This condition is mild and patients do not usually seek out treatment for fright palpitations.

Continuous palpitations (怔忡 *zhēng chōng*): refers to severe throbbing of the heart, which is often felt from the chest down to the umbilicus. It is a further development of fright palpitations and is usually due to internal causes. It is induced or aggravated by exertion. Prolonged duration of this condition is severe and may require medical attention.

(2) Etiology and Pathomechanisms of Palpitations

Palpitations are directly related to the condition of the Heart. Under normal conditions, the spirit resides inside the Heart and is nourished by the blood, qi, essence, and body fluids. When the Heart is attacked by pathogenic factors such as phlegm or blood stasis, or if the Heart is deprived of nutrition due to a deficiency of qi, blood, yin, or yang, then the spirit will be disturbed and restless, which causes fright palpitations. Continuous palpitations represents further exacerbation of the fright palpitations and is viewed as damage to the Heart organ, rather than just a functional pathology.

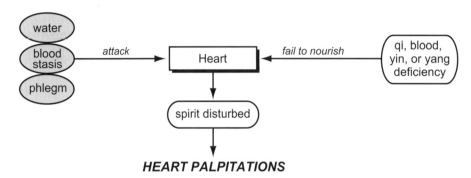

Chart 3.3.18 Pathogenesis of Heart Palpitations

(3) Symptoms and Indications

Signs and Symptoms		Indications
palpitations with paroxysmal pain, pain may be stabbing or colicky in nature, radiation into left arm	excess	blood stagnation
palpitations come and go; induced by anxiety or fright; dizziness, vertigo		phlegm disturbing Heart
palpitations with sudden onset, induced by fright or panic attack		emotion (fright) disturbing the Heart
palpitations with stifling sensation in the chest, shortness of breath, edema in the lower extremities or the face		water attacking the Heart
palpitations with irritability or fright; insomnia, poor memory, dizziness, blurred vision, pale face	deficiency	Heart blood deficiency Heart yin deficiency
palpitations with shortness of breath, palpitations induced or aggravated by exertion or by any physical or mental activity		Heart qi deficiency Heart yang deficiency

Table 3.3.22 Symptoms and Indications of Palpitations

IV. BLOATING AND DISTENTION

(1) Definition

A sensation of bloating (滿 *mǎn*) and/or distention (痞 *pǐ*) in the abdomen. In severe cases there is an enlargement of the abdomen.

Bloating is a subjective sensation of fullness that is only felt by the patient.

Distention means bloating that is both a subjective and objective symptom that may be seen or felt by both the patient and the practitioner.

(2) Etiology and Pathomechanisms of Bloating and Distention

Any disorder in the circulation of qi in the abdominal area can cause qi accumulation. It can be caused by obstruction due to excess pathogens, or by qi deficiency in which the loss of power to move and lead out accumulation is compromised. Pathogens can obstruct the flow of qi, giving rise to bloating and distention. Pathogens such as dampness can come from the exterior. Food stagnation arises from improper diet. Dysfunction of the *zàng fǔ* organs can produce phlegm or blood stasis. Spleen qi deficiency that impedes the transportative and transformative functions is the major endogenous cause of abdominal bloating and distention.

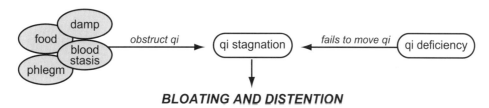

Chart 3.3.19 Pathogenesis of Abdominal Bloating and Distention

(3) Symptoms and Indications

Signs and Symptoms		Indications
abdominal bloating, not relieved by pressure; nausea or vomiting of clear or turbid fluids	excess	cold damp obstruction
		damp heat
abdominal bloating and distention; or pain, symptoms induced by overeating; acid regurgitation, anorexia		food stagnation
abdominal bloating and distention, resistance to pressure, abdominal pain and tightness, constipation		*yáng míng fǔ* pattern (excess heat)
intermittent abdominal bloating; sometimes severe, sometimes mild; desire for and relieved by warmth and pressure, anorexia	deficiency	Spleen and Stomach deficiency with cold

Table 3.3.23 Symptoms and Indications of Bloating and Distention

V. Tingling and Numbness (麻木 *má mù*)

(1) Definition

A group of symptoms that describes abnormal sensations or reduced tactile sensitivity.

Tingling (麻 *má*): a sensation that is neither painful nor itchy. It feels like there are insects crawling inside the muscles. This sensation is not alleviated with pressure and it is aggravated by scratching.

Numbness (木 *mù*): reduced sensitivity to tactile sensation. The patient cannot feel it when you touch, press, or scratch the area of numbness.

Tingling and numbness often arise simultaneously in the clinic. A medical term that spans both *má* and *mù* is "paresthesia."

(2) Etiology and Pathomechanisms of Tingling and Numbness

This (lack of) sensation is due to a loss of nourishment to the muscle. When pathogenic factors block the channels and collaterals, or if *zàng fǔ* organ disorders cause qi and blood deficiency, the muscles will lose their nourishment and this will cause the abnormal sensations of tingling and numbness or paresthesia.

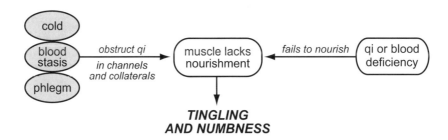

Chart 3.3.20 Pathogenesis of Numbness

(3) Symptoms and Indications

Numbness	Signs and Symptoms	Indications
facial numbness	weak or atrophied muscles, fatigue, pale complexion	qi and blood deficiency
	muscle numbness with twitching or spasms, may have deviated mouth or eye, greasy tongue coating, slippery pulse	wind phlegm obstructs the channels
numbness of the tongue and mouth	numbness and stiffness, difficult speech, headache, wiry and rapid pulse	Liver wind
	numbness and stiffness of the tongue, thick greasy tongue coating, slippery pulse	phlegm obstruction
	tongue numbness, pale tongue body, weak pulse	blood deficiency
scalp numbness	paresthesia that favors numbness	phlegm damp obstruction
	paresthesia that favors tingling, follows severe bleeding or chronic illness	blood deficiency

Numbness	Signs and Symptoms	Indications
half side body numbness	acute onset, body aches, floating and tight pulse	wind cold attack
	acute onset, numbness with some tremors, dizziness, headache, wiry and forceful pulse	Liver wind
	acute onset, numb and heavy sensations, nausea, greasy tongue coating	phlegm damp obstruction
	usually found on the right side, weakness of the limbs, fatigue, shortness of breath, sweating, aversion to wind	middle burner qi deficiency
	usually found on the left side, arises following severe blood loss, dizziness, palpitations, insomnia	blood deficiency
numbness in the extremities	numbness with pain, worse during cold weather, aversion to cold and wind, cold limbs	wind cold attacking the channels
	numbness with distending pain, relieved by movement, dim complexion, purple tongue	qi and blood stagnation
	numbness with tremors, dizziness and headaches, irritability, anger, wiry pulse	Liver wind
	numbness with itchy sensations, possible tremors, dizziness, heavy sensations	wind phlegm blocking channels
	numbness with burning pain in the lower limbs, feels hot to the touch, yellow greasy tongue coating	damp heat
	numbness, weakness giving rise to difficult movement, shortness of breath, pale complexion, thin pulse	qi and blood deficiency
numbness in the fingers and toes	numbness and cold in the fingers and toes, pale color beneath the nails, fatigue, dizziness	blood deficiency
	chronic and stubborn numbness, however sensations are still distinguishable between the individual fingers and toes	damp phlegm stagnation
	chronic and stubborn numbness, may be accompanied by pain, purple color beneath nails	blood stasis

Table 3.3.24 Symptoms and Indications of Numbness

■ Question Five: Symptoms of Ears and Eyes

The ears and eyes are sense organs. The ears manage hearing, and the eyes distinguish color and shapes. Both the ears and eyes are directly connected to the internal organs through the channels and collaterals. Signs and symptoms of the ears and eyes reflect not only pathological changes in the ears and eyes themselves, but also the condition of their associated *zàng fǔ* organs.

I. Physiological Functions of the Ears and Eyes

The normal physiological functions of the ears and eyes rely on the normal functioning of the internal organs and a sufficiency of qi, blood, body fluids, and essence.

The ears are the orifice of the Kidney. Normal hearing depends upon proper nourishment from the essence qi of the Kidney. The ears are also the gathering place of the channels and collaterals, the five *zàng* and six *fǔ*, all of which connect to the ears through the channels.

The eyes are the orifice of the Liver. Normal vision depends on proper nourishment from the blood of the Liver. The eyes are also the gathering place of essence qi from the five *zàng* and six *fǔ* organs. *The Divine Pivot*, Chapter 80 (靈樞。大惑論) says that "The essence from the five *zàng* and six *fǔ* flows upward to irrigate the eyes."

II. Scope of Inquiry

For inquiring about the ears, the following questions should be asked:

- presence or absence of ringing in the ear, whether it is on one side or both sides, its volume and quality, and whether it occurs continuously or intermittently
- presence or absence of hearing impairment or deafness

For inquiring about eyes, the following questions should be asked:

- presence or absence of pain or itching in the eyes, whether or not there is redness, swelling, distention, tearing or secretion
- whether or not the vision is clear, the presence or absence of visual blackouts, and aversion to light

III. Clinical Significance

Inquiring into detailed information about the condition of the ears and eyes can help one:

- understand whether there are any pathological changes in the eye or ears
- recognize pathological changes in the Liver, Gallbladder, and Kidney

IV. Pathological Changes of the Ears and Eyes

(1) Ear Ringing (Tinnitus) and Hearing Loss

— A. Definition

Ear ringing or tinnitus: a buzzing or a ringing sound inside the ear, heard only by the patient, that may sound like cicadas or ocean waves. The ringing may be mild or severe, and is usually perceived as worse when the room's ambient noise is low. In severe cases, it may affect the patient's ability to hear.

Hearing loss and deafness: a diminished or defective sense of hearing.

— B. Etiology and Pathomechanisms of Ear Ringing or Hearing Loss

Loss of nourishment to the ears is the pathomechanism for ear ringing and hearing loss. There are two causes for this loss. The first is that the ear channel is obstructed by pathological factors, either due to *zàng fǔ* organ disorders leading to stagnation of qi, phlegm, and blood stasis, or to exopathogens that directly attack the channels in the area of the ear. The second cause for a loss of nourishment to the ears is insufficient qi, blood, or essence. These deficiencies arise from the *zàng fǔ* organs, especially Kidney and Liver yin deficiency in the aged patient, or from chronic illness that has consumed the qi, blood, and essence.

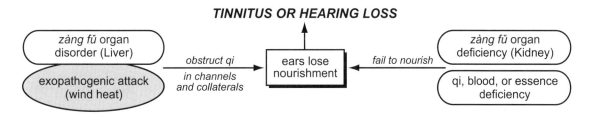

Chart 3.3.21 Pathogenesis of Tinnitus or Hearing Loss

— C. Symptoms and Indications

Signs and Symptoms		Indications	
sudden onset, feeling of distention; constant ringing is low-pitched and loud; and is not relieved by pressing the ears closed	sudden onset, involves one or both the ears, ringing sounds like wind, feeling of congestion or distention in the ear	excess	wind heat attacking the Lungs
	sudden onset, loud ringing that sounds like a storm or ocean waves, possible ear pain or swelling, possible hearing loss, symptoms aggravated by emotional stress		Liver fire
			Liver yang rising
	ringing that sounds like cicadas or crickets, ear feels obstructed, some decrease in hearing		phlegm heat
	tinnitus follows traumatic injury to the ear or head		qi / blood stagnation
Chronic hearing loss; intermittent ringing is high-pitched and soft, worse with stress or exertion; and relieved by pressing ears closed	variable ringing that sounds like cicadas, hearing loss, dizziness, blurred or weak vision, visual floaters	deficiency	Liver blood deficiency
	gradual onset of condition, soft ringing that sounds alternately like rushing water or cicadas, ringing worse at night, poor memory, feeling of emptiness in the head, possible hearing loss or deafness		Kidney qi or yin deficiency; Kidney/Heart disharmony
	intermittent ringing, induced or aggravated by exertion		Spleen and Stomach deficiency

Table 3.3.25 Symptoms and Indications of Tinnitus

(2) Pathological Changes of the Eyes

— A. Definitions

Blurred vision: the loss of visual acuity (sharpness of vision) resulting in a loss of the ability to see small detail.

Floaters: small specks or clouds moving through the field of vision. They are easiest to see when looking at a plain background, like a blank wall or cloudless sky. Floaters may look like specks, strands, webs, or other shapes.

— B. Etiology and Pathomechanisms

When the eyes lack nourishment, pathology will arise. The loss of nourishment can be due to either pathogenic factors attacking the eyes, or an internal deficiency. Pathogenic factors either arrive from the exterior, such as wind, heat, dryness, dampness, etc., or from *zàng fǔ* organ disorders. Loss of proper nourishment is caused either by a deficiency of qi, blood, or essence, or by such pathogenic factors as blood stasis or dampness obstructing the flow of nourishment in the channels.

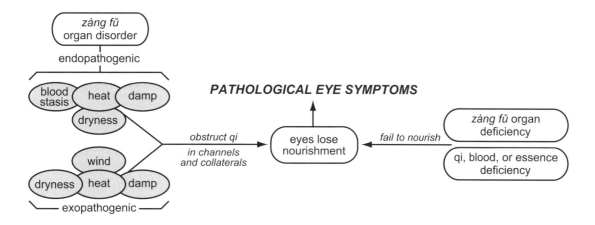

Chart 3.3.22 Pathogenesis of Eye Symptoms

— C. *Symptoms and Indications*

Symptoms	Description	Indications
eye pain	eye pain feels like there is a foreign object inside the eye, or needle-like pain; redness in the eye	fire toxin in Heart channel
	pain, swelling, and redness of the eye	exterior wind heat attack, or Liver fire
	distending pain, or feeling of pressure in the eye	Kidney yin deficiency with Liver yang rising
eye itching	severe itching on eyelid, may include redness and excessive hardened yellow secretions ("sleep")	wind heat
	mild itching, usually occurs in both eyes, intermittent symptoms, dry eyes	blood deficiency
dry eyes	eyes feel dry	Liver and Kidney yin deficiency
tearing	tearing without redness, aggravated when exposed to wind	Liver blood deficiency with exterior wind attack
	frequent clear tearing without redness, may be worse during the winter	qi and blood deficiency, or Kidney and Liver deficiency
	tearing with redness and swelling in the tissues surrounding the eye	Liver fire, or damp heat in the Liver channel
	warm tearing, tearing during the day, dryness during the night	Fire due to yin deficiency
blurred vision	blurred vision with dry eyes, worse after reading	Liver blood deficiency
	blurred vision that gets worse with age	deficiency of Kidney and Liver
	acuity of vision decreases during the night	Liver blood deficiency
floaters	smell specks or filaments floating through field of vision	Kidney essence deficiency, Liver blood deficiency
photophobia	aversion to light, or sensitivity to light; may be accompanied by blurred vision or light headache	Liver blood deficiency

Table 3.3.26 Pathological Symptoms and Indications of the Eyes

■ **Question Six: Inquiring about Dietary Information**

Human life depends on food and drink as the basic materials for maintaining normal physiological functions, growth, and development. Intake and digestion of food and drink mainly depend on the functions of the Spleen and Stomach. These organs are the root of acquired essences, the source of the engendering and transformation of essence and blood. Other organs, such as the Liver, Large Intestine, Small Intestine, and Triple Burner, are also involved in the digestion of food. Gathering information about food, drink, and taste from the patient can help the practitioner assess the functioning of the patient's *zàng fǔ* organs and the condition of the food essences.

Inquiry about dietary information includes thirst, fluid intake, appetite, food intake, and abnormal tastes in the mouth.

I. Thirst and Fluid Intake

Fluid intake is one of the main sources of body fluids. The feeling of thirst and the intake of fluids are closely related to the condition and the metabolism of the body fluids. Thirst, satiety, and water intake tells us about the thermal nature of a disease, as well as the status of the body fluids.

(1) Definition

Thirst: the sensation of dryness in the mouth or the desire to drink fluids.

Thirst and drinking are closely related. Generally speaking, when thirsty, a person will drink more than normal; when not thirsty, she does not like to drink. However, these relationships do not always hold true.

(2) Physiology of Fluid Intake and Metabolism

Water and other fluids are the source of body fluids. When fluids are taken into the body, they are transformed into body fluids through the transportative and transformative functions of the Spleen, as well as the functions of the Lung and Kidney. Body fluids are distributed to the entire body; when they rise to the mouth, it will remain moist. When a person feels thirsty, it is a signal that the body fluids are insufficient.

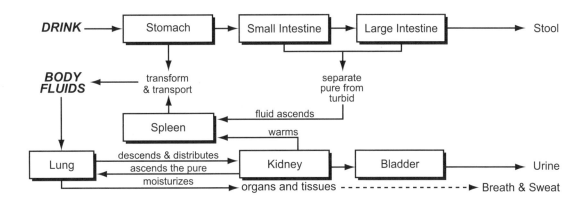

Chart 3.3.23 Fluid Metabolism

(3) Etiology and Pathomechanisms of Thirst

There are two reasons that body fluids may be unable to nourish the tongue and mouth, which leads to a sensation of dryness. The first is due to a deficiency of body fluids, and the second to a disorder in the distribution of body fluids.

Deficiency of body fluids can be caused by either over-consumption or insufficient formation. Pathogenic heat, severe diarrhea, profuse sweating or bleeding can all contribute to the overconsumption of body fluids. Insufficient water intake, or a dysfunction of the Stomach, Spleen, Small Intestine, or Kidney, can all cause insufficient formation of body fluids.

The distribution of body fluids is accomplished mainly by the joint functions of the Spleen, Lung, Kidney, and Triple Burner. A disorder of the distribution of fluids can be caused by either pathogenic factors attacking or by a *zàng fǔ* organ deficiency. When pathogenic cold and dampness impair the Lung or Spleen, or obstruct the Triple Burner's water passages, the body fluids will be unable to distribute in a normal manner. If there is Kidney yang deficiency, there will not be enough power to steam and transform the water into body fluids, which again will impair the distribution and quantity of body fluids.

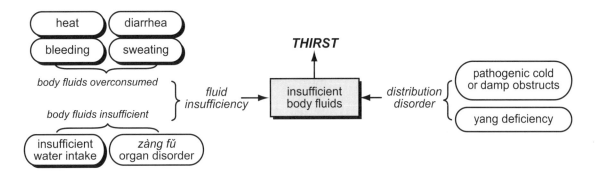

Chart 3.3.24 Pathogenesis of Thirst

(4) Scope of Inquiry regarding Thirst and Drinking

When inquiring about thirst and drinking, the following factors should be considered:

- characteristics: refers to the unique qualities of thirst, such as a thirst with a desire to drink or thirst without a desire to drink
- degree or severity of the thirst
- amount of water intake
- preference for cold or hot drinks
- accompanying symptoms

(5) Symptoms and Indications

Thirst	Pathogenesis	Indications
absence of thirst	body fluids not impaired	cold syndrome; or normal
thirst with copious water intake	body fluids injured or over-consumed by heat, mouth loses moisture	heat syndrome; or following severe sweating, vomiting or diarrhea
thirst with desire to drink, but vomiting immediately afterwards	Fluid retention is a yin pathogen that impairs yang, so water cannot transform into body fluids to moisten the mouth, hence there is thirst. However, because there is adequate fluids already in the body, additional water intake will be expelled.	water, dampness, or phlegm accumulation in middle burner
thirst, without desire to drink	Blood stasis creates heat which injures body fluids, when blood is stagnant, qi movement is blocked, when qi movement is blocked, body fluids cannot be distributed normally.	blood stagnation
	Heat injures the fluids to cause thirst, however when heat invades the nutritive/blood levels, it steams the body fluids within the blood which rise to the mouth to moisten the tongue.	heat in the nutritive or blood level
	Heat injures and damp reduces the efficiency of body fluids formation, both of which cause thirst, meanwhile the fluids have accumulated in the middle burner leading to a lack of desire to drink.	damp heat
	Kidney yang deficiency leads to both a lack of heat to steam the body fluids as well as force to lift the fluids to the mouth, hence there is thirst even though there is no real deficiency of body fluids.	deficiency cold in lower burner

Table 3.3.27 Symptoms and Indications of Pathological Thirst

II. Appetite and Food Intake

Based on one's appetite and food intake the practitioner can assess the condition of the Spleen and Stomach. The Stomach receives food and the Spleen transforms and transports it. Together, they are the acquired root of the human body. Inquiring about appetite and food intake can help the practitioner assess the severity and the prognosis of a disease.

(1) Definitions

Appetite: the physical desire to eat food, felt as hunger.

Anorexia: absence or loss of appetite for food.

(2) Physiology of Appetite and Food Intake

The five *zàng* and six *fǔ* are all involved in the process of digesting food, however appetite and food intake mainly depend on the functions of the Stomach and Spleen. There is a full sensation (satiety) when the Stomach is filled, and there is hunger when the Stomach is empty.

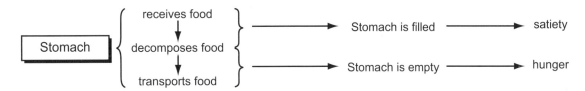

Chart 3.3.25 Physiology and Pathogenesis of Hunger and Satiety

The Stomach is a *fǔ* organ which has "more qi and blood." It prefers moistness and dislikes dryness. It is responsible for receiving, decomposing (rotting and ripening), and descending. Decomposing is the primary digestive process. Food in the Stomach is reduced to chyme by the decomposing and grinding action of the Stomach. Descending means the transmission of incompletely digested food downward to the Small Intestine and then to the Large Intestine to complete the digestion and re-absorption process. The fulfillment of the digestive function is attributed to the joint efforts of the Stomach yang and Stomach yin. Stomach yang supplies the power for this process, and the Stomach yin supplies the body fluids to moisten and dissolve the food.

The Spleen is a *zàng* organ. It is responsible for transporting and transforming the food into food essence, which is sent upward to the Lung to be distributed to the entire body. The Spleen likes dryness and dislikes dampness. Both the Spleen and Stomach are located in the middle burner and are connected by channels, forming an exterior-interior relationship. Physiologically, they share the work and coordinate to maintain normal digestive functions. Pathologically, they readily affect each other. The Stomach's descending function is paired with the Spleen's ascending function. When one organ is impaired, the other will be as well.

The function of the Liver also affects the appetite and food intake. Digestive functions include the processes of receiving and decomposing the food, followed by distributing and absorbing the essential substances. The Liver is the organ that promotes secretion and excretion of bile to assist with the decomposition processes. The dispersing and draining functions of the Liver also maintains the normal ascending and descending functions of the Spleen and Stomach qi.

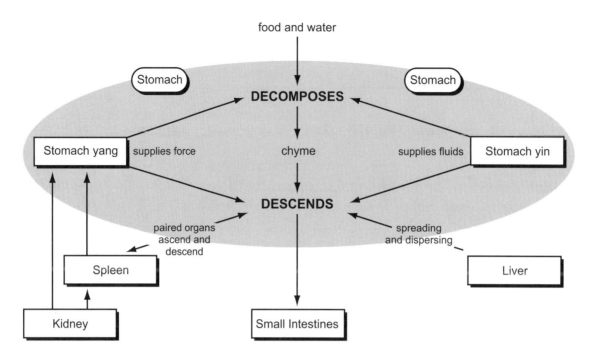

Chart 3.3.26 Physiology of Stomach's Decomposition and Descending Processes

(3) Etiology and Pathomechanisms of Abnormal Appetite and Food Intake

Disorders of the Stomach's decomposing or descending functions are the pathomechanisms underlying abnormal appetite. There are two possible pathological changes for the decomposing function of the Stomach: increased decomposition and decreased decomposition. Generally speaking, when the decomposing process is too fast, it causes an increase in the appetite, a greater tendency to feel hunger, and overeating. When the decomposing process is too slow, it may cause a loss of appetite or anorexia.

The process of *rapid decomposition* is caused by pathogenic heat. The pathogenic heat may come from an exopathogenic heat attack on the Stomach, or from the interior due to *zàng fǔ* organ dysfunction. Endopathogenic heat can arise from either excess or deficiency. Excess heat is due to hyperactivity of the Stomach (Stomach heat); deficiency heat is caused by Stomach yin deficiency, which may result from chronic illness or improper diet.

There are three possible causes for the process of *slowed decomposition*. The first is due to a loss of power resulting from pathogenic cold, which may enter from the exterior as a complication of a direct attack of exopathogenic cold, or arise from deficiency of Stomach yang secondary to deficiency of the Spleen or Kidney yang. The second possible reason for slowed decomposition is overeating, which causes stagnation in the Stomach. The third reason for slowed decomposition is a lack of moisture due to Stomach yin deficiency.

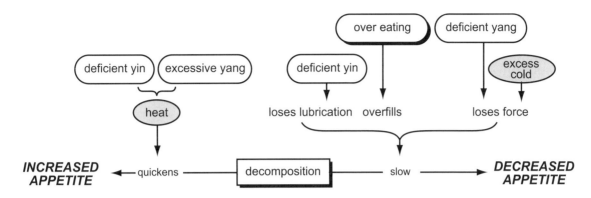

Chart 3.3.27 Pathomechanism of Abnormal Decomposition Processes

The causes of disorders in the descending function include the following: loss of downward force due to yang deficiency (Stomach, Spleen, and Kidney yang); loss of moisture due to Stomach yin deficiency; and stagnation of food, phlegm, dampness, or blood. Impairment of the Stomach's descending function may also be caused by Spleen/Liver disharmony. When the Spleen is deficient or is attacked by dampness, its ascending function will be compromised, which in turn will adversely affect the Stomach's descending function. The Liver is responsible for seeing that qi moves in the right direction. The Spleen's qi ascends and the Stomach's descends. When Liver qi stagnates, the Stomach qi won't descend, and the appetite and food intake will be compromised.

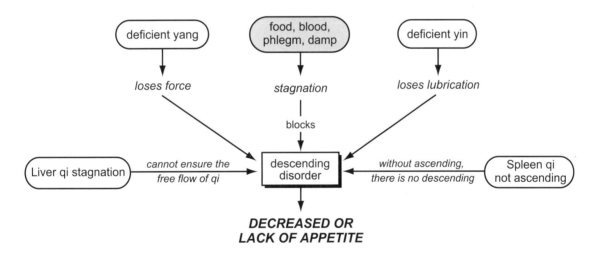

Chart 3.3.28 Pathomechanisms of Functional Stomach Descending Disorders

(4) Scope of Inquiring about Appetite and Food Intake

When inquiring about appetite and food intake, the following should be considered:

- the nature of the abnormal appetite or food intake, such as loss of appetite, overeating, hunger with no desire to eat, or abnormal taste in the mouth

- the degree or severity of the abnormal appetite or food intake, such as a dislike of food, a decrease in appetite, or absolutely no appetite at all

- the amount of food intake

- food preferences, such as cold or warm, spicy, sour, etc.

- accompanying symptoms

(5) Symptoms and Indications

Appetite		Indications	Pathogenesis
decreased appetite	no hunger	Liver qi stagnation	usually induced or aggravated by emotional stress, Liver qi stagnation will affect the ascending and descending function of the Spleen and Stomach
	partial hunger	Spleen and Stomach deficiency	Stomach and Spleen deficiency fails to transport or transform leading to food remaining in the Stomach longer than usual
dislike of food	after overeating	food stagnation	food or dampness stagnates in the middle burner, slows down the decomposition and transportation processes
	specific to greasy food	damp heat in the middle burner	
hunger without desire to eat		Stomach yin deficiency	deficiency heat decomposes food and causes patient to have the sensation of hunger, however because the yin deficiency does not nourish the Stomach, it is unable to receive more food
hunger even after overeating		strong Stomach, weakened Spleen	Stomach fire decomposes food rapidly, but the deficiency of Spleen qi fails to transform the food into essence and thus does not nourish the body
food addiction or craving		parasitic invasion	parasites cause malnutrition leading to a lack of specific nutritional components, patient will then crave or feel addicted to food or non-food materials that contain the lacking nutrient(s)

Table 3.3.28 Symptoms and Indications of Pathological Changes in Appetite and Food Intake

III. Tastes in Mouth

The tongue's sensitivity to taste can affect the appetite. Under normal circumstances, the tongue will taste only what is taken in food and drink. Abnormal tastes in mouth often reflect disease in the *zàng fǔ* organs. Asking questions about abnormal tastes in the mouth can be helpful in diagnosing such diseases.

(1) Definition

Taste: the basic sensations detectable by the tongue. There are five basic tastes that can be distinguished: bitter, sweet, sour, pungent (acrid), and salty.

Abnormal taste: a taste that occurs in the mouth that is unrelated to the intake of food or drink, and refers to the morbid taste of disease.

(2) Physiology of Taste

The tongue is the sense organ that detects taste. All internal organs are directly or indirectly connected to the tongue through the channels and collaterals. The tongue is the sprout of the Heart ("the Heart opens to the tongue"), therefore the tongue directly reflects the condition of the Heart. The Spleen opens to the mouth, and the Spleen channel connects to the root of the tongue and disperses over its underside. The Kidney channel harbors the root of the tongue, and the Liver channel has a channel network in this root. The throat is the gateway to the Lung, hence it connects with the tongue. Thus, abnormal tastes in the mouth can reflect the condition of the *zàng fǔ* organs.

(3) Etiology and Pathomechanism of Abnormal Tastes in the Mouth

As described above, all of the *zàng fǔ* organs have some direct or indirect connection to the tongue via the channels and collaterals. Liver and/or Gallbladder fire can produce a bitter taste in the mouth when bile is regurgitated upward from the Stomach. Sweet is the flavor of the earth element, and can be tasted in the mouth when damp-heat arises from the Spleen and Stomach. The sour taste can arise from heat in either the Liver or Stomach when the Stomach's descending function is compromised.

(4) Scope of Inquiring about Tastes in the Mouth

When inquiring about abnormal tastes in the mouth, the following factors should be considered:

- the nature of the abnormal taste, such as the five flavors
- degree or severity of the abnormal taste
- factors that aggravate or ameliorate the abnormal taste
- food preferences: cold or warm, spicy or sour, etc.
- accompanying symptoms, such as poor appetite, loose stools, etc.

(5) Symptoms and Indications

Signs and Symptoms		Indications	
tastelessness	patient cannot taste food, anorexia, no desire to eat, fatigue, weak pulse	Spleen and Stomach qi deficiency	
	tastelessness when patient eats, chills and fever, nasal congestion, floating and tight pulse	exterior wind cold syndrome	
sweet taste	sweet and sticky feeling in the mouth, heavy sensations in the head and body, dry mouth and thirst	damp heat in the Spleen and Stomach, early stage *xiāo kě*	
sour taste	sour taste in the mouth, hypochondriac distention, emotional distress	heat in the Liver and Stomach	
	acid regurgitation, foul odor in mouth, abdominal distention and bloating	food stagnation	
bitter taste	bitter taste in mouth, irritability, dry mouth, hypochondriac pain and distention, yellow urine	interior heat syndrome	heat in the Liver / Gallbladder
	bitter taste in mouth, palpitations, insomnia, thirst		Heart fire
	bitter taste in mouth, dizziness, low back pain, irritability, thirst, thin and rapid pulse		Kidney yin deficiency heat
salty taste	salty taste in mouth or sputum with salty taste, low back pain, weak knees	Kidney disease	
sticky sensation	sticky sensation in mouth, no desire to drink, poor appetite, abdominal bloating	dampness accumulation in Spleen and Stomach	

Table 3.3.29 Symptoms and Indications of Pathological Changes in Taste

■ Question Seven: Inquiry into Defecation and Urination

Feces and urine are waste matter expelled from the body. This is part of normal physiology, and is the result of the body's metabolism. The metabolism requires that the five *zàng* and six *fǔ* organs function harmoniously. Metabolic wastes are closely related with the transformative and transportative functions of the Spleen and Stomach, the dispersing and draining functions of the Liver, the dispersing and descending functions of the Lung, and the warming function of the Kidney. The functions of the Bladder and Triple Burner also play important roles in this process. Thus, inquiring about the processes of defecation and urination will not only help one assess the functioning of the digestion and condition of water metabolism, but also the thermal nature of disease.

I. Defecation

(1) Definition

Tenesmus: the constant feeling of the need to empty the bowel, accompanied by pain, cramping, and involuntary straining efforts.

Dysentery: severe diarrhea with passage of mucus and blood.

(2) Physiology of Feces Formation

While defecation is controlled directly by the Large Intestine, it is also closely related with other organs. The Spleen and Stomach govern the reception, transportation, and transformation of water and food. The Spleen transports the food essences up to the Lung, from where it is distributed to the entire body. The turbid descends to the Small Intestine, where the clear is further separated from the turbid. The clear is sent back to the Spleen, and then ascends to the Lungs to be distributed, while the turbid is transported to the Large Intestine. The Large Intestine governs the conversion of matter, forming the turbid matter into feces to be eliminated from the body. The dispersing and draining functions of the Liver, and the warming function of the Kidney, also play important roles in this process.

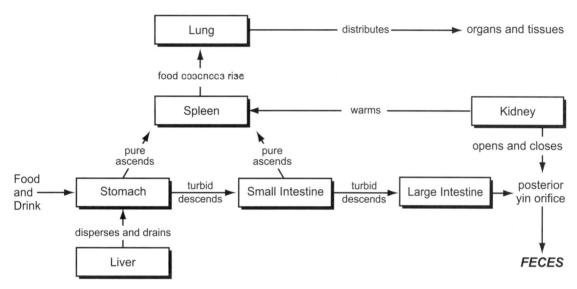

Chart 3.3.29 Physiology of Feces Formation

(3) Normal Defecation

The healthy person defecates every day or every other day. Defecation is smooth, without burning pain or uncomfortable sensation. The stool is brown, soft, and can maintain its own shape. There is no pus, blood, mucus, or undigested food in it.

(4) Scope of Inquiry about Defecation

Inquiry about defecation should include the following:

- form of stool
- color of stool
- smell
- time and frequency of the bowel movements
- quantity of stool

- sensations during defecation

- accompanying symptoms

(5) Pathological Defecation

Abnormal defecation can be classified by frequency, form, color, and sensation into the following categories.

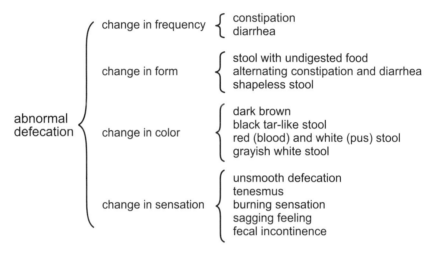

Chart 3.3.30 Abnormal Defecation

— A. Changes in the Frequency of Defecation

Normal frequency of defecation is once per day or every other day. It is a morbid change if the defecation is more than three times per day, or less than once every other day.

⋯ a) Constipation

DEFINITION: difficulty in passing stool, prolonged intervals between stools, or a desire to defecate without the ability to do so, either partially or completely.

ETIOLOGY AND PATHOMECHANISMS OF CONSTIPATION: constipation is associated with the dysfunction of the Large Intestine to transport. This dysfunction can divided into three causes.

The first is when the Large Intestine lacks moisture. This may be due to pathogenic heat in the Large Intestine and Stomach, which consumes body fluids, or to yin or blood deficiency arising from a chronic illness, aging, profuse sweating, bleeding, or other improper treatment.

The second cause of constipation is when the intestines lose their force and power of transportation. This may be caused by qi stagnation arising from emotional stress, or by qi and yang deficiency as the result of a chronic illness or aging.

The third cause of constipation is when the Large Intestine is obstructed by a pathological accumulation, such as food or phlegm stagnation. This may result from improper diet, emotional stress, or dysfunction of a *zàng fǔ* organ.

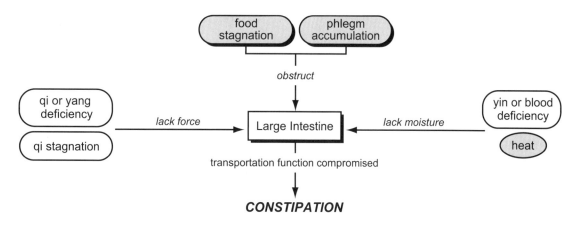

Chart 3.3.31 Pathogenesis of Constipation

SYMPTOMS AND INDICATIONSS

Symptoms		Indications	Pathogenesis
severe constipation, dry stools, abdominal pain and distention, dry mouth, red tongue, rapid pulse	E X C E S S	excess heat in the Stomach and Intestines	excess heat in the Stomach and Intestines injures fluids and causes dry stools
constipation with small stools such as might be left by a goat, stools are not dry, may alternate with diarrhea, symptoms induced or aggravated by emotional stress or lack of physical activity		Liver qi stagnation or Liver attacking Spleen	Liver and Spleen qi stagnation will cause intestinal qi to stagnate, Large Intestine loses its transportation function
dry stool or soft stool, with days between bowel movements, has desire to defecate but lacks energy to complete movement, extremely tired after bowel movement, may include rectal prolapse	D E F I C I E N C Y	Spleen and Lung qi deficiency	Spleen and Lung qi deficiency will cause the Large Intestine to lose force in its transportation
more common among the elderly or post-partum women, round dry stools, normal frequency however difficult passing of stools, dizziness, pale complexion		blood and yin deficiency	blood or yin deficiency fails to moisturize the intestinal tract
difficult defecation, stools may or may not be dry, abdominal pain relieved by warmth, cold limbs, weak or cold knees, pale tongue, deep and slow pulse		Spleen and Kidney yang deficiency	yang qi deficiency causes weakness to the Large Intestine's transportation function

Table 3.3.30 Symptoms and Indications of Constipation

— b) Diarrhea or Loose Stools

DEFINITION: frequent passing of watery or shapeless feces.

ETIOLOGY AND PATHOMECHANISMS OF LOOSE STOOLS: the pathomechanism of diarrhea is usually too much fluids or dampness accumulating in the intestines with increased intestinal peristalsis. The main pathological changes which cause diarrhea occur in the Spleen and Stomach where dampness originates as a pathogenic factor.

Dampness can arise from either the exterior, such as an attack of damp-heat or damp-cold; improper diet; or *zàng fǔ* organ dysfunction. Interior dampness arises from a dysfunction of the Spleen. It is either due to Liver attacking, or to deficiency of the Spleen and/or Kidney. If the Spleen's functions of transformation and transportation fail, dampness will accumulate.

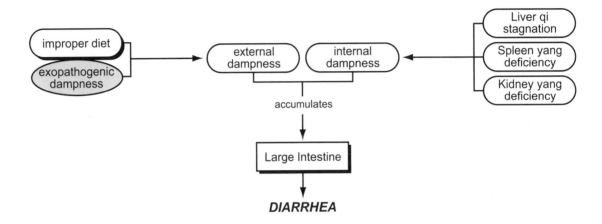

Chart 3.3.32 Pathogenesis of Diarrhea

SYMPTOMS AND INDICATIONS

Symptoms	Indications	
acute onset, foul smelling stools with blood or mucus, burning sensation in the anus, tenesmus	excess type diarrhea: acute onset, short duration, frequent diarrhea	damp heat in the lower burner
diarrhea with watery stools, abdominal pain relieved by warmth, borborygmus, tenesmus		cold damp invasion
diarrhea after overeating, smelly stools with undigested food and copious foul smelling gas		food stagnation
diarrhea with tenesmus, induced or aggravated by emotional stress, alternating with constipation		Liver fire attacking the Spleen
dark green watery diarrhea with foul smell, severe abdominal pain that resists pressure, pain is not relieved following passage of diarrhea		*yáng míng fǔ* pattern
chronic diarrhea or loose stools that contain undigested food, diarrhea worse after eating greasy or cold raw food	deficiency type diarrhea: chronic duration, condition appears intermittently	Spleen deficiency
early morning diarrhea with undigested food, diarrhea immediately follows intestinal borborygmus and abdominal pain which is relieved after passing the diarrhea		Kidney deficiency

Table 3.3.31 Symptoms and Indications of Diarrhea

— B. Changes in the Form of the Stool

The normal form of the stool is soft and moist, with a long oblong shape

Stool Form	Indications
dry stool with dark yellow color	heat in the Intestines
small round stools like that of a goat	Liver qi stagnation
small round stools, very dry	blood deficiency
loose and shapeless stool	deficiency cold in the Spleen and Stomach
initial stool hard followed by loose stools	dampness from Spleen deficiency
randomly alternating loose and dry stools	Liver / Spleen disharmony
loose stools with visible undigested bits of food	Kidney or Spleen yang deficiency
stools with yellow mucus	damp heat in the Large Intestine
yellow sticky stool with putrid odor	food stagnation
stools with pus and blood	dysentery

Table 3.3.32 Abnormal Stool Forms and Their Indications

— C. Changes in the Color of Stool

Normal stool color is brown, but stool color is often affected by food and drugs, which would not otherwise suggest a pathology.

Color of Stool	Indications
dark yellow	heat stagnation in the Intestines
black stool like tar	blood stasis or "far bleeding" (bleeding in upper GI)
red blood in stool	hemorrhoids or "near bleeding" (bleeding in lower GI)
red (blood) and white (pus) in stool	dysentery resulting from damp heat in Large Intestine
grayish white stool	damp heat jaundice (steatorrhea)

Table 3.3.33 Abnormal Color of Stool and its Indications

— D. Abnormal Sensations during Defecation

Under normal circumstances, defecation should occur easily and smoothly without any uncomfortable sensations.

Abnormal Sensation	Description	Indications	Pathogenesis
unsmooth defecation	abdominal pain with defecation, incomplete sensation	Liver attacking Spleen	qi flow in the intestines is obstructed, does not transport the turbid downward
		damp heat in Intestines	
burning sensation	burning sensation in anus during and immediately following defecation	damp heat in Large Intestine	excessive heat in the stool
tenesmus	paroxysmal abdominal pain, frequent and urgent desire to defecate, difficult to completely discharge stools, small quantities of fecal matter, heavy sensation in anus	dysentery due to damp heat	damp heat obstructs qi flow in intestines
fecal incontinence	patient cannot control defecation, stool is discharged spontaneously	Spleen yang deficiency	Spleen and Kidney deficiency cannot control muscles, most likely appearing in elderly, patients with chronic diarrhea or a chronic illness
		Kidney yang deficiency	
sagging feeling in anus	patient feels something sagging from the inner body to the anus, in severe cases, prolapse of rectum can occur	Spleen qi deficiency	Spleen qi deficiency compromises its lifting function

Table 3.3.34 Abnormal Sensations during Defecation and their Indications

II. Urination

(1) Definitions

Urine: the waste of water metabolism.

Excessive urination: significant increase in the volume of urine, possibly accompanied by frequency.

Enuresis: spontaneous urination while sleeping, although good control while awake. This is usually seen in children.

Dysuria (癃 *lóng*): a mild condition that suggests difficult urination. The urine passes only as drops and in small quantity overall. It is usually a chronic condition.

Anuria (閉 *bì*): a severe condition in which there is an absence of discharged urine, even though there is an urge to urinate. It is usually an acute condition.

Although there are some differences between dysuria and anuria, they both refer to difficulty in eliminating urine, and thus the two words together, *lóng bì* (癃閉), are simply translated as urinary blockage.

(2) Physiology of the Formation of Urine

The formation of urine is governed by the Bladder and closely related to the Lung, Spleen, Stomach, Small Intestine, Kidney, Liver, and Triple Burner. The Stomach receives and absorbs the fluids. The Spleen transforms the fluids into water essence and transports it to the Lung, which distributes the water essence to the entire body to nourish the organs and tissues. The water that isn't absorbed by the Stomach is transported to the Small Intestine. This organ separates the clear from the turbid, reabsorbs the clear, and transports it to the Spleen, where it then rises to the Lung. The turbid pours down to the Bladder where it is eliminated. The dispersing and draining functions of the Liver and the warming function of the Kidney also play important roles in the process of water metabolism.

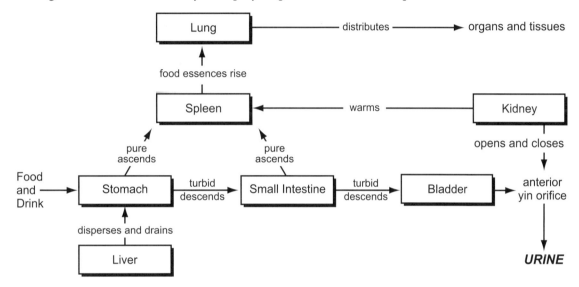

Chart 3.3.33 Physiology of Urine Formation

(3) Normal Urination

A normal person passes urine four to six times during the day and either not at all or just once at night. The amount of urine per day is 1,500 to 2,000 ml., and the color is a clear yellow. The frequency, color, and quantity of urination are influenced by fluid intake, air temperature, sweating, and age.

(4) Scope of Inquiry about Urination

Inquiring about urination should include the following:

- urine color
- odor
- time and frequency of urination
- quantity of urine
- feeling during urination
- accompanying symptoms

(5) Pathological Urination

Abnormal urination can arise due to *zàng fǔ* organ dysfunction, deficiency of body fluids, dysfunction of the functional activity of qi (氣化 *qì huà*), and water retention. The types of abnormal urination can be classified by quantity, frequency, color, or problems of elimination.

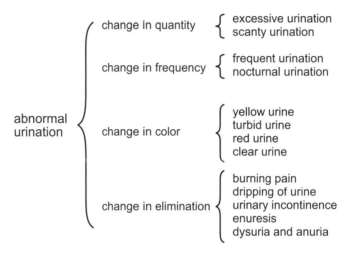

Chart 3.3.34 Abnormal Urination

— *A. Abnormal Quantity of Urine*

The normal amount of urine should be between 1,500 and 2,000 ml. per day. If the body fluids are insufficient, or water cannot transform into body fluids and flow downward to the Bladder, then the quantity of urine will be changed.

	Description	Indications	Pathogenesis
copious urination	copious urine, thirst with abundant water intake	*xiāo kě* pattern (Kidney yin deficiency)	Kidney deficiency fails to transform water into body fluids, and so the water flows downward
	clear and copious urine	Kidney yang deficiency	
scanty urination	scanty yellow urine	excess heat, over-sweating, vomiting or diarrhea	body fluids consumed by heat, or loss of fluids from vomiting or diarrhea
	scanty and clear urine with edema	yang deficiency	Lung, Spleen, and/or Kidney yang deficiency fails to transform body fluids leading to fluid retention

Table 3.3.35 Abnormal Quantity of Urine and its Indications

— *B. Abnormal Frequency of Urination*

A healthy person should feel the need to urinate four to six times per day, and either not at all or just once at night. If urinary frequency exceeds ten times during the daytime, or more than twice at night, it may be considered pathological.

Description		Indications	Pathogenesis
frequent urination	with urgency, dark yellow urine, scanty quantity	painful urinary disorder due to damp heat	damp heat in the lower burner leads to dysfunction of the Bladder, heat pushes out the urine
	with clear urine, usually seen in aged or patients with chronic illness	Kidney qi deficiency	Kidney qi unable to consolidate, leads to Bladder dysfunction
	with passage of only small amounts of urine, aggravated by stress	Liver qi stagnation	qi stagnation disrupts smooth flow of Bladder qi and thus prevents full emptying of bladder leading to frequent passage of small quantities of urine
nocturnal urination	increased frequency at night, often more than three times per night, or the quantity at night is greater than the quantity during the day.	Kidney yang deficiency	Kidney yang deficiency that is unable to consolidate at night, leads to Bladder dysfunction and its inability to store the urine

Table 3.3.36 Abnormal Frequency of Urination and its Indications

— C. Abnormal Color of Urination

The color of urine is related to the cause and thermal nature of the disease. Normal urine is light yellow and transparent. Vitamins, medications, and certain foods may alter the color of urine without indicating pathology.

Color of Urine	Indications
yellow urine	excessive heat
clear urine	deficient cold
turbid urine	damp heat
red urine	collateral impairment due to heat
profuse milky urine with excessive water intake	xiāo kě disease

Table 3.3.37 Abnormal Color of Urine and its Indications

— D. Abnormal Feelings or Changes in Elimination during Urination

Under normal circumstances, urination should be smooth and without pain, burning, or feelings of discomfort. Any abnormal sensation during urination indicates a pathological change.

Description		Indications	Pathogenesis
burning pain	pain with urination and feeling of urgency	painful urinary disorder due to damp heat	heat injures the vessels to cause pain, as well as stimulates the frequency and urgency of the urinary output
dribbling urine	dribbing after urination, usually seen in the aged or chronic illness patient	Kidney qi deficiency	Kidney qi deficiency fails to consolidate the urine and compromises the Bladder's function of storing the urine, also the Kidney loses control over the anterior orifice
urinary incontinence	loss of control of urination while awake, the urine is discharged spontaneously		
enuresis	spontaneous urination while sleeping with normal control during day, usually seen in children		
dysuria and anuria	difficulty in eliminating urine and in severe cases, dripping or a complete absence of urinary flow	Kidney yang deficiency	
		Kidney stone or blood stasis	stone or blood stasis obstructs the urinary track
		damp heat in the lower burner	damp heat impairs the functional activity of the Bladder qi

Table 3.3.38 Abnormal Elimination of Urine and its Indications

■ Question Eight: Inquiry into Sleep

I. INTRODUCTION

Humans spend one third of their lives sleeping; it is an essential physiological activity. Sleeping occurs regularly each day, largely under the influence of the twenty-four hour circadian rhythm. During sleep, other behaviors and physical activities cease, the eyes close, and there is a generalized reduction in sensory awareness.

(1) Sleeping Mechanism and Theory in Chinese Medicine

Traditional Chinese medicine recognizes the relationship between the mechanisms that produce sleep and the law of yin and yang. However, two other perspectives on the mechanisms of sleep have further developed from yin/yang theory. Thus, there are three perspectives about sleep in TCM: yin and yang, the movement of defensive qi, and the governance of the spirit.

Yin/yang theory: The physiological activities of sleeping and waking are produced by changes of yin and yang in the human body. Because nature follows a yin/yang cycle on a daily basis (night and day), human nature also reflects that daily rhythm in which the yang qi increases and decreases, enters and exits. During the day, the human body's yang qi exits to the exterior, which allows one to get out of bed and begin one's daily activities. At noontime, the body's yang qi is most abundant. At dusk, the yang qi gradually declines and ultimately disappears into the body. When yang enters the yin, there is sleep and when yang exits from the yin there is waking.

Defensive qi movement theory: This theory is another expression of yin/yang theory. In defensive qi theory, the defensive qi circulates through the yang channels during the day, which is what keeps one awake, and at night flows through the yin channels to induce sleep.

Spirit governance theory: The spirit governance theory teaches that periods of sleeping and waking are controlled by the activity of the spirit. Spirit refers to the external manifestation of the body's vital activity. The Heart houses the spirit. The activity of the spirit has a certain regularity that changes along with the natural increase and decrease of yin and yang. Daytime is yang, which is characterized by initiative and activity. Therefore the spirit is transported outward, and the individual is awake and active. Night is yin, which is static and calm. The spirit therefore turns inside at night, allowing the individual to rest and sleep.

The three theories of sleep are interdependent, and together comprise the Chinese medicine view of sleep. Yin/yang theory is the general guiding principle behind sleeping and awaking. Defensive qi movement theory is another expression of yin/yang theory. Spirit governance theory can also be expressed in terms of yin and yang.

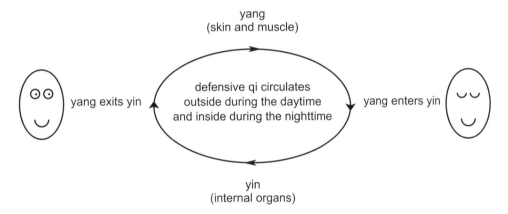

Chart 3.3.35 Mechanism of Sleep according to the Defensive Qi Circulation Theory

(2) The Relationship between Sleep and the *Zàng Fǔ* Organs

Sleep is a complex biological process that likely has multiple purposes. This process involves virtually all the organs and systems of the body. The most important organs related to sleeping are the Heart, Liver, Kidney, Spleen, and Stomach.

Heart: Normal sleeping depends on the function of the Heart. The Heart governs the blood, controls the blood vessels, and houses the spirit. The spirit is the external manifestation of the body's vital activity. Spirit is also the mental activity, which includes conscious and subconscious activity. During the daytime, the yang qi is abundant and the spirit is active exteriorly; one will therefore awaken and become active. During the nighttime, the yin qi dominates, the spirit is stored interiorly, and if it remains peaceful and calm, there will be sleep. The Heart qi and yang promote the activities of the spirit. Heart blood and Heart yin are the substances that nourish the spirit. Therefore, changes to the Heart qi, yang, blood, and yin will affect the status of the Heart spirit; the Heart is thus the major organ directly related to sleep.

Liver: the organ that regulates sleep. The Liver stores the blood, ensures the smooth flow of qi, and houses the ethereal soul (魂 *hún*). Sufficient Liver blood can help anchor the Liver yang, which prevents it from rising up and disturbing the spirit. Liver blood also has the function of nourishing the spirit and ethereal soul. If the Liver blood is insufficient, the ethereal soul will not be anchored and the individual will suffer from dream-disturbed sleep.

Kidney: the congenital root of human life. It stores essence and produces marrow to fill up the brain. The brain is the "sea of marrow" and houses the "primary spirit (元神 *yuán shén*)". It is the organ of spirit, consciousness, and thinking. Kidney yin and Kidney yang are original yin and original yang. Kidney yin is the foundation of the yin fluids of the entire body. Kidney yang is the foundation of the yang qi of the entire body, which provides warmth and promotes growth. The Kidney is the organ that ensures that yin and yang are balanced; it is therefore the organ that ensures normal sleep.

Spleen and Stomach: the acquired root of human life. The transportative and transformative functions of the Spleen and Stomach provide basic nutritional substances to keep and maintain sleeping activity.

(3) Function of Sleep

Sleep functions to provide the body and brain with rest and recovery. It helps one to maintain yin and yang balance and harmony, and to ensure that the normal physiological activities of life can continue.

(4) Normal Sleep

In general, one should be awake during the day and asleep at night. The average amount of sleep for adults is seven to eight hours, but the range of sleep duration experienced by a large majority of people can range from six to nine hours. A small minority of people feel fine with as little as five hours of sleep, while others require more than ten hours to feel refreshed and alert throughout the day. The optimal amount of sleep for the individual is that which allows one to function throughout the day without feeling drowsy when sitting quietly or when trying to pay attention to something.

II. Scope of Inquiry about Sleep:

When inquiring about sleep, one should focus on the following:

- sleeping time and hours: what time one goes to bed, and how many hours of sleep one gets
- state of sleeping: easy or difficult to fall asleep, whether or not sleep is sound, whether there are many dreams, intensity of dreams
- accompanying symptoms: irritability, palpitations, thirst, etc.

III. Clinical Significance

Inquiring about the condition of a patient's sleep can help one understand:

- the condition of the yin, yang, qi, and blood
- the functions of the Heart and Kidney

IV. Sleeping Disorders

(1) Definition

Difficulties related to sleeping, such as difficulty falling or staying asleep, falling asleep at inappropriate times, excessive total sleep time, or abnormal behaviors associated with sleep.

(2) Etiology and Pathomechanisms of Sleeping Disorders

Sleep disorders can be caused by three pathomechanisms: loss of balance between yin and yang, loss of balance between qi and blood, and a *zàng fǔ* organ disorder.

Yin and yang imbalance: When yang enters into yin, there is sleep, and when yang exits from yin there is waking. However, this yin/yang balance can be broken by exopathogens or by *zàng fǔ* organ dysfunctions. When yang is excessive, it becomes difficult for it to enter the yin, therefore the patient will experience difficulty in falling asleep. When yin is deficient, it will be unable to anchor the yang. Yang will escape easily from the yin and the patient may awaken frequently during the night. When yang is deficient, yin will be in relative excess and yang will have difficulty arising from the yin, therefore the patient will suffer from sleepiness.

Qi and blood disorder: During the day, the Heart qi promotes the external activities of the spirit, enabling it to perform physical and mental activities. During the night, the spirit is anchored in the Heart and nourished by blood. Sufficient qi and blood are the basic requirements for normal sleeping. When qi or blood is deficient, the spirit will lack nourishment and thus remain unanchored and the individual will suffer from insomnia. Qi or blood stagnation can also cause the spirit to lose nourishment, or stagnation can create heat which rises to the Heart and disturbs the spirit, leading to insomnia.

Zàng fǔ organ disorder: The Heart stores the spirit, which is nourished by blood. The Liver stores the blood. The Kidney stores essence which transforms into blood. The Spleen and Stomach transport and transform food into food essence, and later into qi and blood. Therefore, a disorder in any of these organs, as well as those that are related to them, may cause a sleeping disorder.

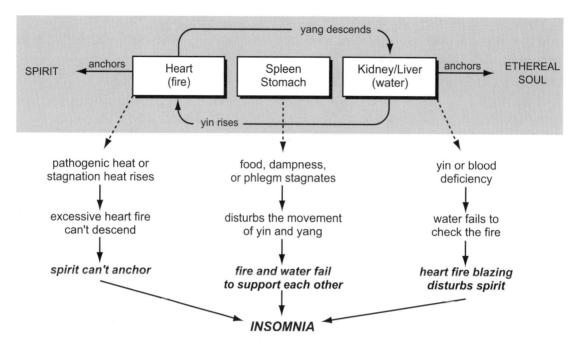

Chart 3.3.36 Etiology and Pathogenesis of Insomnia Related to *Zàng Fǔ* Organs

(3) Sleeping Disorders

Sleeping disorders include insomnia, which means a lack of sleep, and sleepiness, which means over-sleeping or sleeping at inappropriate times.

— *A. Insomnia*

DEFINITION: Insomnia describes a variety of symptoms associated with sleep disturbance, which includes:

- difficulty falling asleep after retiring

- early awakening

- intermittent waking through the period of attempted sleep, or inability to sleep through the night.

- restlessness at night

- dream-disturbed sleep

ETIOLOGY AND PATHOMECHANISMS OF INSOMNIA: The two pathomechanisms of insomnia are pathogenic heat disturbing the spirit, and a loss of nourishment to the Heart. The Heart is the key organ because it stores the spirit.

Pathogenic heat can cause the spirit to become restless. This can be the heat of an external pathogenic factor, or heat which arises from such internal factors as stagnation or deficiency of vital substances, which is often found in the elderly, or in chronic illness or the later stages of a febrile disease.

Loss of nourishment may be attributable to either excess or deficiency. In the case of excess, the stagnation of qi, blood, phlegm, or food can block the flow of qi and blood to the Heart, leading to a shortage of the vital substances necessary for the nourishment of the spirit. Such stagnation can occur because of emotional stress, traumatic injury, or improper diet. With respect to deficiency, the lack of qi, blood, yin, or essence can also deny nourishment to the Heart, which will disturb the spirit. This type of deficiency is usually seen in elderly patients or those with chronic illness.

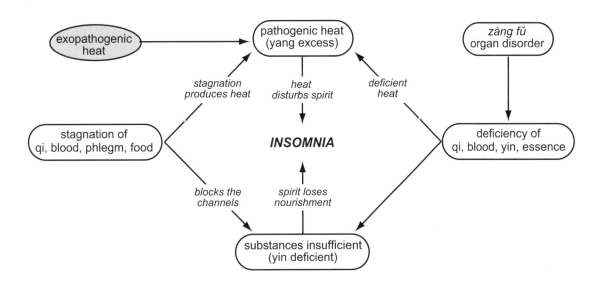

Chart 3.3.37 Pathogenesis of Insomnia

SYMPTOMS AND INDICATIONS OF INSOMNIA:

Main Symptoms	Accompanying Symptoms	Indications	
dream-disturbed or restless sleep, induced or aggravated by emotional stress	irritability, hypochondriac pain and fullness, headache, wiry pulse	excess type insomnia: acute onset, short duration, difficulty falling asleep, active dreams or nightmares, irritability or anxiety	Liver qi stagnation with heat
tossing and turning in bed, excessive dreaming, easily awakened, irritability	fullness and stifling sensation in the chest, profuse phlegm, nausea, slippery rapid pulse		phlegm heat disturbing the Heart
difficulty falling asleep with abdominal discomfort, usually induced or aggravated by overeating or late meals	foul belching, acid regurgitation, bloating, red tongue with yellow greasy coating, slippery pulse		food stagnation
inability to sleep with severe agitation and anxiety, or severe pain	night fever, moodiness, palpitations, manic behavior, a dark purple tongue		blood stagnation
difficulty in falling or remaining asleep, intermittent waking	dizziness, poor memory, tinnitus, weak back, night sweats, five center heat	deficiency type insomnia: chronic onset, long duration, awakens easily or early, difficulty in falling asleep, dreams include sad or depressing content	Heart and Kidney disharmony
easily falls asleep, but sleep is shallow and one is easily awakened during the night	poor memory, palpitations, poor appetite, fatigue, pale tongue with teeth marks, weak pulse		Heart and Spleen deficiency
difficulty falling asleep, dream-disturbed sleep, restlessness, irritability	anxiety, palpitations, night sweats, dizziness, dry mouth and throat, thirst		Liver and Heart blood deficiency
difficult to fall asleep when alone due to fear, easily awakened and frightened, timidity	constant feelings of fright, dizziness, vomiting of bitter fluids, pale tongue, weak pulse		Heart and Gallbladder qi deficiency

Table 3.3.39 Symptoms and Indications of Insomnia

B. Sleepiness (Somnolence)

DEFINITION: also called somnolence or hypersomnia, the state of feeling drowsy, tired, or sleepy.

ETIOLOGY AND PATHOMECHANISM OF SLEEPINESS:

The pathomechanism of sleepiness is that the spirit lacks nourishment, either because of the obstruction of pathogenic factors, or dysfunction of the internal organs resulting from chronic illness or advanced age.

When pathogenic factors such as phlegm, dampness, or blood stasis obstruct the channels and collaterals, the yang qi is unable to rise up to the brain. The brain is the "sea of marrow" and houses the primary spirit (元神). Yang qi is the motive power that maintains activity during the active portion of the day. When the spirit is not motivated by the yang qi, sleepiness will result.

The spirit not only relies on the motivating energies of yang and qi, but also needs the nourishment of blood and essence. When the *zàng fǔ* organs dysfunction, this may result in a deficiency of qi, blood, yin, or essence. When this happens, the spirit is deprived of its nourishment and sleepiness ensues.

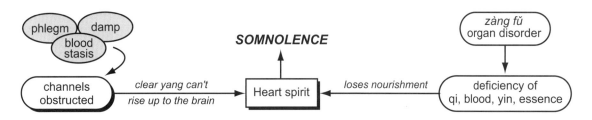

Chart 3.3.38 Etiology and Pathogenesis of Somnolence

SYMPTOMS AND INDICATIONS:

Symptoms	Accompanying Symptoms	Indications
fatigue, heaviness of the head and limbs, sleepiness	poor appetite, abdominal bloating, sticky sensation in the mouth, absence of thirst, loose stools, edema, greasy tongue coating	dampness in the Spleen
usually happens following chronic or severe illness, improper diet, or blood loss; fatigue, hypersomnolence, trance-like staring into space	palpitations, pale face, shortness of breath, poor appetite, irregular menstruation, pale tongue, thin and weak pulse	Heart / Spleen deficiency
fatigue with desire to lay down, listlessness, sleepiness	scanty urine or frequent copious urine, edema, coldness in the lower back and knees, dislike of cold, blue purple lips, dusky tongue with white moist coating, faint pulse	Kidney yang deficiency
mental fatigue, dizziness or vertigo, slow cognitive responses, poor memory, dull facial expression, sleepiness, most commonly found in the aged	tinnitus, deafness, pale tongue, thin and weak pulse	Kidney essence deficiency

Table 3.3.40 Symptoms and Indications of Somnolence

■ Question Nine: Inquiry into Women's Conditions

Menstruation, vaginal discharge, pregnancy, and childbirth are the distinguishing physiological characteristics of the female. Not only are abnormal menstruation and vaginal discharge common symptoms of gynecological illness, they also reflect pathological change in the whole body. Therefore, in addition to the usual questions, inquiry examination must include questions about the circumstances of menstruation, vaginal discharge, and the female's history of pregnancy and childbirth, etc.

I. Inquiry about Menstruation

(1) Definition

Also called the "period," menstruation is the physiological phenomenon of monthly bleeding from the uterus of an adult woman who is not pregnant or lactating.

Menarche: the first menstrual period, or bleeding, as a girl's body progresses through the changes of puberty.

Amenorrhea: pathological absence or cessation of menstruation.

(2) Physiology of the Formation of Menstruation

The major component of menstruation is blood. Blood formation depends on the *zàng fǔ* organs. The movement of blood depends on the function of qi, which also relies on the channels and vessels to transport the blood into the uterus. Thus, menstruation is a product of the joint effort of "heavenly dew" (天癸 *tiān guǐ*), qi and blood, channels and vessels, and *zàng fǔ* organs.

— A. Heavenly Dew and Menstruation

Heavenly dew is the most important material for ensuring sufficiency of blood, essence, and body fluids in the female. Maturity and exhaustion of heavenly dew are related to menarche and menopause, respectively. In women, the heavenly dew arrives at age fourteen and is exhausted at the age of forty-nine.

— B. Qi, Blood, and Menstruation

Female physiology is dominated by blood, the primary ingredient of menses. Blood is generated by the transformation of food essence, ying qi, and essence. The production, movement, and functions of blood depend on qi. Qi and blood travel together within the channels and organs, and are the substantive foundation for the physiological actions of menstruation.

— C. Zàng Fǔ Organs and Menstruation

Blood and qi are generated by the *zàng fǔ* organs. The Heart governs the blood. The Liver stores the blood. The Spleen controls and generates the blood. The Kidney stores essence, and essence transforms into blood. The Lung governs the qi, and qi motivates the movement of blood. Thus, all five *zàng* organs are related to menstruation, but among these organs, the Kidney, Liver, and Spleen play the most important roles.

Kidney: stores prenatal and postnatal essence. The physiology of puberty, fertility, conception, pregnancy, and menopause are greatly influenced by the condition of the Kidney essence. The Kidney's effect on menstruation is reflected in the following two aspects:

- Kidney qi and heavenly dew: heavenly dew is stored inside the Kidney, and the maturity of heavenly dew depends on stimulation from the Kidney qi. Following the lead of the Kidney qi, the heavenly dew either increases or decreases.

- The Kidney stores the essence, and the essence transforms into blood. As we know, blood is the primary ingredient of menses, thus the Kidney essence is one of the fundamental substances in the formation of menstrual blood.

Liver: stores the blood, regulates the sea of blood (*chōng mài*), governs free coursing, and controls the volume of blood.

Spleen and Stomach: Conditions of the Spleen are related to the quantity, quality, and color of the menstrual blood as well as the menstrual cycle.

- The Spleen is the root of the postnatal essence and has the function of generating blood. It is thus the source of the menstrual blood. This function governs the quantity, quality, and color of the menstrual blood

- The Spleen also controls the blood and the raising of qi. The flow of menstrual blood and cycle depend on the functions of the Spleen.

— D. *Chōng Mài, Rèn Mài, Dū Mài, Dài Mài and Menstruation*

Chōng mài (**Penetrating Vessel**): Also known as the "sea of blood" and the "sea of the twelve channels." It is here that the qi and blood of all twelve channels converge, and it is the thoroughfare for the circulation of qi and blood. Menstrual blood comes from this sea of blood. Therefore, when the *chōng mài* is exuberant, the menstrual blood is sufficient.

Rèn mài (**Conception Vessel**): *Rèn* means nourish or conception. The *rèn mài* governs the uterus and fetus; it controls the yin channels and is called the "sea of yin." As such, it exerts an influence on all the yin channels of the body. All yin substances such as essence, body fluids, and blood are controlled by the *rèn mài*. Therefore, when the *rèn mài* is open, menstruation will flow.

Dū mài (**Governing Vessel**): The "sea of yang," this vessel exerts an influence on all the yang channels. Both the *dū mài* and the *rèn mài* originate in the uterus. The yin channel rises up the front of the body while the yang channel rises up the back of the body. Between yin and yang, front and back, the balance of yin and yang is maintained and menstruation is properly regulated.

Dài mài (**Girdle Vessel**): The *dài mài* runs transversely around the waist. All channels and collaterals pass through and are thus controlled by the *dài mài*. This controlling function enables the qi and blood to maintain normal circulation, which in turn enables a healthy menstrual cycle.

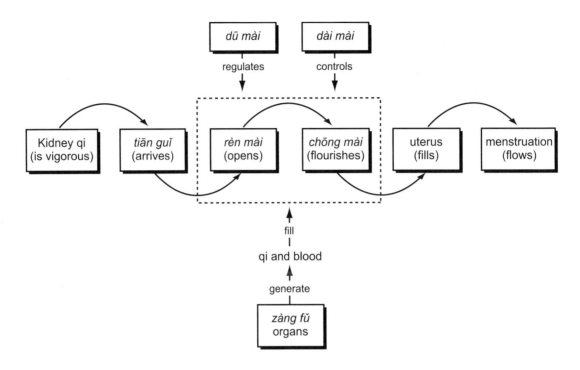

Chart 3.3.39 Physiology of Menstruation Formation

(3) Normal Menstruation and Physiological Variations

The normal menstrual cycle should be around twenty-eight days, with the flow lasting from three to seven days. The quantity of menses averages between 50 and 100 ml. There are differences among individuals based on age, climate, geographic location, and emotional state. The color of the menses should be slightly dark red in the first couple days, and then turn to slightly light red for the remainder of the period. There are no clots, unusual odors, pain, or other accompanying symptoms.

Amenorrhea is a physiological variation that occurs during pregnancy or lactation, as well as after menopause. Irregular menses may also occur following a change of climate, work, or environment.

(4) Scope of Inquiry about Menstruation

Questions about menstruation should focus on the cycle's timing, the quality and quantity of the menses, and accompanying symptoms:

- length of cycle

- days of period

- bleeding

    – quantity (amount)
    – color
    – flow consistency (thick/thin, clots)

- accompanying symptoms:
  - abdominal cramps
  - headache
  - constipation
  - diarrhea
  - insomnia

(5) Pathological Menstruation

Pathological menstruation means an abnormal cycle, flow, or accompanying symptoms that occur before, during, or after the menses.

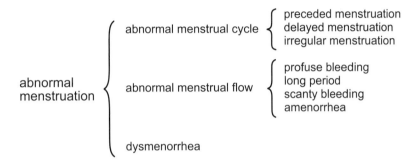

Chart 3.3.40 Abnormal Menstruation

— A. Abnormal Menstrual Cycle

The normal menstrual cycle should be between twenty-eight and thirty-two days. The menstrual cycle depends on the condition of the qi and blood, their ability to circulate, and the health of the *zàng fŭ* organs.

··· a) Preceded Menstruation

DEFINITION: menstrual cycle shortened by more than seven days.

ETIOLOGY AND PATHOMECHANISMS OF PRECEDED MENSTRUATION:

There are two major pathogeneses of preceded menstruation. The first is pathogenic heat invading the uterus, Penetrating Vessel *(chōng mài)*, or Conception Vessel *(rèn mài)*. This injures the vessels and pushes the blood out too early. The other cause is qi deficiency in which the Spleen loses its ability to control the blood. The result is that the blood will spill out of the vessels and cause an early flow.

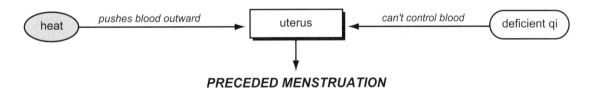

Chart 3.3.41 Pathology of Preceded Menstruation

SYMPTOMS AND INDICATIONS

Main Symptoms	Accompanying Symptoms	Indications	
bright red or dark red color, may include clots, thick viscosity, profuse quantity, may have a foul odor	thirst with desire to drink cold water, irritability, dark yellow urine, red tongue, rapid pulse	heat	excess heat
red or slightly light color, no clots, scanty quantity	dizziness, five center heat, insomnia, red tongue with scanty coating, thin and rapid pulse		deficiency heat
light red color, thin viscosity, profuse quantity	fatigue, lower abdominal sensation of emptiness, poor appetite, palpitations, pale tongue, weak pulse	qi deficiency	

Table 3.3.41 Symptoms and Indications of Preceded Menstruation

··· b) Delayed Menstruation

DEFINITION: menstrual cycle is extended more than seven days. This extension can last for several months.

ETIOLOGY AND PATHOMECHANISMS OF DELAYED MENSTRUATION:

There are two major pathomechanisms of delayed menstruation. The first is blood deficiency in which the *chōng mài* and uterus are unable to fill with blood. The second is blockage in the channels caused by qi or blood stagnation, or attack by pathogenic cold.

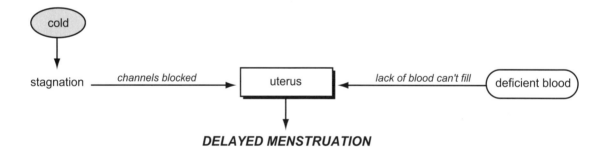

Chart 3.3.42 Pathogenesis of Delayed Menstruation

SYMPTOMS AND INDICATIONS

Main Symptoms	Accompanying Symptoms	Indications	
dark purple color with clots, scanty quantity	severe lower abdominal cramps with sensations of cold, pain relieved by warmth, deep and tight pulse	cold	excess cold
light color without clots, thin viscosity, scanty quantity	dull lower abdominal pain, relieved by warmth and/or pressure, loose stools, deep, slow, and weak pulse		deficiency cold
deep red color with clots, scanty quantity	pain or distention of the lower abdomen, hypochondrium, or breasts; wiry pulse	qi stagnation	
light color without clots, thin viscosity, scanty quantity	no abdominal pain, dizziness, thin and weak pulse, pale tongue, palpitations	blood deficiency	

Table 3.3.42 Symptoms and Indications of Delayed Menstruation

··· c) Irregular Menstrual Cycle

DEFINITION: the menses is sometimes preceded and sometimes delayed. The difference between the first day of two adjacent cycles is more than seven days.

ETIOLOGY AND PATHOMECHANISMS OF IRREGULAR MENSTRUAL CYCLE:

The pathomechanism of the irregular menstrual cycle is related to disorders of qi and blood leading to a disorder in the filling and refilling of the Penetrating Vessel *(chōng mài)* and Conception Vessel *(rèn mài)*. There are three causes for a disorder of qi and blood: Liver qi stagnation, Spleen deficiency, and Kidney deficiency.

The Liver regulates the Penetrating Vessel *(chōng)* and Conception Vessel *(rèn mài)*. The Liver's free coursing allows the blood to fill and refill the Penetrating Vessel *(chōng)* and Conception Vessel *(rèn mài)*. When the Liver is over-coursing, the menstruation comes early, and when the Liver coursing is inadequate, there will be delayed menstruation.

The Spleen qi controls the blood and keeps it inside the blood vessels. When Spleen qi is deficient, this may cause early menstruation. The Spleen is also the source of blood, and thus when Spleen qi is deficient, the blood will diminish, which may delay menstruation.

The Kidney and Liver have a common source. The Liver stores the blood and the Kidney stores the essence. Essence and blood mutually replenish and transform. The Liver is the root of the Penetrating Vessel *(chōng mài)* and the Kidney is the root of the Conception Vessel *(rèn mài)*. When there is Kidney deficiency, the filling and refilling functions of the Penetrating Vessel *(chōng mài)* and Conception Vessel *(rèn mài)* are compromised, which causes an irregular menstrual cycle.

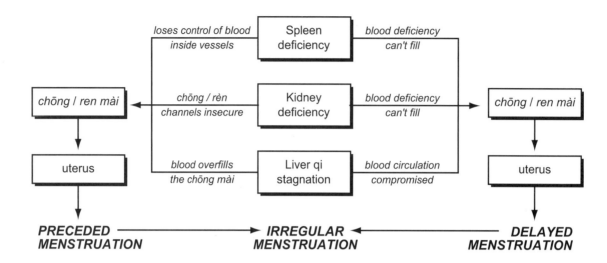

Chart 3.3.43 Pathomechanisms of Irregular Menstrual Cycle

SYMPTOMS AND INDICATIONS:

Main Symptoms	Accompanying Symptoms	Indications
menses with purple color clots, profuse or scanty quantity	lower abdominal distention that can radiate to the chest or hypochondrium, breast distention, irritability, thin tongue coating, wiry pulse	Liver qi stagnation
pale color menses, thin viscosity, scanty quantity	dizziness, tinnitus, lower back pain, frequent urination at night, pale and thin tongue, deep and deficient pulse	Kidney deficiency
pale color menses, thin viscosity, profuse or scanty quantity	fatigue, poor appetite, loose stools, abdominal bloating and distention, pale tongue with teeth marks, white greasy coating, deficient and moderate pulse	Spleen deficiency

Table 3.3.43 Symptoms and Indications of Irregular Menstruation

— B. Abnormal Amount of Menstrual Flow

Under normal circumstances, the menstrual flow lasts from three to seven days. The quantity of menses should be between 50 and 100 ml. The quantity of flow depends on the condition of the qi and blood.

··· a) Profuse Bleeding

DEFINITION: also called heavy periods, the menstruation occurs regularly and lasts the usual three to seven days, but the volume of bleeding is heavier than normal (> 100 ml.).

ETIOLOGY AND PATHOMECHANISM OF PROFUSE BLEEDING:

The pathomechanism of profuse menstrual bleeding consists of three main processes.

- First, the Penetrating Vessel *(chōng mài)* and Conception Vessel *(rèn mài)* are unstable due to qi deficiency, and so the blood is not held inside the vessels but leaks out.

- Second, pathogenic heat injures the vessels and forces blood out.

- And third, blood stasis obstructs the vessels and newly-generated blood has no place to go; it then flows out with the menstrual blood.

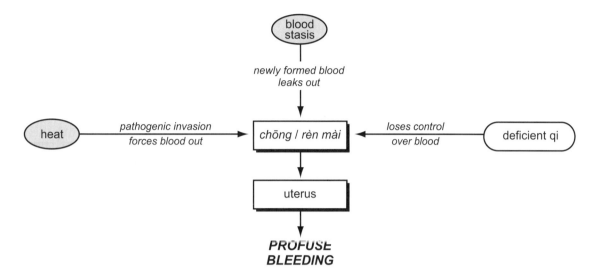

Chart 3.3.44 Pathogenesis of Profuse Menstrual Bleeding

SYMPTOMS AND INDICATIONS

Main Symptoms	Accompanying Symptoms	Indications
menses with a bright red or purple color, thick viscosity, profuse quantity	thirst, irritability, yellow urine, constipation, red tongue with yellow coating, slippery and rapid pulse	pathogenic heat invades the blood
menses with dark purple color and clots, profuse quantity	abdominal pain that is resistant to pressure, purple or dark spots on the tongue, thin and choppy pulse	blood stagnation
pale color menses, thin viscosity, profuse quantity	fatigue, pale face, shortness of breath, palpitations, pale tongue; weak, deficient pulse	qi deficiency

Table 3.3.44 Symptoms and Indications of Profuse Menstrual Bleeding

··· b) Prolonged Period

DEFINITION:

Menstrual flow lasting more than seven days.

ETIOLOGY AND PATHOMECHANISMS OF PROLONGED PERIOD:

There are three major pathomechanisms for a prolonged period:

- Blood stasis obstructing the Penetrating Vessel *(chōng mài)* and Conception Vessel *(rèn mài)*: the newly-generated blood cannot flow into these vessels to fill them, and so it leaks outward.

- Heat due to yin deficiency: the deficiency heat disturbs the Penetrating Vessel *(chōng mài)* or Conception Vessel *(rèn mài)* and pushes the blood out of the channels.

- Spleen qi deficiency: qi is unable to hold the blood within the vessels, leading to prolonged menstrual flow.

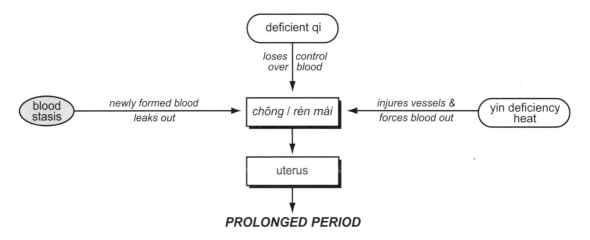

Chart 3.3.45 Pathogenesis of Prolonged Period

SYMPTOMS AND INDICATIONS

Main Symptoms	Accompanying Symptoms	Indications
prolonged periods, dark color blood with clots, scanty flow or spotting	abdominal cramps that are resistant to pressure, purple tongue with spots, choppy pulse	blood stagnation
prolonged periods, red blood, thick viscosity, scanty quantity	dry throat and thirst, hot flashes, five center heat, dry and red tongue body, little or no coating, thin rapid pulse	yin deficiency with heat
spotting between periods, pale color blood, thin viscosity, scanty quantity	easy bruising, bloating, loose stools, fatigue, anorexia, deficient pulse	Spleen qi deficiency

Table 3.3.45 Symptoms and Indications of a Prolonged Period

··· c) Scanty Bleeding

DEFINITION:

Menstrual cycle is normal, but the flow is very light, or extremely sparse, like a small drip. Another definition of scanty bleeding describes a normal flow, but for less than two days in total.

ETIOLOGY AND PATHOMECHANISMS OF SCANTY BLEEDING:

There are two major pathomechanisms underlying scanty bleeding:

- *Chōng mài* (sea of blood) blood deficiency due to Kidney deficiency or qi and blood deficiency

- Penetrating Vessel *(Chōng mài)* and Conception Vessel *(rèn mài)* are blocked by blood stasis or phlegm.

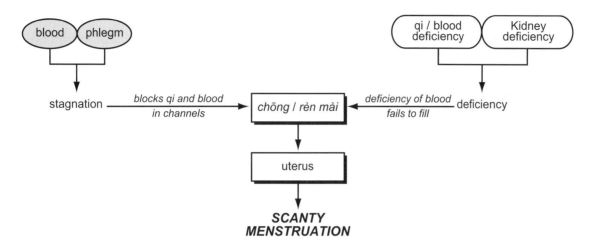

Chart 3.3.46 Pathogenesis of Scanty Menstruation

SYMPTOMS AND INDICATIONS:

Main Symptoms	Accompanying Symptoms	Indications
scanty flow or spotting, pale color, no clots, thin viscosity	dizziness, blurry vision, pale face, palpitations, pale tongue, thready pulse	blood deficiency
scanty flow, pale or dark red color, thin viscosity	dizziness, tinnitus, low back pain, profuse urine at night, deep and deficient pulse	Kidney deficiency
scanty flow, dark purple color with numerous clots, abdominal cramps that are resistant to pressure and relieved after the clots have passed	normal tongue, or with purple spots, wiry and choppy pulse	blood stagnation
scanty flow, pale color, thick and sticky viscosity	obesity, nausea, feeling of oppression in the chest, excessive vaginal discharge, greasy tongue coating, slippery pulse	phlegm stagnation

Table 3.3.46 Symptoms and Indications of Scanty Menstruation

··· d) Amenorrhea

DEFINITION:

Absence or cessation of menstruation. Amenorrhea is conventionally divided into primary and secondary amenorrhea:

- Primary amenorrhea is when menstruation never occurs. It fails to begin at puberty.

- Secondary amenorrhea is the absence of menstrual periods for six months in a woman who had previously been regular, or a lack of periods for twelve months in a woman who had had irregular periods.

ETIOLOGY AND PATHOMECHANISMS OF AMENORRHEA:

Kidney, heavenly dew, Penetrating Vessel *(chōng mài)* and Conception Vessel *(rèn mài)*, and uterus are the major contibutors to the production and generation of menstruation. Dysfunction in any of them may result in amenorrhea.

Primary amenorrhea is usually the result of congenital Kidney qi deficiency. This prevents heavenly dew from developing and maturing. Secondary amenorrhea can be caused by either qi and blood deficiency which cannot fill the Penetrating Vessel *(chōng mài)* and Conception Vessel *(rèn mài)*, or blockage of the Penetrating Vessel *(chōng mài)* and Conception Vessel *(rèn mài)* by pathogenic factors such as blood stasis or phlegm.

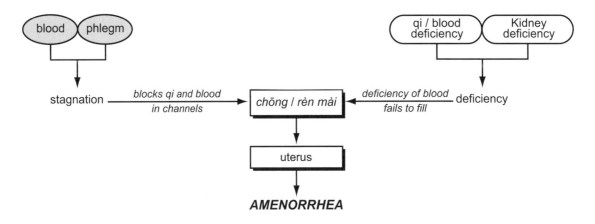

Chart 3.3.47 Pathogenesis of Amenorrhea

SYMPTOMS AND INDICATIONS

Main Symptoms	Indications	Pathogenesis
menstruation suddenly stops, depression, lower abdominal pain and distention that is resistant to pressure	qi and blood stagnation	pathogenic factors (blood stasis and phlegm) obstruct the *chōng* and *rèn mài*
usually occurring in obese patients, begins with scanty quantity and delayed menstruation, gradually develops into amenorrhea	phlegm stagnation	
no menarche by the age of eighteen, secondary sexual characteristics underdeveloped	Kidney insufficiency	Kidney insufficiency prevents the development and maturity of the *tiān guǐ* (heavenly dew)
patient with chronic illness or multiple childbirths, dizziness, weak back and legs, low libido, hair loss	Kidney and Liver deficiency	qi and blood deficiency is unable to fill the *chōng* and *rèn mài*
delayed or scanty menstruation that gradually develops into amenorrhea, may have chronic bleeding, or history of blood loss	qi and blood deficiency	

Table 3.3.47 Symptoms and Indications of Amenorrhea

— C. Dysmenorrhea

DEFINITION:

Cramps or painful menstruation. This includes menstrual periods that are accompanied by either sharp intermittent pain, or dull aching pain, usually in the pelvis or lower abdomen.

ETIOLOGY AND PATHOMECHANISMS OF DYSMENORRHEA:

Stagnation and malnutrition are the two major causes of pain.

Before menstruation, the qi and blood flourish in the sea of blood (*chōng mài*). This flourishing of qi and blood may cause stagnation, which prevents the flow of qi and blood in the Penetrating Vessel (*chōng mài*) and Conception Vessel (*rèn mài*) from entering the uterus. Pathological factors such as cold or damp can generate stagnation as well.

The qi and blood become deficient after menstruation due to the bleeding. During this time, the quantity of qi and blood changes very rapidly and is thus easily affected by pathogenic factors. These factors cause disorders in the movement of qi and blood which in turn can deprive the uterus, Penetrating Vessel (*chōng mài*) and Conception Vessel (*rèn mài*) of nourishment.

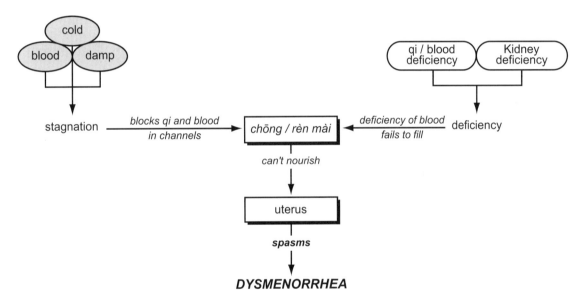

Chart 3.3.48 Pathogenesis of Dysmenorrhea

SYMPTOMS AND INDICATIONS

Symptoms			Indications
abdominal pain and cramps occuring before the menstruation and relieved after menstruation	distending pain related to emotional changes	excess	Liver qi stagnation
	sharp pain with clots, resistant to pressure		blood stagnation
	cold pain with clots, resistant to pressure		cold
dull pain after menstruation	aching pain with empty feeling, symptoms relieved by pressure, usually with a history of blood loss	deficiency	qi and blood deficiency
	dull aching abdominal pain with low back pain, usually found in patients with a history of multiple childbirths		Kidney and Liver yin deficiency

Table 3.3.48 Symptoms and Indications of Dysmenorrhea

II: INQUIRY ABOUT VAGINAL DISCHARGE

In healthy women, starting at puberty, vaginal and cervical glands produce small amounts of clear and odorless fluid that flows out of the vagina daily, taking with it the old cells that line the vagina. We call this vaginal discharge or leukorrhea.

Normal vaginal discharge helps to clean the vagina, as well as keep it lubricated and free of infection and other germs.

(1) Physiology of Vaginal Discharge Formation

Physiological vaginal discharge requires that the heavenly dew reach maturity and that there be an abundance of Kidney qi. Vaginal discharge is mostly essence fluid (精液 *jīng yè*). Vaginal discharge is a body fluid. Essence fluid formation mainly depends on the proper functioning of the Spleen and Kidney. The Spleen is the acquired root of essence. It transports and transforms ingested food and drink into food essence, which nourishes and replenishes the qi, blood, body fluids, and essence. The Kidney is the congenital root of essence. It is also where the essence fluid is stored and maintained.

The Conception Vessel *(rèn mài)*, Governing Vessel *(dū mài)*, and Girdle Vessel *(dài mài)* are also directly associated with the formation of vaginal discharge. As we know, the Conception Vessel *(rèn mài)* is the "sea of yin channels." All yin substances (陰液 *yīn yè*), such as essence, body fluids, and blood, are governed by the Conception Vessel *(rèn mài)*. The Governing Vessel *(dū mài)* is the "sea of yang channels." It warms and regulates the Conception Vessel *(rèn mài)* to maintain the balance of yin and yang. The Girdle Vessel *(dài mài)* controls and keeps the essence fluid inside the body, preventing it from draining away.

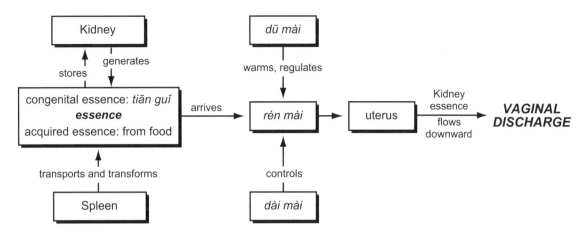

Chart 3.3.49 Physiological Formation of Vaginal Discharge

(2) Normal Vaginal Discharge and Physiological Variations

Normal vaginal discharge appears as a clear, thin mucus which is odorless and in small amounts. The amount and appearance of normal vaginal discharge varies throughout the menstrual cycle. It increases slightly during ovulation or pregnancy. Other factors that may cause changes in the appearance or consistency of physiological vaginal discharge include sexual excitement, breastfeeding, emotional stress, medications and diet.

(3) Scope of Inquiry about Vaginal Discharge

When inquiring about vaginal discharge, the following information should be gathered:

- presence or absence of vaginal discharge
- color of the discharge
- quantity of discharge
- whether the quality of the discharge is clear or opaque, thin or thick, turbid, or sticky
- odor

(4) Etiology and Pathomechanisms of Pathological Vaginal Discharge

Dampness is the major cause of abnormal vaginal discharge. Dampness either comes from the exterior or is generated internally by a functional disorder of the Spleen, Liver, or Kidney. When dampness remains inside the body, it may injure the Conception Vessel *(rèn mài)* and Girdle Vessel *(dài mài),* impairing regulation and control, and resulting in the outward flow of yin essence (陰精 *yīn jīng*).

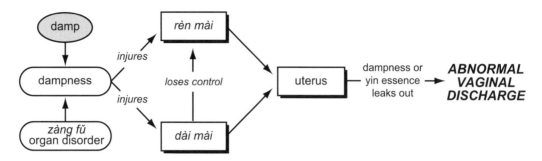

Chart 3.3.50 Etiology and Pathogenesis of Abnormal Vaginal Discharge

(5) Pathological Vaginal Discharge

Abnormal vaginal discharge includes abnormal quantity, color, consistency, odor, or abnormal symptoms that accompany vaginal discharge.

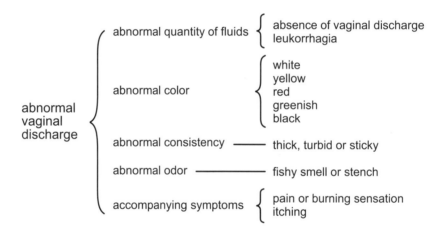

Chart 3.3.51 Abnormal Vaginal Discharge

— *A. Abnormal Volume of Vaginal Discharge*

Symptoms	Description	Indications
profuse vaginal discharge (leukorrhagia)	abnormal increase in vaginal discharge with white or yellow color	dampness invades, or Spleen deficiency, or Kidney deficiency
vaginal dryness	scanty or no vaginal discharge	Kidney deficiency

Table 3.3.49 Abnormal Volume of Vaginal Discharge and its Indications

— *B. Abnormal Colors of Vaginal Discharge*

Color	Description	Indications
white	white color, thin viscosity, odorless discharge, copious quantity	deficiency cold syndrome
yellow	yellow color, thick viscosity, foul odor, large quantity, accompanied by vaginal itching	damp heat
greenish	greenish color, thick and sticky viscosity, strong foul odor	damp heat
red	red color, thick viscosity, slightly foul odor	damp heat, or Liver fire injuring the collaterals
black	dark brown color, slightly foul odor	remants of red discharge

Table 3.3.50 Abnormal Colors of Vaginal Discharge and their Indications

— *C. Abnormal Consistency of Vaginal Discharge*

Viscosity	Description	Indications
thin	vaginal discharge is very thin, like water	normal, or deficiency, cold syndrome
thick	thick, turbid, sticky; may look like cottage cheese, may have a yellow or greenish color	damp heat

Table 3.3.51 Abnormal Consistency of Vaginal Discharge and its Indications

— *D. Abnormal Odor of Vaginal Discharge*

Odor	Description	Indications
odorless	there is no odor associated with vaginal discharge	normal, or deficiency, cold syndrome
foul	vaginal discharge has foul, fishy, or rotten smell; vaginal discharge is yellow or greenish in color, with a thick viscosity	damp heat

Table 3.3.52 Abnormal Odor of Vaginal Discharge and its Indications

— *E. Abnormal Symptoms Accompanying Vaginal Discharge*

Pain, burning, and itching are common symptoms that accompany abnormal vaginal discharge. These symptoms all indicate damp-heat in the lower burner.

◼ Question Ten: Inquiry for Children

The physiology of children is different from that of adults. Children have tender *zàng fǔ* organs, and are full of vitality and rapid growth. Similarly, childhood diseases often present with a sudden onset, quick changes, and a tendency to arise from simple deficiency or excess. Therefore, when inquiring about diseases in children, in addition to the usual questions, the following questions should also be included.

I. Condition Before and After Birth

For infants (< 6 months old): Illnesses are mostly related to congenital factors or childbirth. Therefore, inquiring should include the condition of the mother during the pregnancy and childbirth such as:

- whether there was a normal, full-term pregnancy
- whether the mother had a physical or psychological illness during the pregnancy
- whether the mother took any medication during her pregnancy
- the nutritional status of the mother during pregnancy
- whether there was a difficult or premature labor
- feeding practices: breastfeeding or formula feeding; for breastfeeding, whether the mother is healthy

For toddlers (<3 years old): At this period of time, children grow rapidly and need a lot of nutrition, but the functions of the Spleen and Stomach are not fully developed; thus, illnesses are often closely related to digestive functions. Questions should therefore include the nature of their diet and development.

II. The History of Vaccinations and Infectious Diseases

In children from six months to five years of age, congenital immunity gradually fades away, but acquired immunity has not yet fully developed. Thus, children readily contract infectious diseases such as chickenpox and measles. Asking about the history of vaccination and infectious diseases can help form a quick diagnosis and control infectious disease epidemics.

III. Unique Causes for Children's Illnesses

Climate and environmental changes readily affect children. Because the immune systems in children are still developing, they are apt to suffer from exogenous diseases. Living conditions of children should therefore be queried.

Children readily suffer from indigestion because the functions of the Spleen and Stomach are weaker in children. Vomiting, diarrhea, abdominal distention, and malnutrition frequently result from improper diet. Questions regarding diet and appetite should therefore be asked.

Children are susceptible to fright because their minds and consciousness have not fully developed. They are apt to be frightened, scared, shocked, and to cry. They can also suffer from high fever and convulsions due to a profoundly frightening experience. Hence, whether a child has been deeply frightened or emotionally traumatized should be determined by gentle questioning of the patient or her parent.

Section 4

Questions and Answers for Deeper Insight into Inquiry

1. Why is the inquiry method so important?

Inquiry allows practitioners to determine the onset, development, treatment, presenting symptoms, and other important information.

Disease is a complicated and variable process that can be affected by many factors. The purpose of inquiry is to collect clinical data that the other three methods (inspection, listening and smelling, and palpation) cannot ascertain, such as the onset of the illness, development, treatment, patient's subjective feelings, past medical history, hobbies, living environment, customs, etc. Based on this information, the practitioner can assess the condition of the disease; judge its cause, thermal nature, and location, and ultimately make a differential diagnosis. This method is especially important during the early stage of a disease before signs and symptoms appear. The inquiry method can also help in understanding the patient's emotional status and learn of other illnesses that may be related to the current problem.

2. What is the difference between chief complaints and chief symptoms?

The chief symptom is the major symptom(s) or sign(s) that appears during the disease. It is the external manifestation of internal pathological changes. Every disease has its specific chief symptoms. Chief symptoms may consist of just one sign or symptom, or a group of signs and symptoms. Inquiry should be directed at chief symptoms as the focal points around which one can understand the disease and make a diagnosis.

Chief complaints are the signs and symptoms that the patient feels are most severe and of longest duration. The chief complaint is commonly what brings a patient in for treatment.

Chief symptoms and the chief complaint are often the same, but not always. For example, with the *tài yáng* pattern, a floating pulse, headache, and aversion to cold are the chief symptoms, yet patients who are suffering from an exterior pattern are unlikely to seek treatment because of a floating pulse and aversion to cold. It is more likely that the patient will complain of the headache. Still, to diagnose a *tài yáng* pattern, the patient must have an aversion to cold since that is the chief symptom used in defining the *tài yáng* pattern. Chief symptoms are the objective expression of the essence of a disease, and diagnosis is formed based on the chief symptoms. Chief symptoms are not always the same as chief complaints.

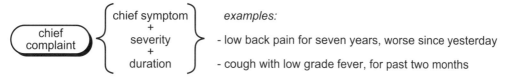

Chart 3.4.1 Chief Complaint and Chief Symptom

3. How is it that an attack of exogenous cold can cause fever?

Basic Questions, Chapter 31 (素問。熱論) notes: "If a man is impaired by exogenous cold, fever may occur." Exogenous cold that invades the body causes aversion to cold, but also fever, headache, body aches, a lack of sweating, and a floating, tight pulse. At this time, the patient may feel a mild fever in the body. Upon palpation, the practitioner may discover that the skin is hot to the touch and the body temperature is indeed running a slight fever. Meanwhile, if exogenous cold is not expelled from the exterior, it can penetrate more deeply into the body and transform into interior heat. This pattern manifests with a high fever, fever without chills, thirst, constipation, and a rapid, forceful pulse. Thus, an attack of exogenous cold is one of the etiologies of febrile disease.

Generally speaking, heat pathogens cause fever, while cold pathogens cause chills. So how is it that pathogenic cold can cause fever? According to Chinese medicine theory, all patterns, regardless of whether they are exterior or interior, hot or cold, involve the entire body's reaction to the struggle between antipathogenic qi and the pathogens. It is the nature of cold to contract and to constrict. When exogenous cold attacks the body, the function of qi is restrained, the interstitial space (腠理 *còu lǐ*) and pores close, and thus there is no sweating. Yang qi then stagnates inside and is unable to radiate outward. Meanwhile, because cold is a yin pathogen, it arouses the defensive yang to launch an attack against the pathogenic factor by increasing the production of heat. Therefore, if the body has a strong constitution, the yang qi is not deficient, and the interstitial spaces and pores close without sweating, then there will be fever even when attacked by pathogenic cold.

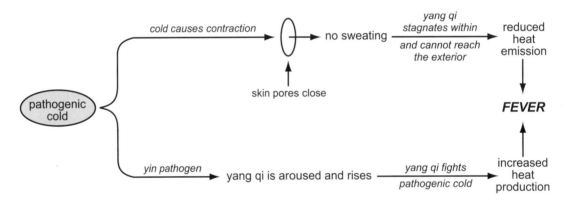

Chart 3.4.2 Pathogenesis of Fever due to Pathogenic Cold

4. Why does yin deficiency cause a fever at night but not during the day?

Under normal physiological circumstances, yin essence and yang qi are balanced and mutually control and generate each other. There are no chills and fever and the body temperature remains in a normal range. If the yin essence is insufficient, it can no longer control the yang qi, which leads to a relative excess of yang. However, this relative excess is not strong enough to cause fever during the day.

Defensive qi pertains to yang. During the daytime it circulates on the surface of the body, and at night it circulates interiorly through the *zàng fǔ* organs. In the late afternoon, defensive qi begins to enter deeper into the body and will be completely inside by evening. Since the internal yang qi is already in a state of relative excess due to the yin deficiency, and the (warm by nature) defensive qi enters the interior in late afternoon and evening, the endogenous internal heat then becomes even more vigorous. This is why a yin deficient patient usually begins to feel warm or hot in the late afternoon and why this becomes even worse during the night.

5. How is it that qi deficiency can cause fever?

Fever caused by qi deficiency is a commonly seen clinical phenomenon, even though it is difficult to explain. Yang governs heat, so there is a fever when yang is in excess. Yin deficiency can cause a relative excess of yang, so a fever may accompany that condition as well. However, qi pertains to yang. How is it that qi deficiency can cause a fever? The answer is that the qi deficiency doesn't directly cause the fever, but the secondary problems do. Qi deficiency can lead to yin deficiency. Qi deficiency can also give rise to qi, blood, food, or damp stagnation, all of which can generate heat. Different pathomechanisms cause qi deficiency fever, and they all present with unique clinical manifestations.

Qi deficiency leading to yin deficiency and causing fever was discussed in *Basic Questions*, Chapter 62 (素問。調經論): "Overstrain can weaken the body and cause qi deficiency in the Spleen and Stomach. The upper burner will then be unable to distribute the food essence, and the lower abdomen will not open. Therefore, the Stomach qi stagnates and creates internal heat." When there is qi deficiency, the Spleen and Stomach lose their motive force for transportation and transformation; food will not transform into food essence, which leads to a lack of nutritive qi, yin, and blood. It also causes a relative excess of yang and thus a low-grade fever. This fever usually arises in the afternoon or evening.

The theory of qi deficiency causing qi stagnation leading to fever was established by Li Dong-Yuan (李東垣 1180–1251) in his book *Treatise on the Spleen and Stomach* (脾胃論). Qi deficiency in this context means Spleen and Stomach qi deficiency. The Spleen and Stomach are located in the middle of the body. The Spleen qi ascends and the Stomach qi descends. The middle is like a pivot for the body, as it keeps the qi circulating properly. When there is qi deficiency, there isn't enough motive power to ensure movement; hence the Spleen qi cannot ascend and the Stomach qi cannot descend. Accumulation and stagnation in the middle generates heat and causes fever. The fever is low-grade and chronic. It may last for weeks or even months. It usually arises in the morning and is aggravated by exertion. It is accompanied by fatigue, poor appetite, frequent colds, shortness of breath, loose stools, and a faint pulse.

Qi is the motive power for blood circulation. When qi is deficient, there is a lack of power to push the blood, which then slows down and eventually stagnates. Similarly, qi deficiency can cause food or damp stagnation. In each of these cases, stagnation generates heat, leading to fever from qi deficiency.

There is another theory about the pathomechanism for qi deficiency fever which occurs during an attack by exogenous pathogenic factors over a preexisting qi deficiency. Defensive qi has the function of protecting the body and preventing pathogenic attacks. Defensive qi is nourished and replenished by food essence, which is the product of the Spleen and Stomach's transportative and transformation functions. When the Spleen and Stomach qi is deficient, defensive qi will lose its strength. Although the defensive qi will generate a fever when it fights exogenous pathogenic factors, it is too weak to generate a high fever.

6. Why does the body temperature increase between 3 and 5 p.m. in the *yáng míng* organ pattern?

Yáng míng means abundance of yang qi. It pertains to these organs: the foot *yáng míng* is the Stomach and hand *yáng míng* is the Large Intestine. The Stomach is located in the middle burner, is associated with earth, and is the "sea of food and water." *Yáng míng* organs have abundant qi and blood, and very strong antipathogenic qi. Thus, when pathogenic factors invade the *yáng míng* organs, it commonly generates a high fever, profuse sweating, great thirst, a forceful pulse, and other symptoms of an excess pattern. Among all the organs, the *yáng míng* organ pattern exhibits the greatest conflict between pathogenic and antipathogenic qi.

The time between 3 and 5 p.m. is the hottest time of the day. Meanwhile, according to the *Shāng Hán Lùn*, it is the time in which the *yáng míng* qi increases to its peak. Abundant yang qi combines with excess pathogenic heat and causes the body temperature to rise higher than at other times.

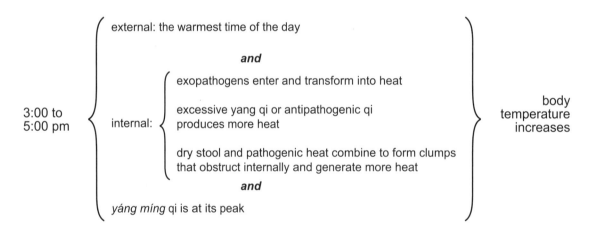

Chart 3.4.3 High Fever in the Afternoon due to *Yáng Míng* Organ Pattern

7. What is unsurfaced fever (身熱不揚 *shēn rè bù yáng*) and what is its pathomechanism?

Unsurfaced fever means that, although the patient feels hot, the skin temperature doesn't feel warm initially, but becomes warmer when contact is maintained with the skin. Another indication of unsurfaced fever is that, although the body temperature may increase, the patient may not feel hot. The fever gets worse in the afternoon, decreases a little after sweating, but then returns to the same degree as before sweating.

Unsurfaced fever is a common symptom unique to damp-warm disease (濕溫病 *shī wēn bìng*). It usually appears when pathogenic damp-warmth is hidden in the qi level or in the middle burner. Dampness prevails at this level. Dampness and heat mix and accumulate with each other. Heat accumulates inside the dampness, and the constraint of dampness causes heat to radiate outward to the surface where it becomes the "unsurfaced fever." Dampness is a yin pathogen; it tends to linger and stick. Hence, the fever is prolonged and stubborn, lingering for a long time. Unsurfaced fever is different from other febrile diseases, which present with an obvious fever and other indications such as red face, irritability and restlessness, thirst, and rapid pulse. Because of the yin characteristic of dampness, with unsurfaced fever there is no obvious signs of heat. The facial color is slightly yellow instead of red. There is no restlessness or irritability. However, potentially there is a sticky sensation in the mouth, little or no thirst, or drinking only small sips, and a soggy and moderate pulse. Other symptoms and signs include heavy-feeling headaches, stifling and oppressive sensations in the chest, heavy limbs and body, fatigue, and a greasy tongue coating.

Unsurfaced fever is also a tidal fever since it rises every afternoon. This phenomenon has two explanations. First, the dominant pathogen is dampness, which is yin in nature, and the afternoon pertains to yin (within yang), thus dampness is more likely to stagnate and accumulate in the afternoon and create more fever. Second, damp-warmth is caused by dampness invading the middle burner, which is associated with the *yáng míng* channel. *Yáng míng* channel qi peaks in the afternoon. Therefore, the fever will increase in the afternoon.

8. What is "Cock's Crow" diarrhea and what is its pathomechanism?

Diseases that appear at certain times of the day may be of internal (biological clock) or external origin (exopathogens). Some diseases, such as tidal fever, have regular times of onset. Everyday between 3 and 5 p.m., the body temperature will rise. Or, in the case of early morning diarrhea, the patient will regularly experience diarrhea between 3 and 5 a.m.

"Cock's crow" diarrhea is also called daybreak diarrhea (五更瀉 *wǔ gèng* xiè*) or early morning diarrhea. Before dawn, between 3 and 5 a.m., the patient starts feeling abdominal pain and an urgent need to defecate. The stool is loose or watery, with visible undigested food. Abdominal pain is relieved following the bowel movement. From the Chinese medicine point of view, "cock's crow" diarrhea is caused by Kidney yang deficiency.

Basic Questions, Chapter 4 (素問。金匱真言論) notes: "From dawn to midday is the yang of the day, and also the yang within yang. From midday to dusk is the yang of the day, and also the yin within yang. From dusk to midnight is the yin of the day, and also the yin within yin. From midnight to dawn is the yin of the day, and also the yang within yin. The physiological nature of man corresponds to this as well." Daytime is yang and nighttime is yin. From dusk to midnight is yin within yin. During this time, the yin qi gradually increases and the yang qi gradually decreases. From midnight to dawn is yang within yin; the yang qi starts to increase.

---

* Wǔ gèng (五更) refers to a traditional Chinese time of the day, from 3 to 5 a.m. "Cock's crow" obviously refers to the time of this diarrhea as being the same as when the rooster rises and begins to make his presence known.

For a normal person, the Kidney yang starts to build at midnight, peaking between 3 and 5 a.m. At this time, Kidney yang will promote, guide, rise, and increase the yang qi throughout the body.

If one has Kidney yang deficiency, there will be insufficient yang qi to motivate or warm, and so in the middle of the night, when yin is at its greatest, the yin and cold will concentrate and the qi will accumulate, and there is no diarrhea. However, in the early morning hours, when the external environment is at its coldest, since the Kidney yang is deficient, it is unable to lift the Spleen yang upward, and this descending causes abdominal pain and diarrhea. Since pathogenic coldness is expelled through defecation, abdominal pain will be relieved after the diarrhea passes. Once the day begins, yang qi is supported by the warmth of the external environment and there will be no more diarrhea until the next morning.

The patient with "cock's crow" diarrhea symptoms may also have accompanying symptoms related to Kidney yang deficiency, such as soreness of the back, aversion to cold, weak legs and knees, impotence, lassitude, profuse urination, edema of the legs, poor appetite, a pale tongue with teeth marks, and a deep and weak pulse.

9. What is the pathomechanism of diarrhea due to excessive heat in the *yáng míng* organ?

Yáng míng organ pattern is a group of pathological phenomena due to excess pathogenic heat invading the Stomach and Large Intestine. It severely injures the body fluids, causes the stools to dry out, and the clumps formed by pathogenic heat and dry stools obstruct any further flow within the Large Intestine.

The *yáng míng* organs (Stomach and Large Intestine) are yang organs which receive, digest, and transmit. They have an affinity for moisture and flow, and dislike dryness and stagnation. When pathogenic heat invades the Stomach and Large Intestine, the *yáng míng* qi will strongly oppose it, which gives rise to excessive pathogenic heat. This heat severely damages the body fluids and causes the stools to dry out. Clinically, we will see high fever, constipation with severe abdominal pain, thirst, profuse sweating, and a deep and forceful pulse.

In *Discussion of Cold-induced Disorders* (傷寒論), section 374 notes: "Diarrhea with delirium, treat by *xiǎo chéng qì tāng* [Minor Order the Qi Decoction]." This diarrhea is also called *yáng míng* organ diarrhea, or "heat accumulation with bypassed fluids" (熱結旁流 *rè jié páng liú*).

Clumps that are formed by pathogenic heat, along with dry stools obstructing the intestines, are the pathomechanism of this diarrhea. Heat clumps and dry stools obstruct the contents of the Large Intestine. Meanwhile, the patient drinks a lot of water due to excessive thirst, which produces water waste. The water waste then passes around the intestinal obstructions and is expelled outside the body as diarrhea. Since the water waste has to pass by the obstruction of dry stool and is consumed by pathogenic heat, it become viscous and turbid. This type of diarrhea is therefore foul-smelling, black-green, and watery. Other symptoms include abdominal distention, fullness and pain which is not relieved after the diarrhea passes, palpable masses in the lower abdomen, and dry mouth and thirst. The tongue is red with a dry, dark yellow or dry, black coating, and a forceful and slippery pulse.

10. What is the difference between diarrhea due to excess heat in the *yáng míng* organ and diarrhea due to damp-heat in the lower burner?

Diarrhea due to both damp-heat in the lower burner and *yáng míng* organ heat manifest with an acute onset, foul-smelling stools, abdominal pain, and a burning sensation in the anus. However, the etiology, pathogenesis, and treatment principles are different.

Diarrhea due to...		Excess Heat in *Yáng Míng* Organ	Damp Heat in Lower Burner
similarities		foul smelling, abdominal pain, burning sensation in the anus	
differences	urgency	not strong	very strong
	abdominal pain	severe, not relieved by passing stools	pain evident, but relieved after passing stools
	stools	watery, black green color	sticky, with blood or mucus
	abdomen	palpable masses in the lower abdomen	no masses found in lower abdomen
	other symptoms	high fever, delirium, coma	may have fever, remains alert
	treatment principle	purging	clear heat, expel dampness, stop diarrhea

Table 3.4.1 Differentiation between the Diarrhea of Excess Heat in the *Yáng Míng* Organ
and the Diarrhea of Damp-Heat in the Lower Burner

11. What is the difference between constipation due to excess heat invading the *yáng míng* organs, and constipation due to heat in the Large Intestine?

Both patterns are located in the Intestines. Both are due to pathogenic heat combining with dry stools to form clumps and obstruction, and both are patterns of excess. Clinically they both present with constipation, abdominal pain which is resistant to pressure, yellow urine, red tongue with yellow, dry coating, and a slippery, rapid, and forceful pulse.

However, constipation due to excess heat in the Large Intestine is an internal disorder. It is usually found in a person with a yang excess-type constitution who is eating too much spicy, hot, and greasy food. The other cause is heat that is transfered from the Lung to the Large Intestine. In this case, the onset is slow over the course of days to weeks. The symptoms last longer and the constipation is not very severe.

Constipation due to excess heat invading the *yáng míng* organs is caused by exopathogens (cold, heat, dryness, etc.) attacking and invading deeper, where they transform into excess heat. This is an external disorder. It usually presents with an acute onset, shorter duration, and more severe symptoms. Patients not only have constipation, abdominal pain, distention, and gastrointestinal symptoms, but also suffer from high fever, delirium, or even coma if excess heat disturbs the spirit.

Constipation due to...	Excess Heat in *Yáng Míng Fǔ*	Excess Heat in the Large Intestine
etiology	exterior pathogenic cold attacks, enters interior and transforms into heat, or exterior heat and dryness attack	yang excess constitution; or over-eating greasy, spicy, or hot food; or Lung heat transmits to the Large Intestine
location	Stomach, Large Intestine	Large Intestine
excess or deficiency	excess type illness	
patho-genesis — similar	pathogenic heat invades the Large Intestine, injures the body fluids and dries out the stool, then pathogenic heat combines with dry stools to form clumps that obstruct the intestines	
patho-genesis — different	exopathogenic factors generate excess heat	internal disorders generate heat
onset, duration, severity	acute onset, short duration, severe	slow onset, long duration, mild
symptoms — similar	constipation, abdominal pain that is resistant to pressure, red face, thirst, yellow urine, red tongue body with a dry yellow coating, slippery, rapid and forceful pulse	
symptoms — different	high fever that is worse in the afternoon, delirium or coma, manic behavior, foul smelling black green watery diarrhea	

Table 3.4.2 Differentiation of Constipation due to Excess Heat in the *Yáng Míng* organs versus the Large Intestine

12. How does one differentiate excess and deficiency type tinnitus?

Tinnitus refers to buzzing or ringing in the ear(s). It is a subjective symptom that only the patient will hear. It may sound like cicadas, or like ocean waves. It may be mild or severe and is more noticeable when there is no ambient sound in the room. In severe cases, it may affect the patient's ability to hear. Tinnitus can be differentiated into excess and deficiency types.

Excess-type tinnitus is usually caused by either an obstruction in the ear channel caused by endogenous pathogenic factors such as blood stasis, phlegm, or qi stagnation, or by an attack of exogenous factors. Clinically, we see sudden onset, a feeling of distention, and constant ringing in the ear. This ringing is low-pitched and loud. It may sound like wind, storms, ocean waves, cicadas, or crickets. It is not relieved by pressing the ears closed. There may also be accompanying symptoms such as ear pain, congestion, or a feeling of obstruction.

Deficiency-type tinnitus is mostly seen in elderly patients. There isn't enough qi, blood, or essence to nourish the ears. This is due to either a deficiency in the internal organs, especially the Kidney and Liver yin in elderly patients, or to chronic illness that has consumed the qi, blood, and essence. Clinically, we see chronic deafness or intermittent ringing that is high-pitched and not too loud. The ringing is aggravated by stress and exertion, and relieved by pressing the ears closed. It is often accompanied by hearing loss.

Tinnitus	Excess Type	Deficiency Type
onset, duration	acute, short term	chronic, long term
age	young	older
pitch and volume	low pitch, loud volume	high pitch, soft volume
sensation in ear	obstructed, congested, painful	none
relieved by pressing ears closed	no	yes
hearing loss	seldom	often

Table 3.4.3 Excess and Deficiency Type Tinnitus

13. How can heat in the Gallbladder cause a bitter taste in the mouth?

Although the Spleen is the only organ that directly opens to the mouth, other organs connect directly or indirectly with the mouth through the channels and collaterals. The Gallbladder channel of foot *shào yáng* originates at the outer canthus. From the retroauricular region it enters the ear, runs downward to ST-5 (*dà yíng*), and meets the Triple Burner channel of hand *shào yáng* in the infraorbital region. Another branch passes through ST-6 (*jiá chē*) where it directly connects to the mouth. Therefore, when there is pathogenic heat in the Gallbladder, the bile will steam upward to the mouth and cause a bitter taste. In the *Golden Mirror of the Medical Tradition* (醫宗金鑑), written in 1739, Wu Qian said: "Bitter taste in the mouth is caused by Gallbladder qi steaming upward."

14. What does it mean to say that "yang added on yin produces sweating"?

"Yang added on yin produces sweating" was originally stated in *Basic Questions*, Chapter 7 (素問。陰陽別論). "Added on" can also mean "more than" or "forced onto." This sentence provides Chinese medicine with a fundamental theory to explain the mechanism and pathomechanism of sweating. *Guidance for Medical Case Study* (臨證指南醫案) notes: "Yang added on yin produces sweating, from this we can see that yang heat added to yin fluids causes the yin to be pushed outside in the form of sweat." Dr. Wu Tang (1758–1836) observed: "The yang qi and yin essence combine and steam out, producing sweat. Sweat is a substance that needs yang qi as the power and yin essence as the material." Therefore, regardless of whether it is physiological or pathological, the balance of yin and yang explains the phenomenon of sweating.

Sweating is affected by the balance of yin and yang. Defensive qi governs, controls, and regulates the secretion of sweat. The physiological functions of sweat include regulating the body temperature, keeping body fluids and yang qi in balance, and expelling pathogens and metabolic wastes. When yin and yang are balanced internally, there is no visible sweat. When yang becomes excessive, sweat enables the venting of heat. If the temperature of the external environment is low, there is no sweating because the body's interstitial spaces are closed to retain the body's heat.

Under pathological circumstances, when the yang qi is more abundant than the yin, or the yang qi is insufficient leading to a deficiency in the ability of defensive qi to regulate the pores of the skin, abnormal sweating will result.

Sweat	Pathogenesis	Indications
spontaneous sweating	skin pores open, body surface loses protection	yang qi deficiency
scanty or no sweat	not enough power to steam body fluids, so none transform into sweat	yang qi deficiency
no sweat, dry skin	insufficient resources to supply sweat	deficiency of body fluids, blood, or essence
night sweats	deficiency heat pushes out body fluids at night	yin deficiency heat
profuse sweating	internal heat pushes out body fluids to enable body to vent out heat	interior excess heat
no sweating	interstitial space closes to protect body heat	exopathogenic cold attacks surface
sweating or spontaneous sweating	defensive and nutritive qi disharmony	exopathogenic wind attacks surface
sweating on half of the body only	channels and collaterals obstructed by pathogens, leads to abnormal qi movement and inability of body fluids to distribute evenly	channels and collaterals stagnated
sticky or yellow sweat	turbid dampness encumbers internally which generates heat and pushes out body fluids	accumulation of turbid damp
cold pearly sweating on head	a critical sign of the separation of yin and yang	yang collapse

Table 3.4.4 Pathological Sweating and its Indications

Understanding the theory of "yang added on yin produces sweating" can help one differentiate physiological and pathological sweating, as well as provide some insight into the mechanisms of sweating.

15. Why does yin deficiency cause sweating at night, but not during the day?

Sweating is both a physiological and pathological clinical phenomenon. Sweating is a form of body fluid. According to *The Divine Pivot–Chapter* 30 (靈樞。決氣), "When the interstitial spaces open, the body fluids come out to form sweat." Sweating is a body fluid which is evaporated and sent to the skin through the pores of the body by the yang qi. The yang qi is the power that pushes the body fluids out of the body as sweat. *Basic Questions*, Chapter 7 (素问。陰陽別論) notes: "Yang added on yin produces sweating."

In this statement, yang means defensive yang, and yin is nutritive yin primarily. During normal physiological activities, nutritive yin and defensive qi are balanced. They mutually control and generate each other. Defensive qi circulates on the exterior of the body during the day to protect the body from attacks of exterior pathogenic factors as well as to adjust the opening and closing of the pores so as to regulate sweating and body temperature.

At night, the defensive qi enters its yin phase and circulates interiorly with the nutritive yin. This allows one to fall asleep. When defensive qi enters the interior, the protection at the exterior is weaker. The interstitial spaces become slightly looser and the skin pores easily open. At this time, a very mild form of heat, like the heat of deficiency or the heat generated by stagnation, may be able to evaporate and push the body fluids outward, causing night sweats.

In the case of yin deficiency, the yin essence is so deficient that it cannot control the yang, which leads to a relative excess of yang qi. This creates endogenous deficiency heat. This pathogenic heat is so mild that it can hardly evaporate the body fluids during the day since the defensive qi is mobilized on the exterior performing its consolidating function. However, during sleep, defensive qi enters the interior. Defensive qi is yang in nature, and when it combines with deficiency heat it produces heat which is strong enough to evaporate and push out the body fluids, thus causing sweat during sleep.

16. How can a nutritive/defensive (營衛 yíng/wèi) disharmony cause sweating or spontaneous sweating?

Yíng means nutritive qi, and *wèi* is defensive qi. Both of them are rooted in the Kidney and are continually nourished by food and water essence. *The Divine Pivot*, Chapter 18 (靈樞。營衛生會) notes: "Humans are endowed with qi from grain. When grain enters the Stomach, the essence is transported to the Lung, and then distributed to the five *zàng* and six *fǔ* [organs]. The refined part of essence forms nutritive qi. The coarser part of essence forms defensive qi. Nutritive qi runs within the channels [and blood vessels]. The defensive qi runs outside the channels. Nutritive qi and defensive qi move unceasingly, and meet once after fifty cycles [one twenty-four hour circulation]."

Defensive qi pertains to yang. It circulates outside the channels, guarding the exterior. Its main function is to protect the body from an attack of exterior pathogenic factors. It warms, moistens, and nourishes skin and muscles. It also adjusts the opening and closing of the skin pores and regulates sweating and body temperature. Therefore, defensive qi tends to warm and strengthen.

Nutritive qi pertains to yin and circulates inside the blood vessels and channels. The main function of nutritive qi is to nourish the internal organs and the entire body, as well as to transform into blood. Therefore, nutritive qi nourishes and transforms.

Under normal circumstances, defensive qi and nutritive qi (*yíng qì*) mutually control and generate each other. They maintain a relative balance, which we call harmonized defensive qi and nutritive qi. Defensive qi strengthens and protects the exterior and keeps the nutritive qi inside. Nutritive qi circulates interiorly and nourishes the internal organs and defensive qi. Defensive qi and nutritive qi are coordinated, harmonized, and in balance.

Defensive qi and nutritive qi not only interact physiologically but also pathologically. No matter which undergoes a pathological change, it will undermine the relative harmonious balance and give rise to disharmony between the defensive qi and nutritive qi. When the defensive qi is weaker than the nutritive qi, it will be unable to keep the nutritive qi inside the body, giving rise to spontaneous sweating. When the defensive qi is stronger than the nutritive qi, there will be fever and sweating. This is because defensive qi, which pertains to yang, is constrained interiorly, and thus the heat steams the nutritive qi and it escapes from the surface of the skin in the form of sweat due to fever.

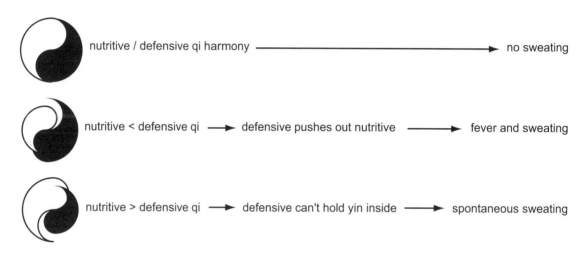

Chart 3.4.4 Sweating due to Nutritive/Defensive Qi Disharmonies

17. Why is there no significant thirst associated with pathogenic heat in the nutritive (*yíng*) or blood (*xuè*) level?

The *Systematic Differentiation of Warm Pathogen Diseases–Upper Burner Chapter* (溫病條辨。上焦篇) notes: "[In] *tài yīn* warm disease, [you will feel the] pulse is big at the distal position, [and see a] dry tongue with a deep purple color. [There] should be severe thirst, but there is not. It is pathogenic heat invading the nutritive level, treat it using *qīng yíng tang* (清營湯) [Clear the Nutritive Level Decoction], omitting *huáng lián* [Coptidis Rhizoma]. Thirst is one of the basic symptoms of warm disease, but it is confusing because the patient doesn't show severe thirst, but [still has] a dry, deep purple tongue and big pulse at both distal positions. This all indicates that it is a warm disease. [However] because pathogenic heat enters the nutritive level and steams the nutritive qi upward, there is no severe thirst."

There are five ways to explain this phenomenon:

  i. Pathogenic heat enters the nutritive and blood levels and steams the nutritive *yíng* upward to the mouth to nourish the oral cavity, so there is no strong sensation of thirst. Just like boiling water inside a pot, the hot steam will rise and moisturize the lid.

  ii. Pathogenic heat in the qi level presents with high fever, profuse sweating, and severe thirst. When pathogenic heat enters the nutritive and blood levels, the body temperature is not as high as when it is in the qi level, therefore the degree of damage to the body fluids is not as severe as when the heat is at the qi level. Additionally, because the heat has already left the qi level, the body fluids have had an opportunity to be replenished.

iii. When there is pathogenic heat in the qi level, it impairs the body fluids, which causes thirst that can be relieved by drinking. When pathogenic heat is in the nutritive and blood levels, it damages the nutritive yin, but drinking water doesn't actually repair this damage, so there is no strong desire to drink water.

iv. When pathogenic heat enters the nutritive and blood levels, the patient will often have mental symptoms or manic behavior. In either case, the patient will be less sensitive to sensations such as thirst and therefore may be unaware of any dryness or thirst.

v. Blood stagnation in the Stomach can be steamed by pathogenic heat, lifting the moisture to the mouth, which prevents thirst. When pathogenic heat enters the nutritive and blood levels, it damages the blood vessels and pushes blood outward. Externally, we can see ecchymosis, skin rashes, and various kinds of bleeding; internally, since the Stomach is a *fŭ* organ which contains a lot of qi and blood, it can readily bleed if attacked by pathogenic heat. Blood escapes from the vessels and accumulates inside the Stomach, creating blood stasis. Pathogenic heat steams the blood stasis and lifts that moisture up to the mouth; therefore, there is no strong sensation of thirst.

18. How does blood stagnation cause thirst without a desire to drink?

Thirst without the desire to drink indicates either slight damage to body fluids or a disorder in the body's distribution of fluids. In the case of blood stagnation, either of these two mechanisms can play a part.

Blood stagnation may produce pathogenic heat, which consumes body fluids and eventually causes thirst. However, the pathogenic heat generated by blood stagnation is usually not very strong. The body fluids may be slightly impaired, therefore the patient feels thirsty but has no desire to swallow. This symptom was described for the first time in *Essentials from the Golden Cabinet* (金匱要略): "Patient feels stifling sensation in the chest, [has] withered lips [and a] green purple tongue, thirst which [is the] desire to drink water, but [the patient] doesn't want [to] swallow down [any fluids], there are no chills or fever ... this indicates blood stagnation." It goes on to say: "If there is mild heat, then there is desire to drink water, but no desire to swallow; if there is severe heat, then the mouth is dry, and [there is] desire to drink water."

Blood stagnation can also impair the distribution of body fluids. Qi is the motive power underlying the distribution of body fluids, and the movement of qi is readily impaired by the obstruction of a pathogenic factor. Internal blood stasis obstruction can lead a disorder of qi movement in which the body fluids are not distributed to the tongue and mouth, resulting in thirst. However, in this situation, the body fluids are not actually impaired, therefore the patient feels thirst and desires to drink water, but doesn't want to swallow it. This mechanism was described in *Discussion of Blood Patterns–Blood Stasis* (血證論。瘀血): "When blood [is] stagnated inside, there is thirst. The reason is that qi and blood are not separate. When there is blood stagnation, there will be a qi circulation disorder, [and so the qi cannot] lead the body fluids upward to nourish the mouth. The result is thirst. It is also called 'blood thirst'. When blood stasis is removed, there is no thirst."

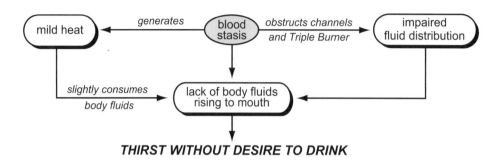

Chart 3.4.5 Thirst without Desire to Drink due to Blood Stasis

19. What are the three theories that explain sleep in Chinese Medicine?

Traditional Chinese medicine theory describes three mechanisms for sleep. These are the yin/yang theory, defensive qi movement theory, and the spirit governing theory.

(1) *Yin/yang theory*: According to this theory, the physiological activities of sleep and waking are produced by the cycles of yin and yang in the human body (growth and decline, exit and enter, etc.) *Basic Questions*, Chapter 5 (素問。陰陽應象大論) notes: "The yin and yang are the law of heaven and earth, the guiding principle of everything, the parents of variations, the root of life and death, and the locus of power in the universe." Yin and yang form a rule of nature. Chinese medicine places sleep and waking under the theory of yin and yang.

Changes in yin and yang have a daily rhythm in the natural world that is reflected in the cycles of the human body. *Basic Questions*, Chapter 4 (素問。金匱真言論) notes: "From dawn to midday is the yang of the day, and also yang within yang. From midday to dusk is the yang of the day, and also yin within yang. From dusk to midnight is the yin of a day, and also yin within yin. From midnight to dawn is the yin of a day, and also the yang within yin. Human nature corresponds to this as well."

Because yin and yang increase and decrease, each day has a daily rhythm. Humanity and nature correspond to each other, therefore the yang qi of the human body also has a daily rhythm that increases and decreases, enters and exits. During the daytime, the human body's yang qi travels to the exterior, one awakens and starts activities. At noon, the human body's yang qi is at its most abundant. At dusk, the yang qi gradually declines and disappears. At night, the yang qi hides inside, and one sleeps. Sleep results from yang entering yin. Waking arrives when yang exits yin. *The Divine Pivot*, Chapter 28 (靈樞。口問) notes: "When the yang decreases to its end and yin is most abundant, one closes the eyes and falls asleep; when yin decreases to its end and yang is most abundant, one awakens."

(2) *Defensive qi movement theory*: This theory is a further development of the yin/yang theory. In defensive qi movement theory, the yang qi that increases during the day and hides at night is referring to the defensive qi. According to defensive qi movement theory, when the defensive qi is circulat-

ing in the yang channels during the day, one is awake. When the defensive qi retreats to circulate through the yin channels and five *zàng* at night, one falls asleep.

Defensive qi originates from the food and water essence, circulates just inside the surface of the body, and is part of the yang qi. *The Divine Pivot*, Chapter 18 (靈樞。營衛生會) notes: "Humans are endowed with qi from grain. When grain enters the Stomach, the [essence] is transported to the Lung. From there it is distributed to the five *zàng* and six *fǔ*. The refined part of essence forms nutritive qi. The coarser part of essence forms defensive qi. The nutritive qi runs inside the vessels. The defensive qi runs outside the vessels. Both move unceasingly and meet once after fifty cycles. The circulation of the nutritive qi and defensive qi through the yin and yang channels is ceaseless, in a loop."

During a twenty-four hour cycle, the defensive qi circulates through the yang channels twenty-five times during the day, and makes twenty-five cycles through the yin channels and internal organs during the night.

In the morning, defensive qi exits the interior from the inner canthus. It circulates through the foot *tài yáng* channel, to the hand *tài yáng*, foot *shào yáng*, hand *shào yáng*, foot *yáng míng*, and the hand *yáng míng* channel. From the hand *yáng míng* it enters the center of the palms, and from the foot *yáng míng* it enters the center of the soles. There it enters internally and exits again from the inner canthus, thus completing one full yang channel cycle.

At night, the defensive qi circulates through the yin channels and internal organs. *The Divine Pivot*, Chapter 76 (靈樞。衛氣行) notes: "After the defensive qi completes its course of the yang portions during the daytime, it [the defensive qi] will undertake the yin portion at nighttime. When it enters the yin, it starts in the foot *shào yīn* channel, from which it then pours into the Kidney organ. From the Kidney it pours into the Heart, from the Heart it pours into the Lung, from the Lung it pours into the Liver, from the Liver it pours into the Spleen, from the Spleen it pours back into the Kidney to complete one cycle." Therefore, the internal cycle of defensive qi inside the organs follows the five phase controlling cycle of Kidney, Heart, Lung, Liver, and Spleen.

During the daytime, defensive qi moves in abundance to the surface where it warms and protects the entire body. While this occurs, one is awake and engaged in activity. At night, defensive qi circulation follows the yin channels and internal organs, which allows one to fall asleep and rest. Defensive qi in the *yīn qiāo* and *yáng qiāo* vessels controls the opening and closing of the eyes. As a result of the daily movements—internal and external—of defensive qi, the body's physiological activities of waking and sleeping are regulated.

DAYTIME CIRCULATION
(twenty-five cycles per daylight period)

UB 1
(*jīng míng*)

↓

head

|

outside of
yang channels

foot *yáng míng* channel   **hand** *yáng míng* channel

↓   ↓

soles   palms

NIGHTTIME CIRCULATION
(twenty-five cycles per nighttime period)

Kidney ——→ Heart ——→ Lung ——→ Liver ——→ Spleen
within yin channels and internal organs

Chart 3.4.6 Defensive Qi Circulation

(3) *Spirit governing theory*: The spirit governing theory teaches that sleep and waking are controlled by activity of the spirit. Zhang Jing-Yue (張景岳) wrote: "Sleeping is based on yin, governed by the spirit. When the spirit is calm, there is sleep. When the spirit is restless, there is no sleep."

Spirit in the human body suggests the external manifestation of vital activity. It also refers to one's spirit, consciousness, and cognitive activity. *The Divine Pivot*, Chapter 8 (靈樞。本神) notes: "The original substance which enables the evolution of the human body is called the essence of life; when the yin essence and the yang essence combine, it produces the activity of life which is called the spirit." Spirit is born along with the congenital essence, gestated by the parents. It then divides into the spirit (神 *shén*), ethereal soul (魂 *hún*), corporeal soul (魄 *pò*), thought/intention (意 *yì*), and will power (志 *zhì*). Each of these five spirits are stored in different organs, but are still governed by the Heart. *The Divine Pivot*, Chapter 71 (靈樞。邪客) notes: "The Heart is the king that dominates the five *zàng* and six *fǔ*; it is the place where the spirit is stored." The Heart governs the spirit, controls and regulates the five *zàng* and six *fǔ* organs, and takes charge of spiritual, mental, and cognitive activities.

The spirit plays an important role in the human body. When the spirit is sufficient, the body is strong. When the spirit fades, the body is weak. The activity of the spirit has a certain regularity just like yin/yang and defensive qi. During the day, the spirit is transported to the surface and one is awake. At night, the [five] spirits retreat to the interior and are stored in the five *zàng* and one can sleep. *Discussion of Blood Patterns* (血證論) notes: "[During] sleep, the [five] spirits return to their homes. Rest means the spirit has returned to its root." It goes on to say: "The Liver stores the ethereal soul. When one is awake, the ethereal soul swims to the eyes. When one is asleep, the ethereal soul returns to the Liver." If the five spirits are peaceful and calm and are able to remain inside the organs, one can easily fall asleep. If the five spirits cannot settle within their organs, but float upward, then one may suffer from insomnia, dream-disturbed sleep, somnambulism (sleepwalking), or somniloquence (sleep talking).

The three sleep theories of TCM are interdependent and together comprise the Chinese medicine system of sleep theory. The yin/yang theory of sleep is the general guiding principle. Defensive qi movement theory is a further development of yin/yang theory, and spirit governing theory views sleep as a function of the vital activity of the spirit in the body.

20. What is the relationship between heavenly dew and Kidney essence?

Basic Questions, Chapter 1 (素問。上古天真論) notes: "For a female, the Kidney qi prevails, the teeth change, and the hair grows when seven years old. When she is fourteen years old, the heavenly dew (*tiān guǐ*) appears. The conception vessel opens, the penetrating vessel becomes exuberant, and menstruation comes regularly so that she can become pregnant and bear a child. At the age of forty-nine, the conception vessel becomes debilitated, and the qi and blood of the penetrating vessel decline and become scanty. The heavenly dew is exhausted, and the menstrual tunnel becomes obstructed. Her physique becomes old and feeble, and she can conceive no more."

Heavenly dew is an invisible liquid material that helps in the development of the human body, sexual functions, and in women, the ability to produce offspring. It is a kind of yin essence, one part of congenital essence that comes from our parents at conception. It is stored inside the Kidney after birth. It is nourished and replenished by the post-natal essence and is stimulated by the Kidney qi to develop and mature. It increases and decreases with Kidney qi.

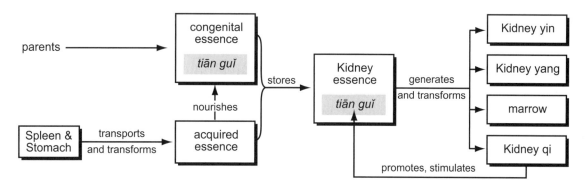

Chart 3.4.7 Relationship between Heavenly Dew (*tiān guǐ*) and Kidney Essence

In the female, heavenly dew is responsible for inducing menarche and other reproductive functions. It assists in stimulating the growth of secondary sexual characteristics such as breast development, pubic hair, armpit hair, and subcutaneous fat deposits in the chest, shoulders, and buttocks. In the male, it is responsible for maturity and sperm production.

The heavenly dew's cycle in the female lasts approximately forty-nine years. From the embryonic stage to seven years old is the early stage when it is almost dormant. Beginning at seven years old, it becomes more active and increases until its peak of activity at the age of twenty-one. This peaking stage lasts fourteen years. Starting at the age of thirty-five, the activity and functions of the heavenly dew begin to gradually decrease until age forty-nine, when it is exhausted. For the male, the heavenly dew cycle lasts approximately sixty-four years and moves in stages of eight years.

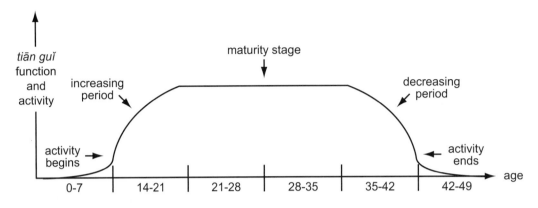

Chart 3.4.8 Female Heavenly Dew's Activity Cycle

21. Why do cramps generally occur only around the time of menstruation?

Dysmenorrhea means cramps or painful menstruation. It describes menstrual periods that are accompanied by either sharp intermittent pain, or dull aching pain, usually in the pelvis or lower abdomen.

The menstrual cycle follows an increase and decrease of yin and yang, storage and expulsion of qi and blood, and the metabolic activities of the female reproductive system. One cycle can be divided into four phases: the menstrual phase, post-menstrual phase, between menstrual phase, and the pre-menstrual phase. The condition and status of the yin and yang, and qi and blood, change during each of the four quarters of the menstrual cycle.

(1) Menstrual phase (days 1–4): The sea of blood *(chōng mài)* is full and yang qi is abundant. The yang qi pushes the uterus open to expel the blood. At this time the qi and blood in the Penetrating Vessel *(chōng mài)* and Conception Vessel *(rèn mài)* decrease dramatically, along with the bleeding.

(2) Post-menstrual phase (days 5–13): The uterus and *chōng mài/rèn mài* are empty. The uterus is closed and the Penetrating Vessel *(chōng mài)* and Conception Vessel *(rèn mài)* start to store the blood. Yin-blood gradually increases.

(3) Between menstrual phase (days 14–15): The yin increases to its maximum during this quarter of the monthly cycle. When yin is excessive, yang begins to generate. Under the power of the Kidney yang, the yin starts to transform into yang, yin-essence transforms to yang qi, and impregnation is possible.

(4) Pre-menstrual phase (days 16–28): The yang qi continues to gradually increase to its maximum. The yin-essence and yang qi have filled the Penetrating Vessel *(chōng mài)*, Conception Vessel *(rèn mài)*, and uterus.

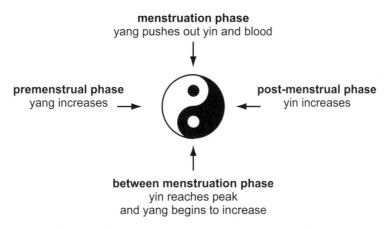

Chart 3.4.9 Yin and Yang of the Menstrual Cycle

When menstruation is not taking place, the qi and blood circulate smoothly and are balanced. Because of this, pathogens do not readily cause stagnation or deficiency of qi and blood. However, around menstruation, the quantity of qi and blood changes very rapidly, and are therefore readily affected by pathogenic factors. These factors can give rise to disorders in the movement of qi and blood, or cause a lack of nourishment in the uterus, Penetrating Vessel *(chōng mài)*, and Conception Vessel *(rèn mài)*. Any stagnation or lack of nourishment will cause pain.

22. How can blood stagnation cause menstrual disorders? What is the pathogenesis?

Blood stasis refers to a state of retarded blood circulation, the unsmooth flow of blood, or the congealing of blood. There are two causes for the formation of blood stagnation: circulatory problems and bleeding. Disorders of the blood circulation can be caused by deficiency of qi, qi stagnation, cold in the blood, or heat in the blood. Bleeding can be caused by blood level heat, local trauma, and qi deficiency.

These two types of blood stagnation can cause various kinds of abnormal menstruation, mostly related to the quantity and duration of menstrual bleeding. Blood stagnation can also give rise to abdominal cramps that are resistant to pressure, or pain that subsides after the passing of clots, a purple tongue with spots, and a choppy pulse.

Abnormal Period	Symptoms	Pathogenesis
profuse bleeding	profuse bleeding (heavy period), the color is dark purple, with clots	blood stasis obstructs the *chōng mài* and *rèn mài*, newly generated blood has no place to go, and thus leaks out
long period	periods that extend more than seven days, scanty flow, dark color, clots	
bleeding between periods	scanty and dark bleeding between periods	
scanty flow	scanty bleeding with dark purple color, many clots	*chōng mài* and *rèn mài* do not fill with blood due to blood stasis obstructing the channels
dysmenorrhea	abdominal pain and cramps before menstruation, relieved after period	*chōng mài* and *rèn mài* do not fill and lose nourishment due to blood stasis obstructing the channels
amenorrhea	menstruation suddenly stops, depression, lower abdominal pain and distention that is resistant to pressure	blood stasis obstructs the *chōng mài* and *rèn mài*, blood cannot flow outward

Table 3.4.5 Abnormal Menstruation caused by Blood Stagnation

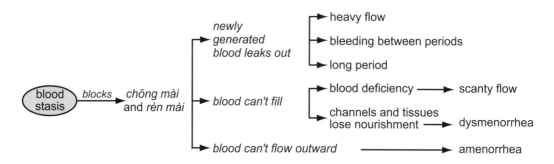

Chart 3.4.10 Abnormal Menstruation due to Blood Stagnation

Chapter Four

PALPATION 切診

■ CONTENTS

PALPATION 切診

Through thousands of years of clinical practice, TCM practitioners have developed a unique diagnostic technique through touching and palpation of certain parts of the body to gather information about the qi and blood, the state of yin and yang, and to assess the condition of the internal organs.

Definition: Palpation technique means that the practitioner uses his hands to touch, feel, press, and palpate certain areas of the patient's body to collect information to help differentiate the pattern. This method includes:

PULSE EXAMINATION: to feel the patient's arterial pulse with the practitioner's fingers to ascertain the condition of the disease by assessing the pulse qualities.

PALPATION: to infer the location, thermal nature, and state of an illness by touching, feeling, pushing, and pressing certain parts of the patient's body to feel for local abnormal changes.

Section 1

Pulse Examination

◼ One: Introduction

Pulse diagnosis is a highly subjective diagnostic procedure. The practitioner must understand the relationship of the qi, blood, and *zàng fǔ* organs to the formation of the pulse. Attention should be paid to pulse-taking methods in order to gather the most accurate information from the patient.

I. DEFINITION

Pulse examination is a special diagnostic method. The practitioner uses his fingers to feel the patient's arterial pulse. Based on the pulse quality, the practitioner can assess the different physiological and pathological states of the patient.

II. RELATIONSHIP AMONG THE PULSE QUALITY, QI, AND BLOOD

The pulse arises mainly from the flow of qi and blood in the vessels. Normal flow and sufficiency of the qi and blood in the vessels creates a normal pulse quality. When the flow of qi and blood is abnormal, or there is insufficient qi and blood in the vessels, a morbid pulse will be formed.

Qi and blood play different roles in the generation of the pulse. Qi is associated with yang and governs movement, while blood is associated with yin and provides the substance that fills the vessels. Blood depends on qi for its movement.

When qi is insufficient and fails to move the blood, the pulse will be forceless or choppy because the blood flow is not smooth. When blood is deficient and fails to fill the vessels, the pulse will be thin or hollow.

Overall, qi and blood are the basic components of the pulse, and qi plays a major role in the pulse quality.

III. RELATIONSHIP BETWEEN THE *Zàng Fǔ* ORGANS AND THE PULSE QUALITY

The substance of the pulse is blood, and the power of the pulse is qi. The Heart, which governs the blood and the vessels, pumps qi and blood into all parts of the body through the vessels. The qi and blood circulate continuously. They enter the *zàng fǔ* organs internally and reach the limbs and skin externally. Qi and blood circulation also depend on other organs which must coordinate with the Heart. The Lung gathers the channels and blood vessels, and governs the qi; hence, blood circulation depends on the distributive function of the Lung.

Blood and qi generation depends on the transportive and transformative functions of the Spleen and Stomach. Spleen qi also controls the blood that circulates inside the vessels. The Liver stores blood and regulates the quantity of blood. It also ensures the smooth flow of qi. The Kidney stores the essence, which is transformed into original qi, and provides the foundation for all the yin and yang energies of the body. Essence can also be transformed into blood. Thus, the pulse quality is a reflection of the condition of the *zàng fǔ* organs.

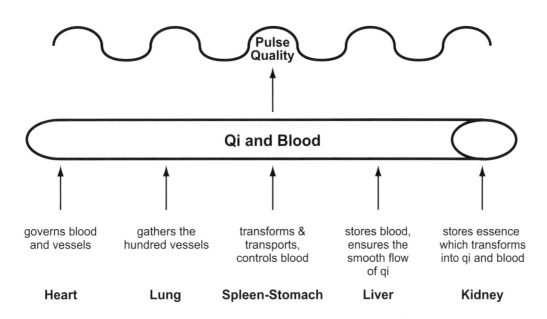

Chart 4.1.1 Relationship between *Zàng Fǔ* Organs and Pulse Quality

IV. CLINICAL SIGNIFICANCE OF PULSE EXAMINATION

Pulse diagnosis is a major tool to help the practitioner gain understanding into the pattern of disharmony and its pathomechanisms.

The pulse quality can help one to:
- differentiate the thermal nature of a disease
- assess the pathogenesis of a disease
- reach a prognosis for the disease

V. WHERE TO TAKE THE PULSE

(1) Systemic Pulse-Taking

Taking the pulse at different places around the body was discussed in *The Yellow Emperor's Inner Classic* (黃帝內經). This technique originally required one to check pulses at three separate locations or "portions" on the body. Each of these locations is associated with three "regions." For this reason, the technique is also called "three portions nine regions" pulse diagnosis (三部九候 *sān bù jiǔ hòu*).

Three Portions	Nine Regions	Channel Diagnosed	Point(s) Used Diagnostically	Relevant Location or Structure
Upper	Heaven	foot *shào yáng*	*tài yáng xué*	front and lateral head
	Earth	foot *yáng míng*	Stomach 3	mouth and teeth
	Human	hand *shào yáng*	Triple Burner 21	ears and eyes
Middle	Heaven	hand *tài yīn*	Lung 8 or Lung 9	Lungs
	Earth	hand *yáng míng*	Large Intestine 4	chest
	Human	hand *shào yīn*	Heart 7	Heart
Lower	Heaven	foot *jué yīn*	Liver 3 or Liver 10	Liver
	Earth	foot *shào yīn*	Kidney 3	Kidney
	Human	foot *tài yīn* or foot *yáng míng*	Spleen 11 or Stomach 42	Spleen Stomach

Table 4.1.1 Three Portions and Nine Regions Pulse Diagnosis

(2) Three-Part Method

This technique was developed by Zhang Zhong-Jing (張仲景) and is a simplified version of the three portion nine region technique. The pulse is assessed at three locations:

- carotid artery pulse at ST-9 (*rén yíng*): Stomach qi
- radial artery pulse (*cùn kǒu*): 12 channels
- dorsal artery of foot pulse at ST-42 (*chōng yáng*): Stomach qi

(3) Radial Artery (寸口 *cùn kǒu*) Pulse Taking

First mentioned in *Basic Questions* (素問), radial artery pulse diagnosis was later organized and further developed in the *Pulse Classic* (脈經) by Wang Shu-He. Because of the accessibility of the radial artery and its clinical accuracy, this method is the most prevalent method used in the modern era.

— A. Definition of cùn kǒu

The *cùn kǒu* pulse refers to the pulse on the radial artery proximal to the crease of the wrist. The distnace from wrist crease to the styloid process of the radius is one *cùn*. *Kǒu* means gate, gap, or pass and in this case suggests the area or gap on the pulse that we palpate.

— B. The Basic Theory of Radial Artery (cùn kǒu) Pulse-Taking

Cùn kǒu is also called *mài* (vessel, channel) *kǒu* (gate, pass), or *qì kǒu*. It is located at the medial aspect of the forearm on the radial artery. The pulse at the radial artery reflects the functional status of the *zàng fǔ* organs. There are two reasons for this:

First, the radial artery is the artery through which the hand *tài yín* channel of the Lung passes. It is the area where qi and blood accumulates. The circulation of qi and blood in all five *zàng* and six *fǔ* organs starts and ends at the Lung. Thus, their functional states are manifest in the Lung. *Classic of Difficulties-First question* (難經。一難) notes: "There are arteries on all twelve channels, why only use the radial artery to determine the condition of the five *zàng* and six *fǔ*? Because the radial artery is the location where all the channels meet."

Second, the Lung channel starts in the middle burner, where the Spleen and Stomach are located. The Spleen and Stomach are the source of acquired qi. They are the source of the production of qi and blood. The Lung channel communicates with the Spleen and Stomach in the middle burner, thus the condition of the qi and blood in all the *zàng fǔ* organs is reflected at the radial artery. As noted in *Basic Questions*, Chapter 11 (素問。五臟別論): "How is it that the radial artery can reflect the five *zàng*'s condition? Because the Stomach is the sea of food and water, and the source of the six *fǔ*. The five tastes enter the mouth and are stored in the Stomach to nourish the five *zàng*. The radial artery also pertains to *tài yīn*, which begins in the middle burner, thus the condition of the *zàng fǔ* [organs] can be shown on the radial artery."

— C. Location and Division of the Cùn Kǒu Pulse on the Radial Artery

Distal (寸 *cùn*): This position is located adjacent and distal to the middle *(guān)* position. It is 6 *fēn* long. (*Fēn* is an ancient unit of measurement equal to one-tenth of a *cùn*.)

Middle (關 *guān*): This position is located medial to the styloid process of the radius at the wrist, and is 6 *fēn* long. *Guān* is the word used to describe a military fort that overlooks a mountain pass. Naming this position *guān* is a reference to the nearby mountain top (the styloid process) that overlooks the valley containing the radial artery.

Proximal (尺 *chǐ*): This position is located adjacent and proximal to the middle position and is 7 *fēn* long.

— D. The Division of Radial Artery Pulse Positions and their Corresponding Zàng Fǔ Organs

There are many opinions about the correspondences between the pulse positions and the internal organs and structures. The table below reflects some of the most common paradigms taught in modern China.

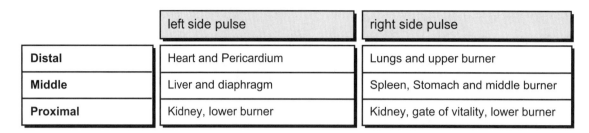

	left side pulse	right side pulse
Distal	Heart and Pericardium	Lungs and upper burner
Middle	Liver and diaphragm	Spleen, Stomach and middle burner
Proximal	Kidney, lower burner	Kidney, gate of vitality, lower burner

Table 4.1.2 Radial Artery Positions and their Corresponding *Zàng Fǔ* Organs

— E. Three Depths

Superficial depth: when the skin is just lightly touched, the pulse is felt at the skin level.

Middle depth: when a moderate amount of pressure is applied, the pulse is felt in the muscle level.

Deep depth: when a heavy pressure is applied, the pulse is felt at the tendon and bone level.

VI. The Method of Pulse Examination

(1) Time

Pulse-taking should be performed at a time when the patient and practitioner are both relaxed and calm, such as in the morning.

(2) Posture

The posture and position of the patient can affect the qi and blood circulation and cause changes in the pulse. The correct posture of the patient during pulse-taking should be sitting straight or lying on his back, with his arms naturally extended at the same elevation as the heart, wrist extended, palm facing upward, fingers slightly bent, and with a soft cushion placed beneath the wrist.

(3) Finger Placement

— A. Finger positions

- *middle*: place the third finger medial to the styloid process
- *distal*: place the index finger distal and adjacent to the middle finger
- *proximal*: place the ring finger proximal and adjacent to the middle finger

— B. Finger location

The distances between fingers are determined according to the patient's height. They should be evenly spaced. The appropriate distance can be determined by placing the finger on the middle position medial to the styloid process, with the distal and proximal positions placed adjacent to the middle. The fingers should be put at a greater distance in the case of an especially tall or long-armed patient.

— *C. Adjusting the fingers*

The fingers should all be on the same line, directly atop the radial artery. The very tip of the fingers should come into contact with the pulse for greatest sensitivity.

(4) Strength of pressure

—*A. Touching* (舉 *jǔ*): palpating with slight pressure. The finger lightly rests on the skin.

—*B. Pressing* (按 *àn*): palpating with heavy pressure. The finger presses down to the bones and tendons.

—*C. Seeking* (尋 *xún*): palpating with moderate pressure. The finger presses into the muscle area, sometimes with light pressure and sometimes with heavier pressure, moving around and searching for the pulse.

(5) Normal breath

—*A. One breath* = one inhalation + one exhalation

—*B. Calm breath:* during pulse-taking, the practitioner should keep his own breathing calm, allowing the breath to be regular and natural. The practitioner can then use his own breath to assess the patient's pulse rate.

(6) Duration

The time spent taking the pulse should not be less than 50 breaths or 2–3 minutes.

■ Two: Normal Pulse (Physiological Pulse)

The normal pulse can be found in a person who has no pathology, slight pathology; or in the very early stages of a pathological process where the pathology has not yet affected the pulse.

I. Characteristics of a Normal Pulse

The normal pulse has an even and gentle pulsation in all three positions, and beats 4–5 times in one breath (of the practitioner). When timed to a clock, the rate will be approximately 60 to 90 beats per minute. The normal pulse is neither deep nor superficial, neither wide nor thin, neither forceless nor forceful, and has equal intervals with a regular rhythm. The features of a healthy pulse can be summarized in three aspects:

(1) The Normal Pulse is full of Stomach Qi (胃氣 *wèi qì*)

DEFINITION OF STOMACH QI: Stomach qi is the physiological functions of the Stomach and Spleen in the middle burner, including the functions of the digestive system. It is the motive force for the generation of nutritive substances in the body, and forms the basis of the pulse.

FORMATION OF THE PULSE BY THE STOMACH QI: Stomach qi forms the pulse by creating the food (*gǔ*) qi. The Stomach and Spleen are the root of acquired qi in the body. Their function is transportation and transformation. Transformation is the changing of food into essential substances such as the qi and blood inherent within the pulse.

CHARACTERIZATIONS OF THE PULSE, WHEN THE STOMACH QI IS FULL: the pulse beats are calm, gentle, steady, and have a regular rhythm with moderate strength. It is neither wide nor thin, long nor short, superficial nor deep, slippery nor choppy.

CLINICAL SIGNIFICANCE: Stomach qi is an important means by which one can determine the prognosis of a disease and whether the pathogen can be eliminated.

(2) The Normal Pulse is full of Spirit (神 *shén*)

DEFINITION OF SPIRIT: Spirit is the vitality and phenomenon of life. Spirit in the pulse refers to a complex reflection of normal functions of the *zàng fǔ* organs and sufficient qi and blood.

FORMATION OF THE PULSE SPIRIT: Spirit arrives with the normal function of a Heart that has a sufficient amount of qi and blood.

CHARACTERIZATIONS OF A PULSE THAT HAS FULL SPIRIT: Generally speaking, a pulse with strength that reflects the smooth flow of qi and blood is regarded as a pulse with spirit. This pulse beats with a moderate strength and even rhythm in a soft vessel.

CLINICAL SIGNIFICANCE: Because spirit is based on the essence, qi, and blood, the status of the essence, qi, and blood can be detected from the spirit of the pulse. The spirit of the pulse is thus related to the prognosis of the disease.

(3) The Normal Pulse is Rooted (根 *gēn*)

DEFINITION OF ROOT: Root means the source of life.

FORMATION OF THE PULSE ROOT: The Kidney qi forms the root of the pulse. This is because the Kidney is the congenital root of human life.

CHARACTERISTICS OF A PULSE THAT HAS ROOT: This has two meanings:

- The pulse can be felt at the deepest depth at all three positions, the distal, middle, and proximal.
- The pulse that can be felt at the proximal position (at any depth) is also considered to be rooted.

CLINICAL SIGNIFICANCE: Detecting whether the pulse has root can help one determine the prognosis of a disease.

	Stomach Qi	Spirit	Root
Pulse Image	pulse is calm, gentle and has a regular rhythm with moderate strength	pulse has moderate strength and a unified rhythm in a soft vessel	pulse can be felt at the deep level of all three positions or at least in the proximal position
Key Points	smooth pulse wave, moderate strength		
Related Organs	Stomach	Heart	Kidney
Relationship	Stomach qi, spirit, and root are three aspects of the pulse that cannot be separated. If the pulse has Stomach qi, it must also have spirit and root.		

Table 4.1.3 Summary of Stomach qi, Spirit, and Root of the Normal Pulse

II. Components of a Normal Pulse and the Mechanism of Pulse Formation

In TCM pulse diagnosis, the width, depth, strength, length, rate, rhythm, tension, and shape of the pulse are the basic components of a normal pulse.

(1) Width (Blood Vessel's Diameter)

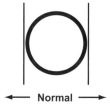

The width of a pulse is the diameter of the vessel. The diameter of the blood vessel is dependent on the qi and blood, which are a reflection of the condition of the *zàng fǔ* organs. When the internal organs are healthy, the blood vessel's diameter is in a normal state. The normal pulse width should be moderate, neither too thin nor too wide.

(2) Depth

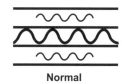

Depth refers to the location where the pulsation is strongest. The normal pulse depth should be mainly felt in the middle depth. This is a manifestation of sufficient Stomach qi and shows that the qi and blood of the body can flow freely from the interior to the exterior as well as to the *zàng fǔ* organs.

(3) Strength

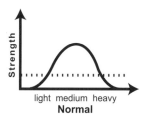

Strength is the beating force beneath the finger. The normal pulse should beat with a moderate strength. It should feel gentle and soft, neither too forceful nor too forceless. The strength of the pulse reflects the condition of the qi and blood.

(4) Length

The length of the pulse is a measure of its length in relation to the three positions (distal, middle, proximal). The normal pulse should be felt at the distal, middle, and proximal positions, and should be neither too long nor too short. Pulse length is determined by the condition of the qi and blood. Since it is qi that makes blood move, qi plays the major role in the length of the pulse.

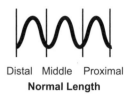

Distal Middle Proximal
Normal Length

(5) Rate

The rate of the pulse is the number of beats per minute. The normal pulse rate should be 4–5 beats per respiratory cycle (one breath) of the practitioner, or 60–90 beats per minute (bpm). Pulse rate is determined by a number of factors, of which the state of the yang plays a leading role because it governs the movement of the blood via the Lung and Heart.

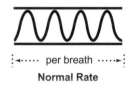

····· per breath ·····
Normal Rate

(6) Rhythm

The rhythm is the pattern of the pulse beats. A normal pulse should beat with a regular rhythm. The rhythm of the pulse is mainly a manifestation of the function of the Heart qi, since the Heart qi commands the blood to move through the vessels. The functions of the other organs play a lesser role in the rhythm of the pulse.

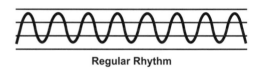

Regular Rhythm

(7) Tension

This refers to the tension of the blood vessel (vasotonia). The normal pulse should be neither too taut nor too slack. The tension of the blood vessel is predominantly a manifestation of the condition of the qi and blood as well as the condition of the blood vessels.

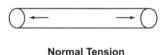

Normal Tension

(8) Shape

Shape refers to the wave form or contour of the pulse. The shape of the normal pulse refers to the rising and falling of the vessel as the blood flows through it. A pulse beat is composed of two periods: ascending and descending. In the normal pulse, the rising and falling of the pulse are about the same. The condition of the blood vessels, qi, and blood determine the pulse shape.

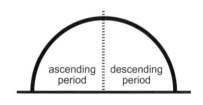

ascending period   descending period

III. Normal Pulse Variations

Physiological variations corresponding with the condition of the external and internal environments will alter the normal pulse qualities, but still within the range of what can be considered normal.

(1) The seasons

Seasonal changes influence the pulse quality.

Season	Spring	Summer	Autumn	Winter
Pulse	Wiry	Flooding	Floating	Deep

Table 4.1.4 The Seasons and Pulse Qualities

(2) Geography and environment

In moist and warm regions, the pulse tends to be soggy and slightly rapid. In dry and cold regions, the pulse tends to be deep and forceful.

(3) Gender

The female pulse may be weaker, thinner, and slightly more rapid than the male pulse.

(4) Age

The qi and blood in the elderly can be weak and deficient, which can make the pulse feel empty and forceless. Conversely, among the young and strong, the qi and blood will be full and exuberant, and the pulse accordingly will arrive full with force.

Age also affects the rate of the pulse.

Age	Beats per Minute	Beats per Breath
Infants	120-140	7
Children	90-110	5-6
Adults	60-90	4-5

Table 4.1.5 Age and the Normal Pulse Rate

(5) Constitution

Each body is unique. Tall, short, fat, and thin bodies may be strong or weak. The relationship between the physiological and pathological pulse is a little different in each individual.

There are also some common physiological pulses that are mistaken for being pathological. The following four constitutional pulses do not indicate pathology:

Six yin pulses (六陰脈 *liù yīn mài*): All six pulse positions are evenly deep and thready, but there is no illness.

Six yang pulses (六陽脈 *lìu yáng mài*): All six pulse positions are evenly forceful and wide, but there is no illness.

Opposite middle pulse (反關脈 *fǎn guān mài*): The radial artery is found on the dorsal side of the radius.

Deviated angle pulse (斜飛脈 *xié fēi mài*): This means that the radial artery isn't found where it is expected to be. This pulse, and the opposite middle pulse, are physiological abnormalities of the blood vessels but do not represent pathologies. Rather, the radial artery may simply not be found where it is normally expected to be.

(6) Mental state

A strong emotional change will temporarily alter the pulse, as shown in the following table; then after the emotion calms down, the pulse will return to normal.

Mental State	Related Organ	Pulse Condition
anger	Liver	wiry or rapid
joy	Heart	slow
melancholy	Spleen	moderate
grief	Lung	short
fear	Kidney	submerged
fright	Gallbladder	moving

Table 4.1.6 Mental States and Pulse Qualities

(7) Physical Labor or Exercise

Physical labor or exercise immediately prior to taking the pulse will cause the pulse to be full and rapid, although this indicates no pathology.

(8) Diet

After taking food and drink, the pulse can become more forceful. Spicy foods can cause the pulse to become slightly rapid. The consumption of alcohol prior to pulse diagnosis may cause the pulse to become rapid and forceful.

Medication and caffeine consumption may also affect the normal pulse qualities.

(9) Pregnancy and Menstruation

This is discussed in detail later in this chapter.

■ Three: Abnormal Pulse (Pathological Pulse)

The pulse found in a person with a disease is called a morbid or pathological pulse. The pathological pulse refers to an abnormality in the pulse that usually manifests in its width, depth, strength, rate, length, rhythm, tension, or shape.

I. COMPONENT CHANGES AND PATHOGENESIS

Qi and blood are the basic components of the pulse; the substance of pulse is the blood, and the power of the pulse is the qi. Qi and blood play different roles in the generation of a pulsation. Qi pertains to yang and governs movement, while blood pertains to yin and functions to fill the vessels. Blood depends on qi for its movement.

The pulse arises mainly from the flow of qi and blood in the vessels. Normal flow and sufficiency of the qi and blood in the vessels is the condition of the normal pulse. When the flow of qi and blood is abnormal or of insufficient volume, the pathological pulse will be formed.

(1) Change in Width

Change in width means that the diameter of the blood vessel has increased or decreased. Since the diameter is dependent on the condition of the qi and blood, it will increase when the qi and/or blood are over filled, and will decrease when there is insufficient qi and/or blood, especially if there is insufficient blood to fill the vessel. A change in the width of the vessel can indicate the following:

Wide width: hyperactivity of yang

- Hyperactivity of yang: excessive heat in the body which raises and moves the qi and blood to expand the blood vessels.

- Hyperactivity of yang due to yin deficiency: outward floating of yang due to the depleted yin failing to control the yang.

Thin width: insufficiency of yin and blood: insufficient yin and blood fails to fill the blood vessels.

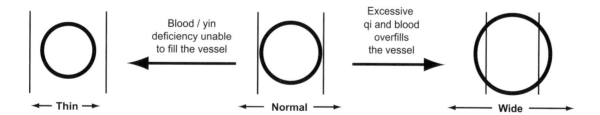

Chart 4.1.2 Pulse Width and its Pathomechanisms

(2) Change in Depth

Change in depth means that the location of the strongest pulsation has changed. Qi moves the pulse; when qi moves, blood moves. The pulse moves to the superficial depths when there is excessive or relatively excessive yang qi (floating yang). The pulse moves to the deeper depths when the yang qi is debilitated, and the pushing movement lacks force and is unable to move the blood to the exterior. A change in depth can indicate the following:

Superficial depth: the qi and blood are moving outward toward the superficial layers

- exterior pattern: the defensive yang and pathogens battle, and the qi and blood amass in the exterior

- hyperactivity of yang due to insufficient yin/blood: when yin blood is insufficient, it is unable to constrain the yang, which then floats to the surface.

Deep depth: the failure of qi and blood to flow outward from the interior of the body due to internal pathogens obstructing the flow of qi and blood; or the deep pulse represents a deficiency of qi and blood which inhibits their ability to flow outward from the interior.

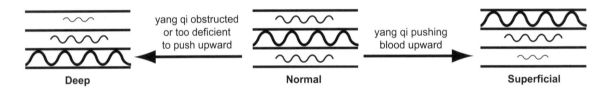

Chart 4.1.3 Pulse Depth and its Pathomechanisms

(3) Change in Strength

The strength of the pulse depends on the qi and blood, especially the qi. Qi moves the blood, and when the qi is strong and exuberant, the blood will move normally and the pulse will be balanced and have force. A change in strength may indicate the following:

Forceful: strong qi and blood fighting off an invasion of pathogenic factors, or a stagnation of qi and blood.

Forceless: deficiency of qi and blood, especially deficiency of qi, which fails to fill and move the blood in the vessels.

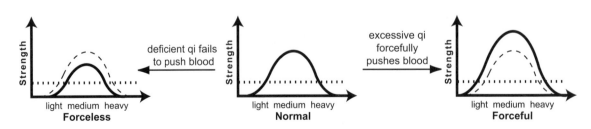

Chart 4.1.4 Pulse Strength and its Pathomechanisms

(4) Change in Rate

Pulse rate is determined by a number of factors, of which the state of the yang qi plays a leading role because it governs the function of the movement of blood via the Lung and Heart. A change in rate can indicate the following:

Increased rate: the yang governs movement, and yang hyperactivity, or the relative hyperactivity of yang qi, may cause the qi and blood to circulate more quickly inside the vessels.

Decreased rate: obstruction of the yang qi by pathogenic cold, or deficiency of yang, may prevent it from promoting the normal circulation of qi and blood.

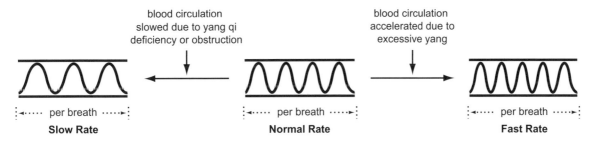

Chart 4.1.5 Pulse Rate and its Pathomechanisms

(5) Change in Length

A normal pulse should be felt at all three positions (distal, middle, proximal). The length of the pulse depends on the condition of the qi and blood. A change in length can indicate the following:

Increased length: excessive qi and blood filling the vessels.

Decreased length: qi deficiency, which fails to activate the flow of blood, or a pathogenic factor that has obstructed the vessels and prevented the qi and blood from filling the pulse to its normal length.

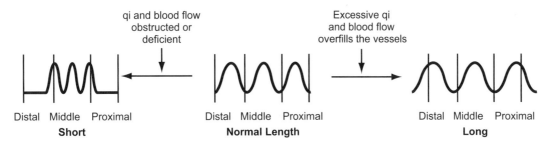

Chart 4.1.6 Pulse Length and its Pathomechanisms

(6) Change in Rhythm

The rhythm of the pulse mainly depends on the Heart qi, since the Heart qi commands the blood to move through the vessels. The pulse beats with a regular rhythm when the qi and blood move smoothly. When qi is deficient, or excessive pathogenic factors (blood stasis, phlegm, food, etc.) obstruct the qi, the pulse will beat with an irregular rhythm.

Arrhythmic pulse: Heart yang qi fails to keep the blood moving constantly in the vessels; or qi exhaustion in other organs affects the Heart yang qi.

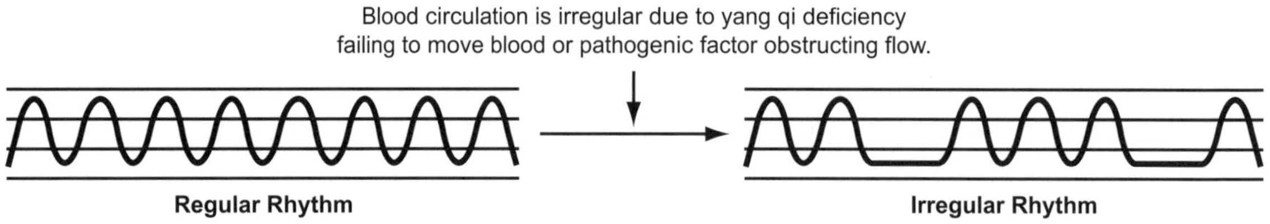

Blood circulation is irregular due to yang qi deficiency
failing to move blood or pathogenic factor obstructing flow.

Regular Rhythm   **Irregular Rhythm**

Chart 4.1.7 Pulse Rhythm and its Pathomechanisms

(7) Change in Tension

Tension refers to the tension of the blood vessels (vasotonia). It is the pulling force of the blood vessels. The tension of the vessel depends on the qi and blood, as well as the condition of the blood vessels. A change in tension may indicate the following:

Taut: the blood vessel feels tight and hard under the fingers due to qi stagnation or to blood vessel constriction.

Slack: the blood vessel feels soft and loose due to qi and blood deficiency failing to fill up the vessels.

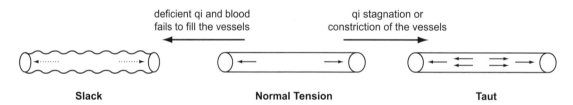

deficient qi and blood   qi stagnation or
fails to fill the vessels   constriction of the vessels

Slack   **Normal Tension**   **Taut**

Chart 4.1.8 Pulse Tension and its Pathomechanisms

(8) Change in Shape

The normal shape of the pulse should be smooth and gentle, reflecting the smooth flow of the qi and blood inside the vessel. There are two possible causes for disruption of the smooth flow of blood:

- Excess pathogenic factors obstruct the flow within the vessel, or excess qi and blood fails to flow smoothly.

- Severe qi, blood, or essence deficiency, which fails to fill the vessel and causes the shape of the vessel to change.

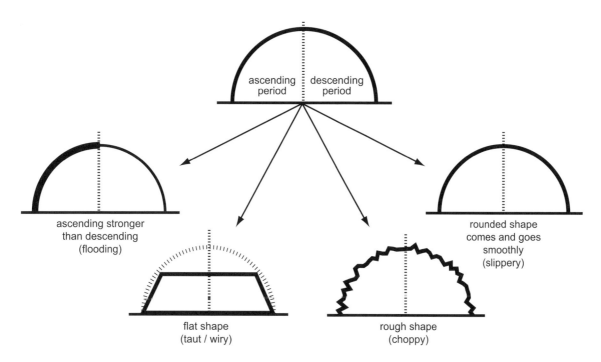

Chart 4.1.9 Pulse Shape and its Pathomechanisms

II. PATHOLOGICAL PULSES

In order to understand pathological pulse qualities, practitioners throughout history have taken the several types of pathological pulses and categorized them in different ways to make them more helpful in the clinic.

(1) Pathological Pulses Categorized by Yin and Yang

All pathological pulses can be divided into the categories of yin and yang. The pulses with forceful strength, or superficial depth, rapid speed, or long length are associated with yang, while those that are forceless, deep, slow, or short are associated with yin.

Pulse Name	Yin / Yang Quality
floating	yang
rapid	yang
excess	yang
large	yang
long	yang
rapid irregular	yang
moving	yang
wiry	yang
racing	yang
slippery	yang within yin
tight	yang within yin
moderate	yang within yin
confined	yang within yin

Pulse Name	Yin / Yang Quality
submerged	yin
slow	yin
deficient	yin
thin	yin
short	yin
slow irregular	yin
choppy	yin
scattered	yin
frail	yin
faint	yin
soggy	yin
leather	yin
hidden	yin
hollow	yin
consistently irreg.	yin
flooding	yin within yang

Table 4.1.7 Pulses According to Yin/Yang (Beinfield and Korn, 1992)

Pulse Name	Yin / Yang Quality
flooding	yang
tight	yang within yin
moderate	yang within yin
confined	yang within yin

Pulse Name	Yin / Yang Quality
leather	yin within yang
hollow	yin within yang
wiry	yin within yang
slippery	yin within yang

Table 4.1.8 Pulses According to Yin/Yang (*Bīn Hū Mài Xué*; Li Shi-Zhen)

(2) Pathological Pulses Classified by Component Changes

Width, depth, strength, rate, length, rhythm, tension and shape are the basic components of the pulse quality, and they all depend on the condition of the qi and blood. If there is any alteration in these components, the pulse will change from a physiological to a pathological state. Based on the number of the components involved, pathological pulses can be divided into two categories: simple pulses and complex pulses.

— A. Simple Pulses

The simple pulse is one in which only one component, such as the rate, is in a pathological state. Otherwise, the pulse is normal.

Simple Pathological Pulses		
Pulse	**Component**	**Description**
floating	depth	Pulse is felt with light touch but loses force with increased pressure.
submerged		Pulse is felt only deeply, beneath the muscle level, but atop the bone.
hidden		Pulse is deeper than deep, fingers will need to push the tendons away to find the pulse atop the bone.
rapid	rate	Over five beaths per breath, or 90-140 beats per minute.
racing		Over seven beats per breath, or over 140 beats per minute.
slow		Less than three beats per breath, or less than 60 beats per minute.
excessive	strength	Pulse is strong and forceful against the fingers at all depths.
deficient		Pulse is weak and forceless at all three depths.
large	width	Pulse is wider than normal.
thin		Pulse is thinner than normal.
long	length	Pulse extends beyond the distal and proximal positions.
short		Pulse can only be felt at one or two positions.
slippery	shape	Pulse comes and goes smoothly.
consistently irregular	rhythm	Pulse misses a beat on a regular basis.

Table 4.1.9 Simple Pulses

— B. Complex Pulses

This refers to pulses in which more than one component is pathological. They are typically combinations of two or more simple pulses.

Complex Pathological Pulses		
Pulse	**Components**	**Description**
choppy	rate, strength, shape	irregular speed, amplitude, shape or strength overall inconsistent feeling to the pulse.
flooding	depth, strength, width, shape	superficial, forceful, wide, the wave arrives stronger than it leaves
moving	speed, length, shape, strength, position	fast, short, slippery, forceful in the middle (guan) position
rapid irregular	rate, rhythm	fast, irregular rhythm
slow irregular	rate, rhythm	slow, irregular rhythm
soggy	strength, width, depth	forceless, thin, superficial
scattered	depth, width, strength	superficial, wide, forceless
faint	width, strength shape	very thin, forceless, vague shape
frail	depth, width, strength	deep, thin, forceless
hollow	depth, width, strength	superficial, wide, forceless at the middle depth
leather	depth, width, tension, strength	mostly superficial. but partially deep, wide, taut superficially, forceless at the middle depth
wiry	strength, length, shape, tension	forceful, long, flat, taut
tight	strength, tension vibration	forceful, taut, vibrating
confined	depth, width, length, shape, strength	deep, wide, long, taut, forceful
moderate	strength, rate	slow to the touch, but not by the clock.

Table 4.1.10 Complex Pulses

— C. The Six Categories of the Pulse

One method of categorizing the many pulse qualities in TCM is by the so-called "six categories." These are: superficial or deep, fast or slow, and forceful or forceless. See the Q&A portion of this chapter for a set of descriptive tables on this topic.

■ Four: Twenty-Nine Common Pathological Pulses

Throughout history, there have been many schools of thought which have developed different pulse qualities. What follows is the most common set of qualities used during the past few hundred years.

I. FLOATING PULSE (浮脈 *Fú Mài*)

DESCRIPTION: The pulse is felt distinctly at the superficial depth. The force decreases slightly at the deeper depths, but without feeling empty.

TRADITIONAL DESCRIPTION: like wood floating on the surface of water

KEY POINTS: forceful on the superficial depth, decreasing in strength with depth

OTHER TRANSLATION: superficial

	exterior syndrome (exterior wind)		deficiency syndrome	
Indications	floating+ forceful	floating+ moderate	floating+ forceless, thin	floating+ forceless
	exterior excess	exterior deficiency	yin, blood exhaustion	yang exhaustion
Pathogenesis	When exogenous factors invade the exterior of the body, the defensive yang (qi) rises against it. The yang pushes the qi and blood to the surface to perform this defensive task, therefore the pulse is mostly felt at the superficial depth		yin is deficient and cannot anchor the yang, or the yang is nearing exhaustion and is too weak to match the yin, so the yang will float to the body's surface as separation of yin and yang begins.	
Remarks	The floating pulse can arrive in the autumn or in a thin individual. Then, the pulse is considered normal. The floating pulse can also be seen in the patient taking vasodilating pharmaceuticals.			

Table 4.1.11 Floating Pulse and its Indications

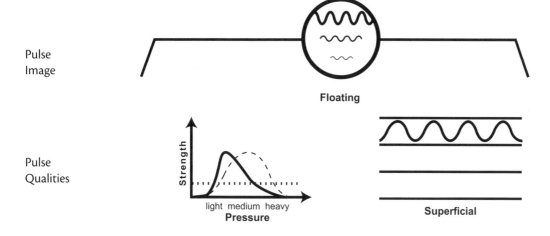

Pulse Image

Floating

Pulse Qualities

light medium heavy
Pressure

Superficial

II. Submerged Pulse (沉脈 *Chén Mài*)

DESCRIPTION: Located deep, next to the bone, it can barely be felt with light or moderate pressure. It is distinct only when pressing down to the bones and tendons.

TRADITIONAL DESCRIPTION: Like a stone thrown into the well, it must sink to the bottom.

KEY POINTS: absent on the superficial depth, increasing in strength with depth

OTHER TRANSLATIONS: deep, sunken

	interior syndrome	
Indications	submerged and forceful	submerged and forceless
	interior excess	interior deficiency
Pathogenesis	Pathogenic factors accumulate in the body, obstructing the outward movement of the qi, blood and yang.	Qi and blood deficiency cannot fill the channels or viscera and thus the pulse remains submerged.
Remarks	The submerged pulse can arrive in the winter or in a heavy person and represent a normal pulse.	

Table 4.1.12 Submerged Pulse and its Indications

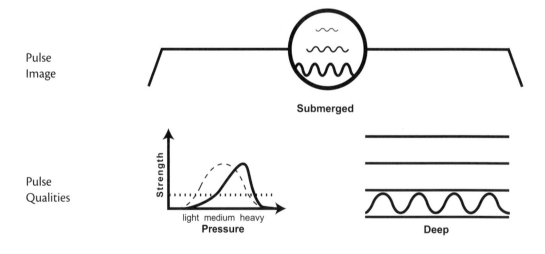

Pulse Image

Submerged

Pulse Qualities

Pressure

Deep

III. Slow Pulse (遲脈 *Chí Mài*)

DESCRIPTION: The pulse beats less than three times per (practitioner's) breath, about 40 – 60 bpm, but with a regular rhythm.

KEY POINTS: Pulse frequency is less than three beats per breath (< 60 bpm).

Indications	cold syndrome		qi deficiency
	slow+forceful	slow+forceless	
	cold accumulation	deficiency cold	
	Biomedicine: Intracranial hypertension, obstructive jaundice, rheumatic heart disease, viral myocarditis, coronary heart disease,and digitalis poisoning.		
Pathogenesis	Cold causes contraction. When cold invades the body, or a deficiency of yang produces cold, the qi and blood become stagnant. Thus the qi and blood circulation in the vessels slows down as does the rate of the pulse.		qi commands the blood and when qi is deficient, the pulse will move slowly.
Remarks	The slow pulse is seen in some healthy persons, specifically athletes or those who engage in daily physical labor.		

Table 4.1.13 Slow Pulse and its Indications

Pulse
Image

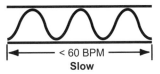

IV. Rapid Pulse (數脈 *Shuò Mài*)

DESCRIPTION: The pulse is rapid and beats over five times per (practitioner's) breath (90–140 bpm), with a regular rhythm.

KEY POINTS: The pulse frequency is more than five beats per breath (90–140 bpm).

OTHER TRANSLATION: fast

Indications	heat syndrome		
	rapid+forceful	rapid+thin	rapid+hollow
	excess heat	yin deficiency	blood deficiency
	Biomedicine: febrile disease, various anemias, acute hemorrhagic shock, acute myocardial infarction, acute pericarditis, congestive heart failure, acute rheumatic fever, myocarditis and hyperthyroidism.		
Pathogenesis	Excessive pathogenic heat increases the circulation of the qi and blood which causes the pulse to quicken.	yin or blood deficiency causes a relative hyperactivity of yang which causes the pulse to quicken.	
Remarks	Physical or emotional activities can temporarily increase pulse rate.		

Table 4.1.14 Rapid Pulse and its Indications

Pulse
Image

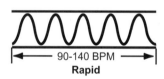

90-140 BPM
Rapid

V. Excessive Pulse (實脈 *Shí Mài*)

DESCRIPTION: The pulse can be felt at all three positions and at all three depths. It is long, wide, and forceful, giving rise to a sense of fullness.

KEY POINTS: long, wide, and forceful

OTHER TRANSLATIONS: full, replete

Indications	excess syndrome
	Any excess syndrome which includes: pathogenic cold accumulation, food stagnation, phlegm retention, qi or blood stagnation.
	hyperactivity of pathogenic factors / strong antipathogenic qi
	Biomedicine: febrile disease, acute hemorrhagic shock, acute myocardial infarction, acute pericarditis, congestive heart failure, acute rheumatic fever, myocarditis and hyperthyroidism.
Pathogenesis	The conflict between hyperactive pathogenic factors and strong antipathogenic qi results in accumulation of qi and blood filling the blood vessel, then the excess type pulse will consequently occur.
Remarks	The excess pulse can also be felt in the normal person. When the pulse is strong and calm it indicates that the person has sufficient antipathogenic qi and *zàng fǔ* organ functions.

Table 4.1.15 Excessive Pulse and its Indications

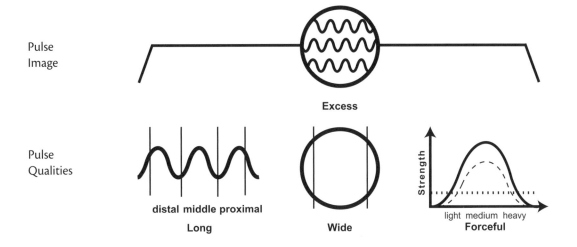

VI. Deficient Pulse (虛脈 *Xū Mài*)

DESCRIPTION: The pulse shape is wide, but without strength. It is forceless at all three positions with either light or heavy pressure. There is a sense of emptiness in this pulse.

KEY POINTS: wide, forceless, and slack

OTHER TRANSLATIONS: empty, vacuous

	deficiency syndrome				
Indications	floating + deficient	submerged + deficient	choppy + deficient	rapid + deficient	slow + deficient
	qi deficiency	internal deficiency	blood deficiency	yin deficiency	yang deficiency
Pathogenesis	If yang and qi are deficient, the pulse will be forceless. If yin and blood are deficient, the vessel will not fill up. So any deficiency (yin, yang, qi, blood) may lead to a deficient pulse.				
Remarks	The deficient pulse may be at any position or depth. It may also be rapid or slow. The deficient pulse is also a group of pulses. These pulses beat without strength, and indicate deficiency conditions. Examples include frail, soggy, and faint pulses.				

Table 4.1.16 Deficient Pulse and its Indications

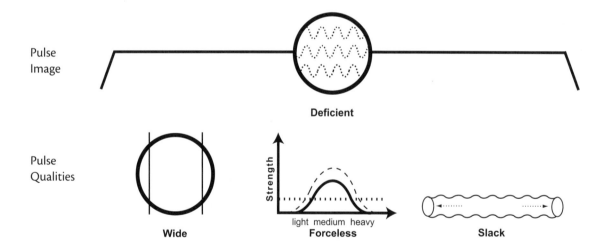

Pulse Image

Deficient

Pulse Qualities

Wide

Strength

light medium heavy
Forceless

Slack

VII. Large Pulse (大脉 *Dá Mài*)

DESCRIPTION: This pulse is wide. The vessel is wide and thick.

KEY POINTS: wide

OTHER TRANSLATION: big

Indications	wide and forceful	wide and forceless
	excess heat	deficiency
Pathogenesis	Excessive pathogenic heat in the interior dilates the blood vessels and accelerates the qi and blood circulation, thus producing a wide and forceful pulse.	Extreme deficiency of essence or yin cannot anchor the yang, and so yang floats to the lateral margins of the vessel.
Remarks	The "large" pulse is not commonly mentioned in Chinese textbooks.	

Table 4.1.17 Large Pulse and its Indications

Pulse
Image

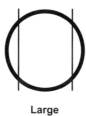

Large

VIII. THIN PULSE (細脈 *Xì Mài*)

DESCRIPTION: The pulse width is very thin and feels like a fine thread, but is very distinct and clear without interruption of rhythm when pushing on the pulse.

KEY POINTS: small and thin, clear and distinct

OTHER TRANSLATIONS: fine, thready. This is also called the "small" pulse and is regarded as the opposite of the "big" or "large" pulse.

		deficiency		excess
	qi	blood	yin	dampness
Indications	**Biomedicine:** heart failure, early stage of shock, neurasthenia, severe hemorrhage of upper digestive tract, serious nosebleed, serious hemoptysis, hemorrhage of intestinal tract, hemorrhage due to rupture of ectopic pregnancy.			
Pathogenesis	Blood or yin deficiency fails to fill the blood vessels. Deficient qi is unable to promote blood circulation, which also prevents the blood from filling the vessel.			Dampness accumulates around the vessel compressing its width.
	Biomedicine: insufficient blood volume reduces effective volume of blood in circulation, so that the vascular bed is contracted through the regulatory function of the neurohumoral mechanism. Another potential explanation is a fall in the cardiac stroke volume which cuts down intravascular pressure and makes the small and medium-sized arteries contract.			
Remarks	The thin pulse is more commonly encountered in the female than the male. In those of a smaller constitution, a thin pulse is not considered pathological.			

Table 4.1.18 Thin Pulse and its Indications

Pulse
Image

Thin

IX. Long Pulse (長脈 *Cháng Mài*)

DESCRIPTION: The pulse is smooth and straight. It can be felt to extend distally and proximally beyond the usual three positions. This pulse can be either normal or pathological.

KEY POINTS: long and straight

Indications	excess syndrome	
	Liver yang rising	excess interior heat
Pathogenesis	Internal excess heat can increase the movement of qi and blood, which causes a fullness of the blood vessels. The pulse will extend beyond the usual pulse locations along the radial artery, thus forming the long pulse.	
Remarks	The long pulse when moderate in strength can also be a sign of health in the normal person.	

Table 4.1.19 Long Pulse and its Indications

Pulse
Image

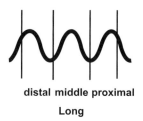

distal middle proximal
Long

X. SHORT PULSE (短脈 *Duǎn Mài*)

DESCRIPTION: The pulse cannot be felt in all three positions. It is absent in the distal and/or proximal positions.

KEY POINT: short

	qi disease	
Indications	short and forceful	short and forceless
	qi stagnation	qi deficiency
	Biomedicine: aortic stenosis of rheumatic heart disease.	
Pathogenesis	Qi stagnation fails to move the blood, and so the vessel is not stretched, the pulse is short.	Qi drives the pulse, when qi is too weak to move blood, blood circulation will slow and the blood in the vessels will stagnate. The pulse will feel short and forceless.
	Biomedicine: Aortic stenosis causes the blood vessels to thin and weaken, in which case blood will be hindered from flowing into the vessels.	
Remarks	Short pulse can be seen in cases where there is profuse sweating but little intake of fluid.	

Table 4.1.20 Short Pulse and its Indications

Pulse
Image

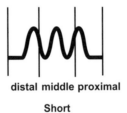

distal middle proximal

Short

XI. Slippery Pulse (滑脈 *Huá Mài*)

DESCRIPTION: The pulse feels quick (though it is not rapid), slippery, and smooth. It is rounded inside the vessel.

TRADITIONAL DESCRIPTION: like a pearl rolling on a plate

KEY POINTS: smooth, slippery

OTHER TRANSLATION: rolling

Indications	food stagnation	phlegm or dampness	excess heat
Pathogenesis	When excessive pathogens enter the body, the antipathogenic qi rises against the pathogens, the qi and blood are mobilized and become entangled with the pathogenic factors in the blood vessels. The pulse becomes plump and slippery. Or dampness or phlegm causes an increase in blood viscosity and a decrease in pulse wave flexibility, hence the smooth pulse without corners.		
	Biomedicine: fine elasticity of blood vessels, smoothness of internal wall, normal or lowered peripheral resistance.		
Remarks	The slippery pulse is considered normal for pregnant women in whom it indicates sufficient and harmonious qi and blood. In the absence of any pathogenic changes the slippery pulse can be found in the normal person.		

Table 4.1.21 Slippery Pulse and its Indications

Pulse
Image

Pulse
Quality

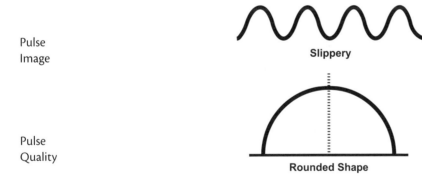

Slippery

Rounded Shape

XII. Choppy Pulse (澀脈 *Sè Mài*)

DESCRIPTION: The pulse seems to be slow and not smooth. The vessel is thin. The rhythm is irregular in force and in fullness.

TRADITIONAL DESCRIPTION: The feeling of the pulse is uneven and sluggish, like that of scraping bamboo with a little knife.

KEY POINTS: unsmooth, short and mutable, (changes rapidly, both in rate and strength).

OTHER TRANSLATIONS: rough, hesitant, sluggish

	excess syndrome			deficiency syndrome			
Indications	choppy and forceful			choppy and forceless			
	qi & blood stagnation	food stagnation	phlegm retention	blood deficiency	essence deficiency	threatened abortion	seminal emission
	Biomedical: arteriosclerosis, hyperlipidemia, severe vomiting and diarrhea, chronic cor pulmonale and polycythemia vera						
Pathogenesis	Excess pathogens block the vessels and impair the circulation of blood.			Blood and body fluid deficiencies cannot fill up the vessels which leads to an uneven flow of qi and blood in the vessels.			
	Biomedical: any mechanism that leads to an increase in blood viscosity which results in an increase in blood adhering to the vascular wall which increases friction and causes a deceleration of blood flow						

Table 4.1.22 Choppy Pulse and its Indications

Pulse Image

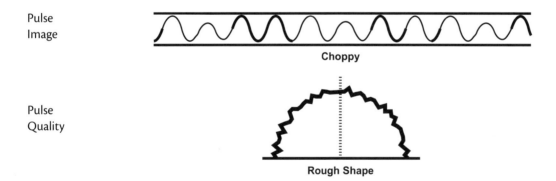

Choppy

Pulse Quality

Rough Shape

XIII. FLOODING PULSE (洪脉 *Hóng Mài*)

DESCRIPTION: The pulse is wide and forceful, although it fades gently. The vessel is wide and thick.

TRADITIONAL DESCRIPTION: like the ocean wave that comes strongly, but leaves calmly

KEY POINTS: easily felt at superficial depth, wide and forceful, arrives with more power than when it leaves

OTHER TRANSLATIONS: overflowing, surging

Indications	excess heat on the qi level
	Biomedicine: various acute infectious diseases, severe pyrogenic bacterial infection or other disease, also may be found in patients with adverse flow of blood caused by aortic insufficiency.
Pathogenesis	Excessive pathogenic heat in the interior dilates the blood vessels and accelerates the qi and blood circulation, thus producing a flooding pulse.
Remarks	Flooding pulse can be a normal pulse during the summer.

Table 4.1.23 Flooding Pulse and its Indications

Pulse Image

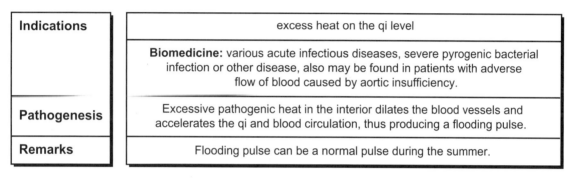

Flooding

Pulse Qualities

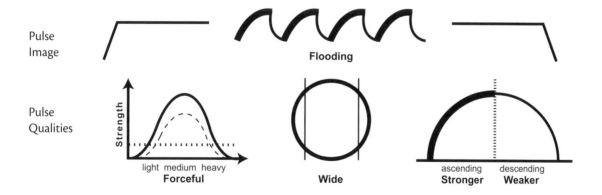

XIV. RAPID IRREGULAR PULSE (促脈 *Cù Mài*)

DESCRIPTION: The pulse beats rapidly with irregular pauses.

TRADITIONAL DESCRIPTION: It feels very agitated and urgent, like a man running and suddenly falling down.

KEY POINTS: rapid, irregular pauses

OTHER TRANSLATIONS: hasty, abrupt, skipping

Indications	excess syndrome		deficiency of *zàng fǔ* organs
	rapid irregular + forceful		rapid irregular + forceless
	excess heat	stagnation	yin and yang disharmony
	Biomedicine: excitation of sympathetic nerve, infectious or viral pathological changes in the myocardium, or sinus tachycardia accompanied with obvious sinus irregularity.		
Pathogenesis	When excessive heat accelerates the blood circulation, the pulse will be rapid, when stagnation of pathogens causes blockages, the pulse will be irregular. Excess heat can give rise to stagnation and stagnation can cause heat.		Yin deficiency gives rise to a rapid pulse. In time this leads to a deficiency of yang which limits the Heart's ability to push the blood, resulting in irregular pauses.
Remarks	In cases of congenital variation, this pulse could prove to be the normal pulse for some individuals.		

Table 4.1.24 Rapid Irregular Pulse and its Indications

Pulse
Image

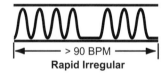

> 90 BPM
Rapid Irregular

XV. Slow Irregular Pulse (結脈 *Jié Mài*)

DESCRIPTION: The pulse is slow with irregularly missed beats. After the missed beat, the pulse immediately resumes.

KEY POINTS: slow, irregular pauses

OTHER TRANSLATIONS: knotted, bound

Indications	excess syndrome			deficiency syndrome
	stagnation	cold	tumor or mass	Heart qi deficiency
	Biomedicine: coronary heart disease, rheumatic heart disease, hypertensive cardiopathy, pulmonary heart disease, and myocarditis.			
Pathogenesis	Pathogenic factors stagnate within the vessels which block blood circulation, thus keeping the pulse slow and intermittent.			If the qi and blood are not sufficient to fill the vessels, the pathogen will insert itself into vessels and cause the pulse to slow and miss beats irregularly.
Remarks	In cases of congenital variation, this pulse could prove to be the normal pulse for some individuals.			

Table 4.1.25 Slow Irregular Pulse and its Indications

Pulse
Image

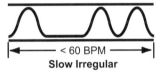

Slow Irregular

XVI. Consistently Irregular Pulse (代脈 *Dài Mài*)

DESCRIPTION: The pulse pauses at regular intervals. After the pause, the pulse will then resume.

KEY POINTS: regularly missed beat, long pauses

OTHER TRANSLATIONS: intermittent, regularly intermittent

	excess syndrome			deficiency syndrome	
Indications	consistently irregular and rapid			consistently irregular and forceless	
	wind syndrome	pain	emotional shock	qi and/or blood deficiency	*zàng fǔ* organ qi deficiency
	Biomedicine: arrhythmia caused by myocardiac infarction, coronary heart disease, cardiomyopathy, myocarditis, hypertensive heart disease, pulmonary heart disease, cardiac insufficiency, coupled rhythm of extrasystoles or atrioventricular block.				
Pathogenesis	Pain, emotional shock or pathogenic factors cause qi stagnation resulting in the intermittent pulse.			The declining *zàng fǔ* organ qi and blood cannot form a successive flow in vessels, so the pulse is forceless and a beat is regularly missed.	
Remarks	In cases of congenital variation, this pulse could prove to be the normal pulse for some individuals. This pulse can also be found during the second and third month of pregnancy at which time, it is again considered normal.				

Table 4.1.26 Consistently Irregular Pulse and its Indications

Pulse
Image

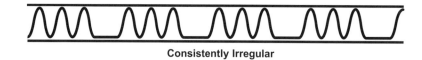

Consistently Irregular

XVII. Soggy Pulse (濡脈 *Rú Mài*)

DESCRIPTION: The pulse is superficial, thin, and forceless. If pressed, it becomes weaker and weaker.

TRADITIONAL DESCRIPTION: Like a strand of cotton floating on the water, it feels very thin and indistinct. It is like a bubble, which bursts when pressure is lightly increased.

KEY POINTS: superficial, thin, forceless

OTHER TRANSLATIONS: weak-floating, soft

Indications	dampness	deficiency syndrome
Pathogenesis	Dampness depresses the vessels. Qi and blood cannot easily flow through the vessels. So, the pulse is thin and soft.	Yang loses its root when qi, yin or blood are deficient. If the pulse disappears when pressed, the yang is expiring.
Remarks	If this pulse is present in a young or otherwise strong patient, the prognosis is not good. Excessive diseases with deficient pulses do not suggest a good prognosis.	

Table 4.1.27 Soggy Pulse and its Indications

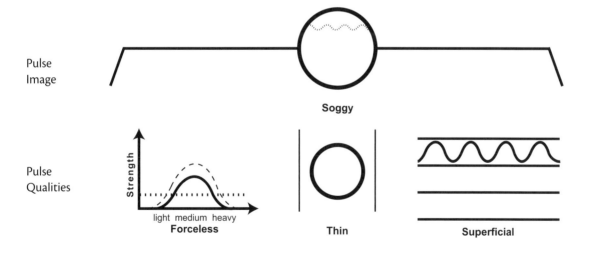

XVIII. Frail Pulse (弱脈 *Ruò Mài*)

DESCRIPTION: The pulse is forceless, deep, and thin. It can only be felt on the deep depth by pressing. If more pressure is applied, the pulse is lost.

KEY POINTS: deep, thin, and forceless

OTHER TRANSLATION: weak

Indications	yin, yang, qi or blood deficiency syndrome
Pathogenesis	The frail pulse is a sign of qi and blood deficiency. The qi and blood are too weak to fill up and drive the pulse. So it is a sign of decline. If the pulse sensation is lost at the superficial level, this indicates that yang is in decline. If heavy pressure causes the pulse to be lost, it indicates an exhaustion of yin.
	Biomedicine: severe vomiting, profuse sweating, or blood loss can cause this condition.

Table 4.1.28 Frail Pulse and its Indications

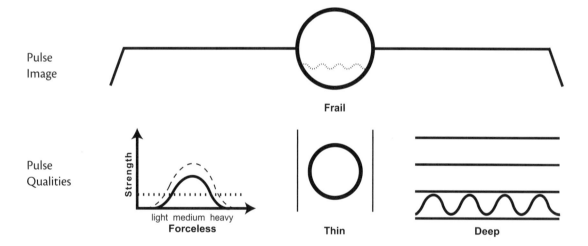

XIX. Hollow Pulse (芤脈 *Kōu Mài*)

DESCRIPTION: The pulse is wide and soft when touched lightly, and hollow when seeking. With pressure, the edges of the vessel are clearly felt but the center is obscure.

TRADITIONAL DESCRIPTION: The hollow pulse feels like a scallion or green onion stalk which has an edge but is hollow on the inside.

KEY POINTS: floating, wide, and slack, with an obscure center

OTHER TRANSLATION: scallion stalk

Indications	hollow and forceless	hollow and rapid
	loss of blood	yin depletion
Pathogenesis	The pulse shows a solitary yang without yin. After loss of blood, the yin and blood cannot fill up the vessel and contain the yang qi. The yang loses its anchor and floats to the superficial layers.	
	Biomedicine: sudden and severe bleeding reduces circulatory blood volume, but blood vessels have not yet contracted leading to the hollow pulse.	
Remarks	The pulse is categorized as a yang pulse, but because it is not rooted, it is a sign of severe deficiency.	

Table 4.1.29 Hollow Pulse and its Indications

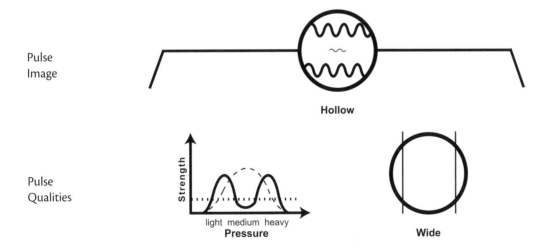

Pulse Image

Hollow

Pulse Qualities

Pressure

Wide

XX. Leather pulse (革脈 *Gé Mài*)

DESCRIPTION: The pulse is large (thick and wide), rapid, and forceful when lightly touched, but hollow when pressed deeply.

TRADITIONAL DESCRIPTION: This pulse is said to feel like the surface of a drum: thick on the surface and hollow beneath.

KEY POINTS: superficial, forceful, taut, wide, and hollow

OTHER TRANSLATIONS: tympanic, drum-skin

Indications	blood loss	essence exhaustion	abortion	metrorrhagia and metrostaxis
Pathogenesis	The wide and taut sensations when touching lightly are due to qi floating which is caused by the deficiency of the essence and blood. The hollow character at the deep depth is a sign of depletion of qi and/or blood.			
	Biomedicine: consumptive diseases, such as aplastic anemia, liver disease, uterine bleeding due to retained placenta, serious dehydration caused by inadequate circulatory blood volume.			

Table 4.1.30 Leather Pulse and its Indications

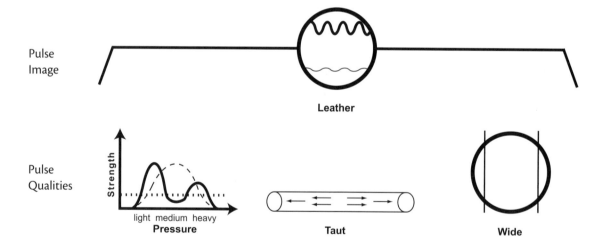

XXI. Scattered Pulse (散脈 Sàn Mài)

DESCRIPTION: The pulse is wide, superficial, forceless, and slack (opposite of "taut") when touched lightly. It has an indistinct and unclear feeling. "Scattered" means diffuse. The boundary of the vessel is vague. When seeking or pressing, the pulse disappears, so much so that the rate is hard to count.

TRADITIONAL DESCRIPTION: like flower blossoms lightly scattering to the ground

KEY POINTS: superficial, scattered without root, uneven rhythm

OTHER TRANSLATION: dissipated

Indications	exhaustion of qi, functional failure of the *zàng fǔ* organs
	Biomedicine: arteriosclerosis, cardiopathy, rheumatic heart disease, mitral stenosis or incompetence, serious cor pulmonale. Insufficiency of effective blood volume or other reduction of the cardiac output.
Pathogenesis	antipathogenic qi is exhausted, dispersion of the yang qi due to dissociation of yin and yang
Remarks	This pulse indicates a critical condition. When this pulse appears in a pregnant woman during the third trimester of pregnancy, labor is imminent. If this pulse is present during the second trimester of pregnancy, it indicates a potential miscarriage.

Table 4.1.31 Scattered Pulse and its Indications

Pulse Image

Pulse Qualities

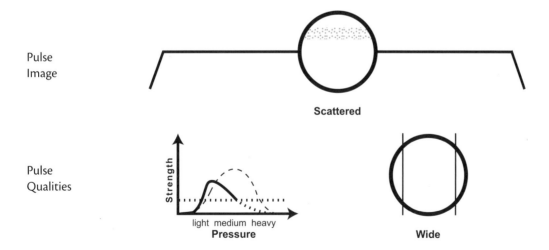

Scattered

Pressure — light medium heavy (Strength)

Wide

XXII. Hidden pulse (伏脉 *Fú Mài*)

DESCRIPTION: The pulse cannot be felt when touching, seeking, or pressing. Only by pressing very heavily to the bone can it be felt. The pulsation seems to come from beneath the tendons and bone.

KEY POINT: very deep

Indications	pathogens obstructing the interior	syncope (yang deficiency)
Pathogenesis	Excessive pathogens obstruct the yang and qi. The qi and blood cannot flow to the exterior or superficial portions of the body through vessels.	Yang is too weak to push the qi and blood to flow outward to the exterior of the body.
	Biomedicine: cardiogenic shock, toxic dysentery, profuse hemorrhage, and severe pain can give rise to the hidden pulse. It is caused by a dramatic reduction of blood volume resulting in a fall of blood pressure.	
Remarks	During pregnancy, a woman may have a hidden pulse. In the absence of other signs and symptoms this pulse would not indicate any pathological changes.	

Table 4.1.32 Hidden Pulse and its Indications

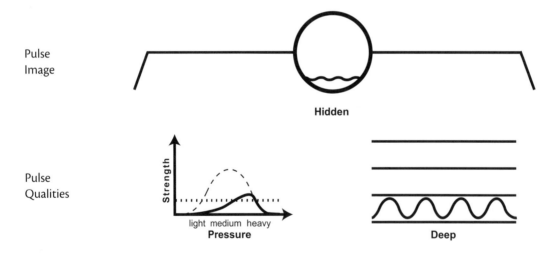

Pulse Image

Hidden

Pulse Qualities

Strength

light medium heavy
Pressure

Deep

XXIII. CONFINED PULSE (牢脈 *Láo Mài*)

DESCRIPTION: The pulse is deep, taut, long, wide, and forceful. Deeply located, it cannot be felt by light or moderate pressure.

KEY POINTS: deep, forceful, wide, taut, long, stable

OTHER TRANSLATION: firm

Indications	Interior excess cold syndrome (hernia, lumps, and masses)
	Biomedicine: arteriosclerosis and chronic nephritis.
Pathogenesis	Because of accumulation of yin cold, it traps the yang qi within, hence the qi and the blood cannot move to the surface, and so the pulse feels confined.
	Biomedicine: the elasticity of blood vessels is reduced but the blood volume remains full and the blood pressure high, so the firm pulse occurs.

Table 4.1.33 Confined Pulse and its Indications

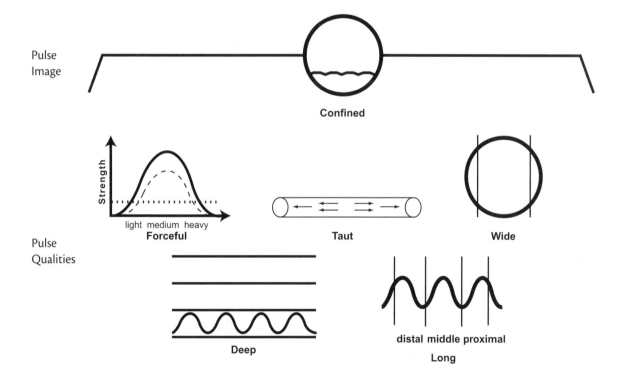

XXIV. Faint Pulse (微脈 *Wēi Mài*)

DESCRIPTION: The vessel is extremely thin and forceless. It seems to be felt, and then not felt. When pressing deeply, the vessel and pulse become vague.

KEY POINTS: thin, forceless, and vague

OTHER TRANSLATION: minute

Indications	yin, yang, qi or blood deficiency syndrome
	Biomedicine: severe vomiting, profuse sweating, blood loss
Pathogenesis	The faint pulse is a sign of qi and blood deficiency. The qi and blood are too weak to fill up and drive the pulse. So it is a sign of decline. If the pulse sensation is lost at the superficial depth, this indicates that yang is in decline. If heavy pressure causes the pulse to be lost, it indicates an exhaustion of yin.

Table 4.1.34 Faint Pulse and its Indications

Pulse Image

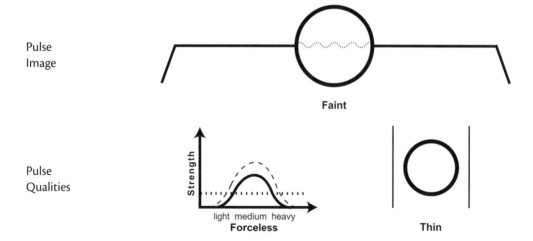

Pulse Qualities

XXV. WIRY PULSE (弦脈 *Xián Mài*)

DESCRIPTION: The pulse feels taut, long, and forceful, whether under pressure of the fingers or not. It maintains a straight line beneath the fingers.

TRADITIONAL DESCRIPTION: like a string stretched on a musical instrument

KEY POINTS: long, taut, stable (not vibrating)

OTHER TRANSLATIONS: string-taut, taut, string-like

Indications	Liver/Gall Bladder disease	phlegm	pain	malaria
	Biomedicine: arteriosclerosis; increase of arterial pressure, peripheral resistance, or vasotonia; hepatitis, cirrhosis, hepatocarcinoma, hypertension.			
Pathogenesis	Wiry pulse is the manifestation of tense vascular qi. The Liver is chiefly responsible for the dispersion and regulation of the flow of qi. When the Liver fails to disperse and govern the flow of qi, it accumulates and strongly pushes the blood which increases the vasotonia and gives rise to the wiry pulse.	Wiry pulse belongs to the condition of yin hidden within yang. The pulse is caused by qi and blood stagnation. Phlegm, pain and malaria result in the imbalance between yin and yang, and this increases the tension of vascular qi. Since all of these pathologies are yang in nature, they tend to increase the vasotonia and give rise to the wiry pulse.		
Remarks	Wiry is a normal pulse during the springtime.			

Table 4.1.35 Wiry Pulse and its Indications

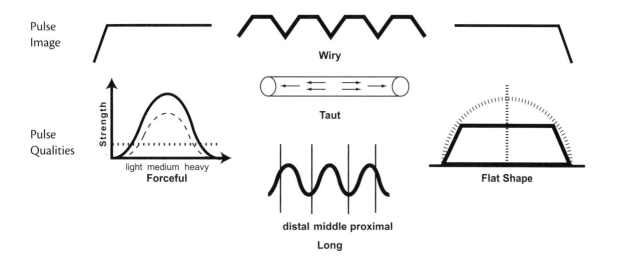

XXVI. TIGHT PULSE (緊脈 *Jǐn Mài*)

DESCRIPTION: The pulse rises and falls with strength and vibrates to the left and right.

TRADITIONAL DESCRIPTION: like fingers on a tightly stretched and twisted cord, snapping back and forth

KEY POINTS: tense and taut, forceful, vibrating (unstable, movable)

OTHER TRANSLATION: tense

Indications	cold pattern	food stagnation	pain
Pathogenesis	Cold causes contraction. Cold in body makes the vessel contract and the pulse becomes tight.	Cold accumulates in the middle burner causing food stagnation which obstructs the movement of qi.	Pain syndrome is mostly due to obstruction. Obstruction causes the vessel to spasm and feel tight.
	Biomedicine: this pulse can be caused by vasotonic increase, blood volume increase or an increase in cardiac stroke volume.		

Table 4.1.36 Tight Pulse and its Indications

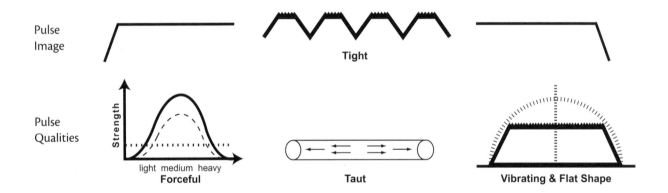

XXVII. MODERATE PULSE (緩脈 *Huǎn Mài*)

DESCRIPTION: The pulse beats four times per practitioner's breath, faster than the slow pulse.

• *Normal pulse*: The pulse is vigorous with equal intervals, moves smoothly, and is the same in all three positions.

• *Morbid pulse*: The pulse is sluggish; its movement feels slow. It is usually accompanied by other pulse qualities.

KEY POINTS: feels slow, though normal in rate when timed

OTHER TRANSLATIONS: slowed-down, lax, retarded, leisurely

Indications	dampness syndrome	Spleen and Stomach deficiency
Pathogenesis	Dampness is sticky and easily collects in the vessels; it then obstructs qi and blood flow.	Spleen and Stomach deficiency causes a retention of water and dampness.
Remarks	If the moderate pulse is present in a patient who is suffering from a prolonged or critical disease, it is a sign of the restoration of antipathogenic qi. Although this pulse indicates a pathology, compared to a critical disease, it is still a positive sign. This pulse may also indicate a normal physiological pulse.	

Table 4.1.37 Moderate Pulse and its Indications

Pulse
Image

Pulse
Qualities

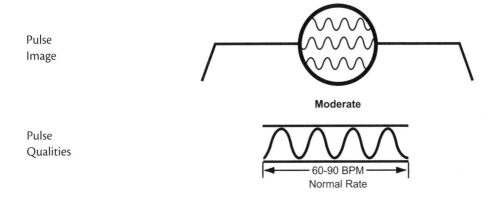

Moderate

60-90 BPM
Normal Rate

XXVIII. Moving Pulse (動脈 *Dòng Mài*)

DESCRIPTION: The pulse is rapid and slippery. At the middle portion, the pulsation is forceful.

TRADITIONAL DESCRIPTION: like a bean bouncing in the vessel, with well-defined peaks, but without head or tail

KEY POINTS: shape is short and round, slippery and rapid, forceful in the middle position

OTHER TRANSLATIONS: stirred, spinning bean, bouncing

Indications	pain	fright
Pathogenesis	The moving pulse is a sign of struggle between yin and yang.	
	Qi and blood stagnation causes pain. yin and yang fight and cause a disharmony of the ascending and descending of the qi and blood. The pulse follows this violent up and down movement.	Emotional shock causes qi and blood disturbance and confusion. This leads to the pushing outward of the qi and blood leading to the moving pulse.
Remarks	The moving pulse can be seen in pregnant women in their first trimester, at which time this is considered a normal pulse.	

Table 4.1.38 Moving Pulse and its Indications

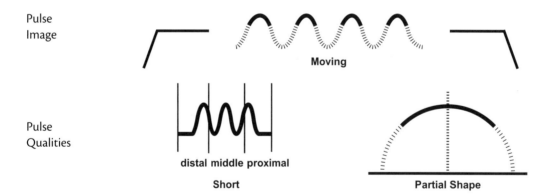

Pulse Image

Moving

Pulse Qualities

distal middle proximal

Short

Partial Shape

XXIX. Racing Pulse (疾脈 *Jí Mài*)

DESCRIPTION: The pulse is rapid and beats more than seven times per practitioner's breath (140–180 bpm). It is the extreme version of the rapid pulse. Its rhythm is generally regular.

KEY POINTS: extremely rapid

OTHER TRANSLATIONS: hurried, urgent, swift

Indications	racing and forceful	racing and forceless
	hyperactivity of yang and excessive heat	yin exhaustion and antipathogenic qi collapse
	Biomedicine: hypertensive cardiopathy, coronary heart disease, hyperthyroidism, myocarditis and pericarditis. Auricular flutter accompanied with regular 2:1 atrioventricular block or functional tachycardia.	
Pathogenesis	Yin exhaustion with hyperactivity of yang or excessive pathogenic heat causes acceleration of the blood flow and a high pulse rate.	
Remarks	This is a critical pulse, however this pulse rate is considered normal for the healthy infant.	

Table 4.1.39 Racing Pulse and its Indications

Pulse
Image

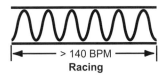

Racing

■ Five: Distinguishing Among Pathological Pulses

Some pulses share components such as length, width, etc., but indicate different pathological changes. In order to make an accurate diagnosis, it is essential that one distinguish between the similar-feeling pulses.

The following charts help differentiate pulses with similar components, but sometimes very different indications.

I. Hollow and Leather

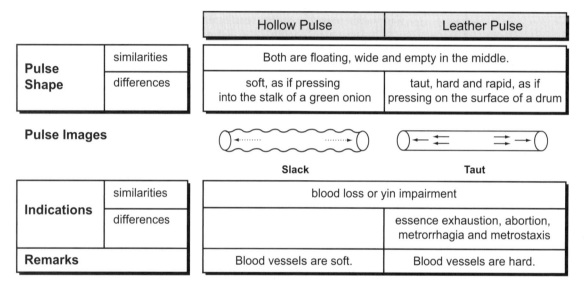

		Hollow Pulse	Leather Pulse
Pulse Shape	similarities	Both are floating, wide and empty in the middle.	
	differences	soft, as if pressing into the stalk of a green onion	taut, hard and rapid, as if pressing on the surface of a drum
Pulse Images		Slack	Taut
Indications	similarities	blood loss or yin impairment	
	differences		essence exhaustion, abortion, metrorrhagia and metrostaxis
Remarks		Blood vessels are soft.	Blood vessels are hard.

Table 4.1.40 Comparison of Hollow and Leather Pulses

II. Large and Flooding

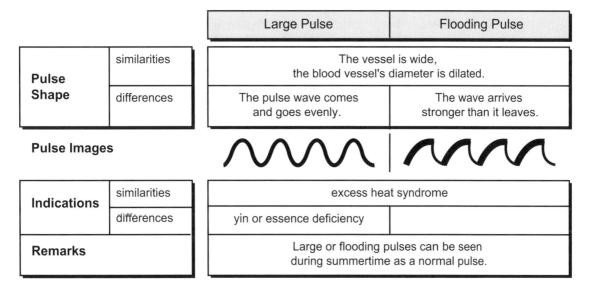

		Large Pulse	Flooding Pulse
Pulse Shape	similarities	The vessel is wide, the blood vessel's diameter is dilated.	
	differences	The pulse wave comes and goes evenly.	The wave arrives stronger than it leaves.
Indications	similarities	excess heat syndrome	
	differences	yin or essence deficiency	
Remarks		Large or flooding pulses can be seen during summertime as a normal pulse.	

Table 4.1.41 Comparison of Large and Flooding Pulses

III. Excessive and Flooding

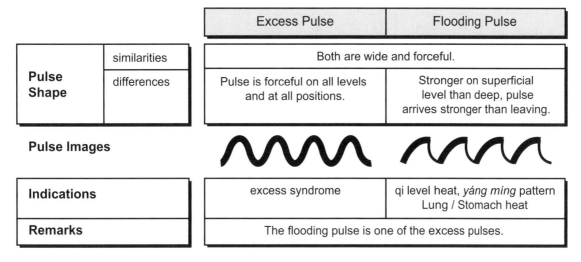

		Excess Pulse	Flooding Pulse
Pulse Shape	similarities	Both are wide and forceful.	
	differences	Pulse is forceful on all levels and at all positions.	Stronger on superficial level than deep, pulse arrives stronger than leaving.
Indications		excess syndrome	qi level heat, *yáng míng* pattern Lung / Stomach heat
Remarks		The flooding pulse is one of the excess pulses.	

Table 4.1.42 Comparison of Excess and Flooding Pulses

IV. Short and Moving

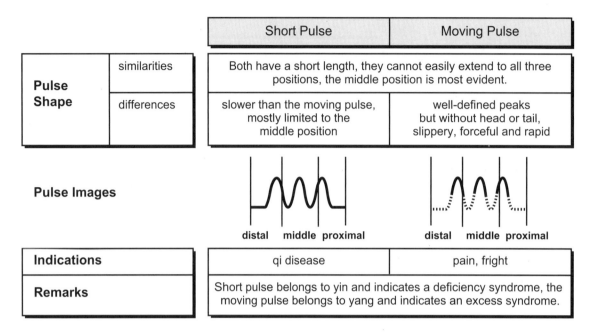

		Short Pulse	Moving Pulse
Pulse Shape	similarities	Both have a short length, they cannot easily extend to all three positions, the middle position is most evident.	
	differences	slower than the moving pulse, mostly limited to the middle position	well-defined peaks but without head or tail, slippery, forceful and rapid
Pulse Images		distal middle proximal	distal middle proximal
Indications		qi disease	pain, fright
Remarks		Short pulse belongs to yin and indicates a deficiency syndrome, the moving pulse belongs to yang and indicates an excess syndrome.	

Table 4.1.43 Comparison of Short and Moving Pulses

V. Moderate and Slow

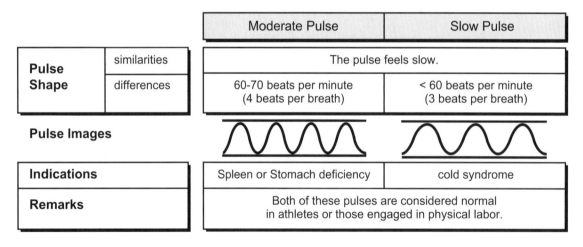

		Moderate Pulse	Slow Pulse
Pulse Shape	similarities	The pulse feels slow.	
	differences	60-70 beats per minute (4 beats per breath)	< 60 beats per minute (3 beats per breath)
Pulse Images			
Indications		Spleen or Stomach deficiency	cold syndrome
Remarks		Both of these pulses are considered normal in athletes or those engaged in physical labor.	

Table 4.1.44 Comparison of Moderate and Slow Pulses

VI. WIRY AND TIGHT

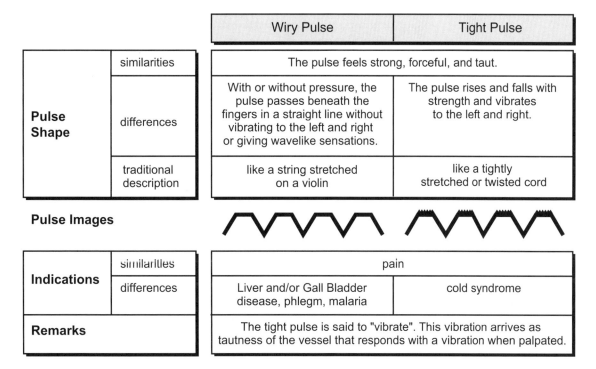

Pulse Shape		Wiry Pulse	Tight Pulse
	similarities	The pulse feels strong, forceful, and taut.	
	differences	With or without pressure, the pulse passes beneath the fingers in a straight line without vibrating to the left and right or giving wavelike sensations.	The pulse rises and falls with strength and vibrates to the left and right.
	traditional description	like a string stretched on a violin	like a tightly stretched or twisted cord

Pulse Images

Indications	similarities	pain	
	differences	Liver and/or Gall Bladder disease, phlegm, malaria	cold syndrome
Remarks		The tight pulse is said to "vibrate". This vibration arrives as tautness of the vessel that responds with a vibration when palpated.	

Table 4.1.45 Comparison of Wiry and Tight Pulses

VII. SOGGY AND FRAIL

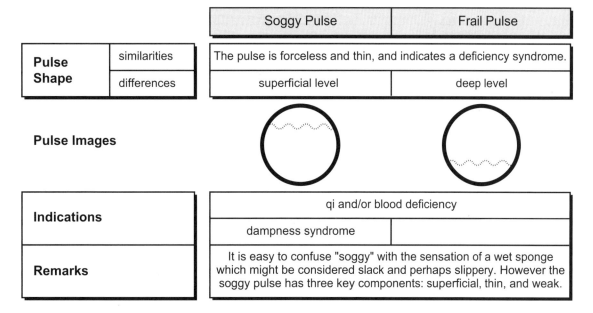

Pulse Shape		Soggy Pulse	Frail Pulse
	similarities	The pulse is forceless and thin, and indicates a deficiency syndrome.	
	differences	superficial level	deep level

Pulse Images

Indications	qi and/or blood deficiency	
	dampness syndrome	
Remarks	It is easy to confuse "soggy" with the sensation of a wet sponge which might be considered slack and perhaps slippery. However the soggy pulse has three key components: superficial, thin, and weak.	

Table 4.1.46 Comparison of Soggy and Frail Pulses

VIII. Submerged, Hidden, Confined

		Submerged	Hidden	Confined
Pulse Shape	similarities	The location is deep.		
	differences	deep	deeper than both submerged and confined	between submerged and hidden in depth, wide, forceful, taut, and long
Pulse Images				
Indications		interior syndrome	obstruction, pain	excess cold, mass, or hernia

Table 4.1.47 Comparison of Submerged, Hidden, and Confined Pulses

IX. Rapid Irregular, Slow Irregular, Consistently Irregular

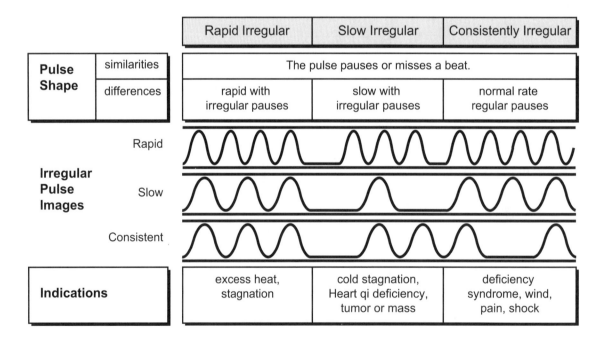

		Rapid Irregular	Slow Irregular	Consistently Irregular
Pulse Shape	similarities	The pulse pauses or misses a beat.		
	differences	rapid with irregular pauses	slow with irregular pauses	normal rate regular pauses
Irregular Pulse Images	Rapid			
	Slow			
	Consistent			
Indications		excess heat, stagnation	cold stagnation, Heart qi deficiency, tumor or mass	deficiency syndrome, wind, pain, shock

Table 4.1.48 Comparison of Rapid, Slow Irregular, and Consistently Irregular Pulses

X. Scattered, Faint, Deficient

		Scattered	Faint	Deficient
Pulse Shape	similarities	All are forceless in strength.		
	differences	vague, difficult to count pulse waves		Forceless on all depths, but vessel is still thick, pulse still feels clear and countable with pressure.
		Superficial without root, it is a vague pulse wave that is uncountable, with an uneven rhythm.	Independent of depth at which it can be felt, it is extremely thin, forceless, vague and uncountable with pressure.	
Pulse Images				
Indications		qi exhaustion, *zàng fǔ* organ failure	severe deficiency	deficiency syndrome
Remarks		This pulse indicates a critical condition.		

Table 4.1.49 Comparison of Scattered, Faint, and Deficient Pulses

■ Six: Female Pulses

Women undergo unique physiological and pathological changes, such as those affected by menstruation, pregnancy, and childbirth. The pulse will reflect changes that arise during these times. In general, in contrast to the male pulse, the female pulse will be thinner, weaker, and slightly faster. In general, the male pulse will be stronger in the distal position and weaker in the proximal position, while the female pulse will be weaker in the distal position and stronger in the proximal position. Other differences are described below.

I. Menstruation Pulse

(1) Premenstrual or During Menstruation

Left hand middle and proximal pulse positions will suddenly feel slippery and full, or stronger than the right hand pulses, but without a bitter taste in the mouth, fever, or abdominal bloating. This suggests that menstruation is either occurring or is imminent.

(2) Irregular Menstruation

The pulse is slightly sluggish or frail in the proximal position but normal in the other two positions.

(3) Amenorrhea

- If the proximal pulse position is deficient, thin, and choppy, it indicates qi and blood deficiency.

- If the pulse is submerged, wiry, and choppy, or the proximal pulse position is slippery and intermittent, it indicates excess.

II. Pregnant Pulse

During pregnancy, the mother's pulses often become slippery and rapid, especially in the proximal position.

III. Antepartum Pulse

Labor and delivery can be predicted when any of the following pulses appear:

- rapid and tight in proximal position

- floating, rapid, and scattered

- deep, thin, and slippery

IV. Fetal Viability Pulse

During pregnancy, the condition of the fetus can also appear in the mother's pulses:

- living fetus: the pulse is deep and surging

- dead fetus: the pulse is sluggish and tight

Section 2

Palpation

Palpation is a diagnostic technique used to understand physiological changes by touching, feeling, pushing, and pressing certain parts of the patient's body in order to find the location, characteristics, and severity of a disease.

■ One: Methods of Body Palpation

I. Methods of Palpation

(1) Touching

The practitioner uses the fingers or palm to lightly touch areas of the patient such as the forehead, limbs, chest, or abdomen. The main purpose is to assess the temperature and moisture of the skin as well as whether the patient is sweating.

The data collected with this method will help distinguish whether the disease resides internally or externally, whether there is sweating, and the condition of the yang qi and body fluids.

(2) Seeking or Stroking

Using fingers to palpate the patient's body with more strength than is used in touching, this method is mainly used in palpating the chest, abdomen, points, and swollen tissues. The purpose is to detect if there is tenderness or swelling, as well as the shape and size of the swelling when applicable.

Information collected with this method will help distinguish the location and the excessive or deficient nature of an illness.

(3) Pressing

Palpation of the patient's body with heavy pressure is used to probe for masses or pain in the deep part of the body or abdomen. Pressing is also used to determine the size, shape, texture, and mobility of palpable masses.

Information collected from this method will provide insight into the condition of the *zàng fǔ* organs and the status of the pathogenic factor(s).

	Touching	**Seeking or Stroking**	**Pressing**
Pressure Force	light	medium	heavy
Depth	skin	flesh and muscles	bones and internal organs
Findings	temperature, moisture, sweating	tenderness, swelling; size and shape of swelling	pain, mass; size, texture, shape, and mobility of mass
Clinical Significance	interior/exterior location of disease, condition of yang qi and body fluids	illness' location and pattern of excess or deficiency	*zàng fǔ* organ's condition and status of pathogen

Table 4.2.1 Touching, Seeking, and Pressing

II. Cautions in the Use of Palpation

- Manual pressure should gradually increase; sudden or rough manipulation should be avoided.

- Warm the hands before touching the patient.

- Observe the patient's changes in expression while pressing.

- Encourage verbal feedback from the patient so that one can quickly determine the location of the patient's pain and/or other sensations brought on by the palpation.

◼ Two: The Scope of Palpation

Palpation of the body includes palpation of the skin, hands and feet, acupuncture points, and the chest and abdomen.

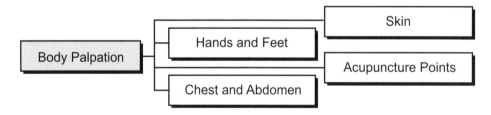

Chart 4.2.1 Scope of Palpation

I. Palpation of the Skin

The purpose of skin palpation is to ascertain whether the skin is cold or hot, moist or dry, swollen or distended. This information further clarifies the nature of pathological change in the body.

(1) Detecting Skin Temperature

Skin temperature reflects the cold and heat in the body. Heat is mainly due to excessive heat while declining yang usually causes cold.

— A. Warm Skin: Yang Excess or Yin Deficiency

Characteristics	Indications
pernicious heat is intense upon initial pressure, but becomes mild after prolonged pressure	exterior heat
pernicious heat is mild upon initial pressure, but becomes intense after prolonged pressure and spreads outward	internal heat
the skin is not hot, but the patient feels hot; or the skin feels hot on heavy pressure when pushing down to the bone	deficiency heat
the skin does not feel hot, but sticky; or the skin feels warmer with prolonged pressure.	damp heat
skin over a blood vessel feels hot with medium pressure, but not with heavy pressure	interior heat in the middle burner or Heart

Table 4.2.2 Warm Skin and its Indications

— B. Cold Skin: Yang Deficiency or Yin Excess

Characteristics	Indications
icy cold hands and feet which extend above the knees and elbows	yang deficiency
icy cold extremities with oily sweating, pale face and feeble pulse	yang collapse
cold extremities, but abdominal temperature is warm or hot	true heat, false cold
cold fingers and toes that are easy to warm up	yang stagnation
skin is not cold, but patient feels cold	exterior cold
cold felt in the loins, lower abdomen and lower back	Kidney yang deficiency

Table 4.2.3 Cold Skin and its Indications

(2) Detecting Moisture and Dryness

The moisture or dryness of the skin reflects the sweating function and the state of the body fluids.

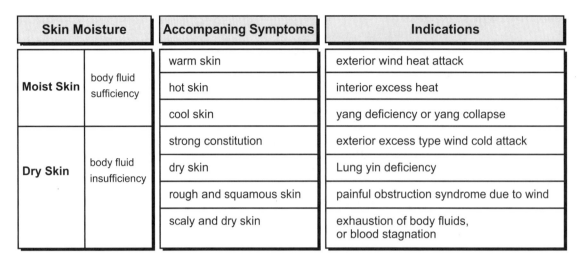

Skin Moisture		Accompanying Symptoms	Indications
Moist Skin	body fluid sufficiency	warm skin	exterior wind heat attack
		hot skin	interior excess heat
		cool skin	yang deficiency or yang collapse
Dry Skin	body fluid insufficiency	strong constitution	exterior excess type wind cold attack
		dry skin	Lung yin deficiency
		rough and squamous skin	painful obstruction syndrome due to wind
		scaly and dry skin	exhaustion of body fluids, or blood stagnation

Table 4.2.4 Skin Moisture and Dryness and its Indications

(3) Detecting Skin Texture

The texture of the skin reflects the condition of the qi and blood.

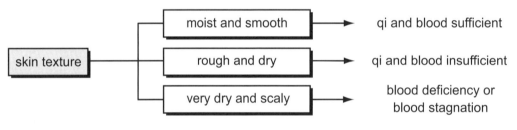

Chart 4.2.2 Skin Texture

(4) Examining Swellings

QI-SWELLING: Pitting is formed when pressed, but returns to normal soon after release of pressure. This indicates local qi stagnation.

EDEMA (WATER-SWELLING): Pitting is formed when pressed, but does not return to normal soon after release of pressure. This indicates dampness or water retention.

(5) Examining Sores or Boils

Sores and boils are palpated to determine if there is pus, and whether its type is yin or yang.

Signs and Symptoms	Indications
swollen and hard, but neither hot nor painful	cold syndrome
swollen, painful, and hot	heat syndrome
sores or boils are flat	deficiency syndrome
swollen with root	excess syndrome
boils or sores are hard upon palpation	no pus
boils or sores are hard on the edges but soft on top	pus formed

Table 4.2.5 Swellings and Boils and their Indications

II. Palpating the Limbs (Hands and Feet)

The four limbs are the terminuses of all the yang channels. The temperature of the hands and feet reflect the state of the yang and qi, as well as the development of disease. The main purpose in palpating the hands and feet is to assess their temperature in order to determine whether the pattern is one of exterior or interior, deficient or excessive, hot or cold.

The temperature of the limbs can also help in making a prognosis. If the limbs are still warm in a yang exhaustion pattern, the patient can survive; otherwise, the prognosis is bad.

Generally speaking, cold hands or feet are associated with a pattern that is caused by yang deficiency and yin predominance; warm or hot hands and feet reflect yin deficiency or yang predominance.

(1) Distinguishing Heat and Cold, Excess and Deficiency

Signs and Symptoms	Indications
hands and feet are cold, sensation of cold can extend above the elbows and knees	Kidney yang deficiency (deficiency cold)
cold only on hands and feet, or to below the elbows and knees	excess cold or qi stagnation
hands and feet are warmer on the dorsum	excess heat
hands and feet are warmer on the palms	deficiency heat

Table 4.2.6 Heat, Cold, Excess, and Deficiency and their Indications

(2) Distinguishing Interior and Exterior

Signs and Symptoms	Indications
dorsal aspect of hands and feet is hotter than the palmar aspect	exterior heat
palmar aspect of hands and feet is hotter than the dorsal aspect	interior heat
forehead is hotter than palm	exterior heat
palm is hotter than forehead	interior heat

Table 4.2.7 Interior and Exterior and their Indications

(3) Palpating the Hands of Children

Signs and Symptoms	Indications
cold finger tips	convulsions
middle finger is hot, but others are normal	wind cold attack
end of middle finger is cold, but others are normal	measles

Table 4.2.8 Children's Hands Palpation and their Indications

III. PALPATING THE CHEST

The chest houses the Heart and Lung. We can assess the condition of these organs by palpating the chest.

Signs and Symptoms	Indications
lifted anterior chest, if accompanied by shortness of breath aggravated by pressure	Lung distention [1]
pain occurs when pressing	water or qi accumulation in chest
chest pain radiates to back, shoulders and medial aspect of arm, pain worse with pressure	chest bì

Table 4.2.9 Palpating the Chest and its Indications

---

1. Lung distention: Retention of pathogenic factors results in stagnation of Lung qi. This manifests as a feeling of oppression over the chest, cough, dyspnea, and pain over the supraclavicular region. In biomedicine, this could be emphysema or pleurisy.

(1) *Xū lǐ* 虚里(Apical Pulse)

In ancient times, palpation of the *xū lǐ* position was the most important diagnostic technique for assessing the condition of the Heart qi.

Location: The the *xū lǐ* position is situated beneath the left breast, between the fourth and fifth ribs, and at the site of the left ventricle apex of the heart where the pulsation of the heart can be felt and sometimes even seen.

Xū lǐ is the region where all the channels meet. It is connected with the great collateral of the Stomach channel, and is the place where the gathering qi gathers.

Clinical significance: Palpating *xū lǐ* can help one assess the condition of the gathering qi, and the deficiency or excess of a disease; it can also help in making a prognosis. It is especially important in serious conditions, e.g., when the pulse cannot be found at the radial artery.

Normal condition: The pulse at *xū lǐ* should be rhythmic, neither rapid nor slow, and with moderate force that can be felt with the fingers. It should have a diameter of 2 to 2.5 cm. This is the sign of abundant Heart qi and gathering qi in the chest.

Physiological variation: The *xū lǐ* pulse may react to certain conditions in the external and internal environments such as shock, fright, panic, anger, exercise, or obesity.

Abnormal condition and indication: The abnormal state of *xū lǐ* can manifest with abnormal findings for strength, rate, and size in the area of the pulsation.

Signs and Symptoms		Indications
Strength of Heartbeat	pulse feels weak beneath the fingers	gathering qi deficiency
	excessively forceful beating that can even be seen through the clothes	gathering qi leaking
	easily distinguished pulse with light pressure, weak pulse with heavy pressure	qi deficiency
	pulse covers a large area with light pressure, but a smaller area with heavy pressure	blood deficiency
	forceful beating that lifts the fingers, with audible sound	Heart and Stomach failure
Rate of Heartbeat	rapid beating with irregularly missed beats	middle burner qi deficiency
	slow beating	Heart yang deficiency
Region of Heartbeat	beating is focused on a small area approximately the width of a fingertip, it is "gathered"	abundant true qi, disease is mild
	"gathered" and forceful beat	extreme heat in exogenous febrile disease or measles eruption
	beating is scattered throughout a large area	deficient *zàng* organ qi
	scattered pulse with rapid beating, lifted chest and shortness of breath	Lung and Heart qi exhaustion

Table 4.2.10 Palpating the Heartbeat at *Xū Lǐ* and its Indications

Signs of heart failure (a critical condition) include a forceful pulse that may actually lift the finger, a forceless pulse that is hard to locate, or a scattered pulse. (The source text for *xū lǐ* is *Basic Questions*, Chapter 18 (素問。平人氣象論).)

IV. PALPATING THE HYPOCHONDRIUM

The hypochondrium is located bilaterally on the sides of the chest from the axillary fossa to the costal margin (see Illustration 4.2.1). The right hypochondrium houses the Liver and Gallbladder. The Liver channel passes through the hypochondrium bilaterally. Palpating the hypochondrium will help assess the condition of the Liver and Gallbladder.

(1) Distention and Pain

Signs and Symptoms	Indications
distending pain in the hypochondrium radiates bilaterally to the lower abdomen	Liver qi stagnation
pain is aggravated by pressure and is hot to the touch	Liver fire
swollen red skin is tender and resistant to touch or pressure	Liver abscess
pain alleviated by pressure	Liver deficiency
sensation of fullness and distention below costal margin	*shào yáng* pattern

Table 4.2.11 Distention and Pain and their Indications

(2) Lumps and Masses

Signs and Symptoms	Indications
lump found below costal margin, with stabbing pain	blood stasis
fluid may be audible when pressed	fluid retention

Table 4.2.12 Lumps and Masses and their Indications

V. PALPATING THE ABDOMEN

Palpation of the epigastrium and abdomen is performed to assess the temperature and texture of the abdomen, and to locate any distention, pain, or masses in the abdominal area. The information collected from this examination will assist the practitioner in distinguishing the location and thermal nature of the pathological change. It also provides insight into the condition of the *zàng fǔ* organs.

(1) Abdominal Divisions

According to traditional Chinese medical theory, the abdomen can be divided into six areas.

Upper abdomen: This includes the region between the xiphoid process and umbilicus (areas 1, 2, and 3).

Epigastrium: In the upper abdomen, the upper half of the stomach region is also called the epigastrium (areas 1 and 2).

Big abdomen: The lower part of the upper abdomen is called "bigger abdomen" (area 3).

Lower abdomen: The abdomen below the level of the ASIS (areas 4 and 5).

Little abdomen: In the central area of the lower abdomen, also called the central lower abdomen (area 4).

Junior abdomen or lateral lower abdomen: The lateral areas of the lower abdomen (area 5).

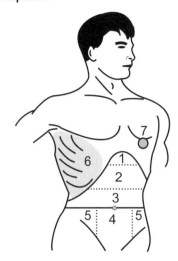

1. Heart
1 + 2. epigastrium
1 + 2 + 3. upper abdomen
3. big abdomen
4 + 5. lower abdomen
4. little (*xiǎo*) abdomen
5. lateral (*shào*) abdomen
6. hypochondrium
7. *xū lǐ*

Illustration 4.2.1 Abdominal Divisions and *Xū Lǐ*

(2) Abdominal Divisions Correspond to the *Zàng Fǔ* Organs

In the abdominal divisions shown above, each area reflects a unique *zàng fǔ* organ.

Abdominal Area	Zang Fu Organ
epigastrium (areas 1 + 2)	Stomach
big abdomen (area 3)	Spleen
area around umbilicus	Small Intestine
little abdomen, area under umbilicus (area 4)	Urinary Bladder, uterus
junior abdomen or lateral lower abdomen (area 5)	blood chamber (ovaries and uterus)

Table 4.2.13 Abdominal Divisions

(3) Palpation and Indications

Parameter	Signs and Symptoms	Indications
Temperature	cold with desire for warmth	cold syndrome
	hot with desire for cold	heat syndrome
Texture	soft and flaccid epigastrium	Stomach and Spleen deficiency
	soft and flaccid lower abdomen	Spleen and Kidney deficiency
	hard and tense (tight) abdomen	excess syndrome
Pain	pain aggravated by pressure	excess syndrome
	pain alleviated by pressure	deficiency syndrome
Masses	fixed and immovable, associated with pain	blood stasis
	come and go, no fixed location, movable	qi stagnation

Table 4.2.14 Palpation and Indications

VI. Palpating the Acupuncture Points

Pressing the acupuncture points and observing objective or subjective reactions is useful for detecting pathological changes in the *zàng fǔ* organs.

Acupoints are places where the qi passes, hence diseases in the interior often manifest with sensitivity to pressure at specific points.

The main pathological changes found at these acupoints are pain, hypersensitivity, sensitive skin, and hardened nodules or cord-like nodules beneath the skin.

Generally speaking, any point can be used in diagnosis. However, certain points are particularly useful in diagnosis. These points are listed in the table below.

Organ	Transport Point	Alarm Point	Source Point	Lower Sea Point	Ashi and Other Points
Lung	BL-13	LU-1	LU-9		BL-43, ST-14, ST-13, ST-16, GB-22, CV-18
Heart	BL-15	CV-14	HT-7		CV-17
Liver	BL-18	LR-14	LR-3		
Spleen	BL-20	LR-13	SP-3		KI-18, CV-19, ST-21
Kidney	BL-23	GB-25	KI-3		BL-53, CV-6, *dān tián*
Large Intestine	BL-25	ST-25	LI-4	ST-37	
Small Intestine	BL-27	CV-4	SI-4	ST-39	
Gall Bladder	BL-19	GB-24	GB-40	GB-34	M-LE-23 *(dán náng xuè)*
Stomach	BL-21	CV-12	ST-42	ST-36	ST-20, KI-17
Urinary Bladder	BL-28	CV-3	BL-64	BL-40	
Appendix					M-LE-13 *(lán wěi xué)*
Reproductive System					BL-31, BL-32, BL-33, BL-34

Table 4.2.15 Palpation of Acupuncture Points

Section 3

Questions and Answers for Deeper Insight into Palpation

1. What is the difference between the pulse, pulse examination, and pulse quality?

The pulse is the rhythmic throbbing of the arteries produced by the regular contractions of the heart. The Chinese character for pulse (脈 *mài*) in ancient times was written as: 𧘂 This character's literal meaning suggests a riverbed within flesh.

Pulse examination (脈診 *mài zhěn*) is a diagnostic method whereby the practitioner places her fingers on the patient's radial artery. This allows the practitioner to inspect the pulse quality or image (脈象 *mài xiàng*) in order to distinguish the different physiological and pathological states of the patient.

Pulse image may also be translated as pulse quality. It is the image or quality of the patient's pulse beating beneath the fingers of the practitioner. It is the combined manifestation of the pulse rate, rhythm, shape, position, width, strength, etc. Since it is felt and interpreted by the practitioner's fingers, the ascertained pulse quality can vary among practitioners.

Summary: *Pulse* is the actual force and substance passing through the arteries of the patient. *Pulse examination* is the diagnostic activity of the practitioner. *Pulse quality* is the perception of the pulse formed by the practitioner when she assesses the pulse of the patient.

2. What are the components of the pulse quality?

The pulse quality is the feeling of the pulse beating beneath the fingers. The formation of the pulse quality is most directly related to the contraction of the Heart. The pulse quality is also related to the condition of the Heart qi, blood vessels, and volume of qi and blood. The blood vessels connect the entire body and the qi and blood circulate continuously inside of them. The blood vessels enter the *zàng fǔ* organs internally and reach the limbs and skin externally. Only through the blood vessels can the qi of the *zàng fǔ* organs perform their functions throughout all parts of the body. Hence the pulse quality will reflect the functions of the *zàng fǔ* organs, the condition of qi and blood, and the state of yin and yang.

In particular, the pulse quality is generated by the following factors:

(1) Heart and blood vessels are the key organs involved with the formation of the pulse quality. The contractions of the Heart are the most obvious sign of life and vitality in the body, and they are the power behind the formation of the pulse quality. The rate of the pulse is not only correlated with the Heart's contraction and rhythm, but is also affected by the Heart qi and blood. Heart blood and Heart yin together form the material basis of the Heart's physiological activities. Heart qi and Heart

yang represent the state of the Heart functions. When Heart qi is exuberant and Heart blood is abundant, Heart yin and Heart yang are balanced and harmonized. The Heart's contractions will be gentle, but with adequate strength and an even rhythm. Therefore, the pulse quality will be gentle, with adequate force, and have an appropriate rate with a regular rhythm.

The Heart governs the blood and blood vessels. The blood vessels house the blood. Qi and blood circulate inside the blood vessels. The blood vessels and Heart are not only connected to each other structurally to form the circulatory system, but are also functionally coordinated as well. In *The Divine Pivot* (靈樞) it is written: "[The vessels] are like a dam that protects the qi and blood from running freely about [the body]"

The blood vessels are not only a necessary pathway for the circulation of qi and blood; they also contain the qi and blood within the vessels, and push the qi and blood throughout the body.

(2) Qi and blood are the material basis in the formation of a pulse quality.

The substance of the pulse is the blood, and the power of the pulse is the qi. Qi plays the greatest role in the formation of the pulse quality. As a function of Heart qi and gathering qi (宗氣 *zōng qì*), the Heart's contractions pump blood into the blood vessels to form the pulse.

(3) Other organs and pulse quality formation

Pulse quality formation is not only related to the Heart, blood vessels, qi and blood, but also to the functions of other organs.

The Lungs govern the qi and respiration. Qi has the function of pushing, controlling, and regulating the blood. The Lungs govern qi and respiration, therefore the Lungs are an important factor in the production of the pulse.

When one's breathing is calm, the pulse is gentle and calm. When breathing is rapid, the rate of the pulse beat increases. Pulse beats follow the breath continuously until the breath stops, at which time the heartbeat will stop as well. The Lungs have the function of gathering the channels and blood vessels, so the Lung qi is closely related to the blood vessels. When breathing is smooth and deep, the pulse quality will be smooth and have a healthy force. When the breathing is shallow and rapid, or there is difficult breathing due to Lung qi accumulation, then the pulse quality will be thin and choppy. In brief, the Lung qi has a significant effect on the rate and shape of the pulse quality.

The generation of qi and blood depends on the transportive and transformative functions of the Spleen and Stomach. Spleen qi also controls the blood to keep it inside the blood vessels. The condition of the qi and blood and the sufficiency of food essence can manifest on the pulse as the Stomach qi.* The Stomach qi of the pulse directly reflects the status of the body's vital substances. A pulse quality that is full of Stomach qi represents a normal and healthy pulse, while one that lacks Stomach qi is a pathological pulse. When the pulse completely lacks Stomach qi, this is a death pulse. Stomach qi is the foundation of the pulse.

The Liver stores the blood and regulates the amount of blood in circulation. It also ensures the smooth flow of qi. When Liver function is impaired, it can have an effect on the circulation of qi and blood and accordingly cause pathological changes in the pulse quality.

---

* In pulse diagnosis, the presence of Stomach qi refers to a gentle harmonious pulse quality, while in internal medicine, Stomach qi refers to the function of the *fŭ* organ called the Stomach.

The Kidney stores the essence, which is transformed into source qi, providing the foundation for all the yin and yang energies of the body. Essence can transform into blood. It is one of the basic materials involved in the production of blood. Essence can also transform into qi. It is the root of yang qi and the source for all energy in the body. When the Kidney qi is sufficient, the pulse quality will have root.

3. What is the relationship among qi, blood, and the pulse quality?

The pulse arises mainly from the flow of qi and blood in the blood vessels. A smooth flow of sufficient qi and blood in the vessels gives rise to a normal pulse. When the flow of qi and blood in the vessels is abnormal or insufficient, a pathological pulse quality will be formed.

Qi and blood play different roles in the generation of the pulse. Blood is the substance of the pulse and qi is the power of the pulse. Qi pertains to yang which governs movement, while blood pertains to yin, which functions to fill the blood vessels.

When qi is deficient, it will fail to move the blood and the pulse will become forceless, or even choppy if the movement of blood is not smooth. When there is blood deficiency, the blood vessels will not be filled and the pulse quality will be felt as thin or hollow.

Qi and blood are the basic building blocks of the pulse. Qi plays a major role in the formation of the pulse quality.

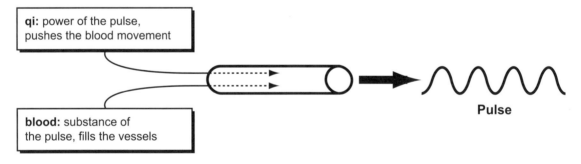

qi: power of the pulse, pushes the blood movement

blood: substance of the pulse, fills the vessels

Pulse

Chart 4.3.1 Relationship among Qi, Blood, and the Pulse Quality

4. How is it that the location of the pulse on the radial artery can reflect pathological changes and conditions in all the *zàng fǔ* organs? And why is it that we use this pulse location for diagnosis?

The location of the radial artery is called inch pass or gate (寸口 *cùn kǒu*). It is also known as the gate or pass of the vessels, channels, and collaterals (脈口 *mài kǒu*) or the gate or pass of qi (氣口 *qì kǒu*). It is located on the medial aspect of the forearm's radial artery. *Cùn kǒu* reflects the functional state of the *zàng fǔ* organs for the following reasons:

(1) The hand *tài yīn* Lung channel passes through the radial artery. The Lung governs the qi of the entire body and "gathers the hundred vessels and channels."* The circulation of qi and blood begins and ends at the Lungs. The radial artery is where the qi and blood accumulate. The location of *cùn kǒu* is a gathering point for the arteries and veins, thus the functional states of the five *zàng* and the six *fǔ* organs are manifested in the Lung. *Classic of Difficulties –First Question* (難經。一難) notes: "There are arteries on all twelve channels, why do we use only the radial artery to assess the condition of the five *zàng* and six *fǔ*? Because the *cùn kǒu* is the location where all channels and blood vessels accumulate, and it is the artery on the hand *tài yīn* [Lung] channel."

(2) The Lung channel starts in the middle burner where the Spleen and Stomach are located. The Spleen and Stomach provide the acquired root of human life. They are the source for the production of qi and blood. The Spleen and Lung are both *tài yīn;* thus the Lung channel communicates with the Spleen and Stomach channels in the middle burner. Because of this connection to the acquired root of life, the quality of qi and blood in the five *zàng* and six *fǔ* organs can be reflected at the pulse location on the radial artery.

Basic Questions, Chapter 11 (素問。五臟別論) asks: "How can the radial artery reflect the condition of the five *zàng*? Because the Stomach is the sea of food and the grand source of all five *zàng* and six *fǔ*, when food of the five flavors enters the mouth, it is stored in the Stomach to supply the five *zàng* with qi. *Qì kōu* [*cùn kǒu*] pertains to *tài yīn*, thus the qi of all five *zàng* and six *fǔ* comes from the Stomach and is manifest in the *qì kōu*."

(3) There are other reasons to use the radial artery to check the pulse. The artery is obvious and easy to assess. It is covered by only a thin layer of tissue, which makes the arterial pulse clear and easy to find.

It is very convenient to check the pulse at the radial artery. The patient needn't remove any clothing, and the practitioner needn't touch the patient on other, less accessible or uncomfortable parts of their body, such as the carotid artery or the dorsal artery of the foot.

Compared with other pulse locations, such as the carotid artery (at ST-9 *rén yíng*) and the dorsal artery (at ST-42 *chōng yáng*), the distance to the Heart is well situated. At the carotid artery, the force of the pulse is much stronger than the volume of blood, while at the dorsal artery point on the foot, the force of the pulse is much weaker than the volume of blood. Only at the point on the radial artery is the force of the pulse about equal to the amount of blood in circulation, hence a more accurate reading of the body's qi and blood is possible.

---

*"Gathers the hundred vessels and channels" is a statement of fact that essentially says that all of the arteries (and channels) of the body pass through or connect with the Lung.

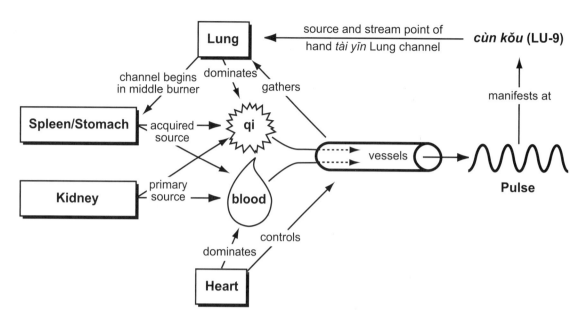

Chart 4.3.2 *Zàng* Organ Relationship to Pulse Formation

5. What is the procedure for pulse examination?

There are three steps in performing a complete examination of the pulse. First, assess the pulse quality; second, determine the pulse position; and third, evaluate the severity of morbidity of the pulse.

The pulse quality is comprised of four parameters: depth, rate, shape, and strength. If one is very clear about these parameters, one can obtain a complete understanding of the twenty-eight morbid pulse qualities.

Depth (位 *wèi*): This refers to the depth of the pulse. Depth is described as superficial (heaven 天 *tiān*), middle (human 人 *rén*), and deep (earth 地 *dì*). When the pulse is easily felt by touching at the superficial depth, and its force decreases as the fingers press more deeply, this is a floating pulse. A pulse that can only be felt by seeking is called a submerged pulse. This parameter is helpful for locating the location of the disease as well as for differentiating deficiency and excess.

Rate (律 *lù*): The pulse rate and rhythm is the number of beats per breath or per minute, which is how we can assess the slow, rapid, moderate, racing, slow irregular, rapid irregular, and consistently irregular pulse qualities. A normal pulse rate is four beats per breath (60–90 beats per minute). A rapid pulse is one that beats more than five times per breath (90+ bpm). A pulse rate that is less than three times per breath (<60 bpm), is called a slow pulse.

Shape (形 *xíng*): Shape includes the width, length, and tension of the pulse. This wave form or contour of the pulse depends on the condition of the blood vessel and of the the blood circulation. If the width of the blood vessel is smaller than normal, it is either a thin or faint pulse; when the diameter is larger than normal, it is either a large or flooding pulse. If the tension of the blood vessel is very taut, it is either a wiry or tight pulse. If the tension of the blood vessel is slack, it is either a frail or soggy pulse. If the blood circulation is smooth, the pulse is slippery. When blood circulation is stagnated, the pulse will feel rough and is called a choppy pulse.

Strength (勢 *shi*): This refers to the movement and force of the pulse. If the pulse is forceless, it is called a deficient pulse. If the pulse is forceful, this is called an excessive pulse.

The second step in pulse examination is determining its position: Where is the morbid pulse most evident? It is this position that is used to determine which organ or which of the three burners is suffering from the morbidity described by the previous components.

The third step in pulse examination is assessing the degree of morbidity. We define morbidity as mild or severe, from which we infer the seriousness of a disease. Clinically speaking, this is the difference between a pulse that is slightly thin or very thin; slightly forceless or very forceless; slightly slippery or very slippery.

To review, the first step in examining the pulse tells us *what* the morbidity is. The second step describes *where* the morbidity can be found. And the third step tells us *how* serious or intense is the morbidity.

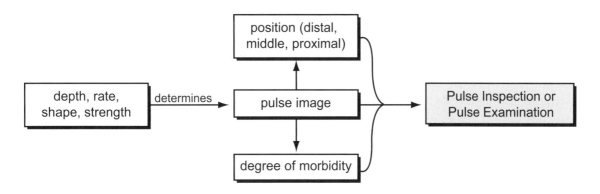

Chart 4.3.3 Pulse Examination Components

6. How do seasonal changes affect the pulse quality, and what are the mechanisms behind these changes?

According to the holistic theories of TCM, there is a correlation between nature on the one hand, and the human body and its physiology on the other. As the seasons change, so does the quality of the pulse.

During the spring, the weather begins to warm up, yang qi begins to increase, and all things on earth begin to grow. The springtime is yang within yin; as such, there is still some coldness remaining from the winter . Cold causes the blood vessels to contract and increase in tension, and the growth of yang qi causes the qi and blood to expand. This expansion presses against the restraining action of the cold on the blood vessels, which causes the hard tension of the wiry pulse, which is associated with springtime.

During the summer, the weather is hot and the yang qi is excessive. This is yang within yang. All things on earth are full of vigor and vitality. The human body is influenced by this as well. The skin and muscles loosen and the blood vessels dilate. The excessive yang qi of the summer strongly pushes the qi and blood inside the blood vessels, and thus the normal pulse quality during the summer will tend toward a flooding pulse quality.

During the autumn, the predominant qi is dryness. The weather is getting colder and the yang qi is decreasing. The vigor and vitality of all things on earth begin to weaken and decline. The power of the pulse also decreases, but there is still some heat remaining from the summer, and so all that is palpable is the floating portion of the wave form. With force, the heat of summer causes a flooding pulse; without force, the heat of summer causes a floating pulse. Autumn is a time of declining force. This is yin within yang.

Winter is the coldest time of the year. This is yin within yin. All things on earth tend toward storage and hiding. Affected by the weather, human physiology will likewise reflect this storage and hiding of the yang qi deep within the body. Since the yang qi governs the pulse, the normal pulse quality in winter will be deeper than in other seasons.

7. Why is the morning the best time to examine the pulse? How should the pulse be inspected at other times of the day?

The yang qi is the precursor to defensive qi and is the force behind antipathogenic qi. It is movable in nature and is thus prone to be disturbed by physical or emotional activity. The yang qi is also the force of the pulse, so when the yang qi is disturbed, it can readily affect the quality of the pulse.

In the morning, the yang qi is just rising and the yin has not become stirred. Both the external and internal environments of the body are in a calm and quiet state. The qi and blood have not been disturbed. At this time, the pulse quality will reflect the true physiological state, including its pathological changes.

Basic Questions, Chapter 17 (素問。脈要精微) notes: "Pulse taking should be carried out in the morning. At this time, the yin has not stirred and the yang has not acted, food has not been taken, and the channels have not yet been filled up. The circulation within the collaterals remains smooth, the qi and blood have not been disturbed, and thus morbid change is easy to recognize."

When examining the pulse at other times of the day, the patient should sit or lie in a quiet and calm environment. The patient should rest and calm down both physically and emotionally before the pulse is examined.

8. Why is it said that the patient will live if the pulse quality has Stomach qi and will die if the pulse quality lacks Stomach qi?

In *Basic Questions*, Chapter 18 (素問。平人氣象論) it is written: "The pulse of the healthy person is endowed with Stomach qi. The Stomach qi is the normal pulse qi of the healthy person. If one's pulse has no Stomach qi, it is unfavorable, and the patient will die."

There are five criteria involved in assessing the Stomach qi in the pulse quality: (1) depth: the pulse appears at the middle depth, neither floating nor deep; (2) rate: the pulse is neither rapid nor slow; (3) strength: the force of the pulse is neither too strong nor weak; (4) width: the blood vessel is neither too wide nor too thin; (5) strength and shape: the pulse is gentle, mild, calm, and regular.

No matter what physiological or pathological differences in the pulse, if the pulse quality is gentle, mild, and smooth, and the blood vessel has elasticity, it indicates the presence of Stomach qi.

Stomach qi represents the physiological functions of the Stomach and Spleen in the middle burner, including all of the functions of the digestive system. It is the motive force for the generation of nutritive substances (qi and blood) and it is the acquired root of the human body. The body that is full of Stomach qi will live well; the body with little Stomach qi will be ill; and the body with no Stomach qi will die.

As we know, blood is the substance of the pulse and qi is the power of the pulse. Stomach qi is the foundation of the pulse quality. When the Stomach qi is full, it can generate sufficient qi and blood, thus the beating of the pulse is calm, gentle, and steady, with a regular rhythm and moderate strength. It is a sign of health.

During an illness, even though the Stomach qi may be deficient, as long as it still exists it will be able to produce qi and blood and keep the antipathogenic qi strong. As a result, the prognosis will usually be favorable.

When the pulse quality lacks Stomach qi, it means that the acquired root function of the Stomach and Spleen are failing, and thus the qi and blood will not be able to regenerate, leading to the exhaustion of antipathogenic qi and therefore a poor prognosis.

9. What does it mean to say that the pulse quality should have spirit (神 *shén*)?

The pulse that beats with moderate strength and a unified rhythm in a supple blood vessel is considered to have spirit. There are two criteria used to assess spirit in the pulse: (1) strength: the pulse beating beneath the fingers is strong, but remains gentle; and (2) rhythm: the pulse beats with a regular rhythm.

The Heart governs the blood and houses the spirit; the blood vessels house the blood. Spirit is the external expression of human vital activity. While qi and blood are abundant, the Heart spirit is vigorous and healthy. Heart contractions will have strength and an even rhythm, and the pulse beating beneath the fingers will therefore have moderate force and a regular rhythm. The spirit of a pulse quality reflects the Heart's spirit, which manifests in the vitality of the qi and blood.

The Heart is the major organ that reflects the spirit of the pulse, but other organs such as the Kidney, Liver, Lung, Stomach, and Spleen also play important parts in the formation of pulse spirit.

In some of the morbid pulse qualities, such as the faint pulse, frail pulse, and soggy pulse, the pulse beneath the fingers is very weak or forceless. However, a gentle pulse still can be felt in a supple blood vessel. This indicates that the pulse quality still has spirit. In some of the pulse qualities, such as the wiry pulse, or the tight pulse, the blood vessel feels very taut or tight, but the pulse still has a gentle and supple feeling. This too indicates that the pulse quality still has spirit.

10. What is meant by "root" (根 *gēn*) of the pulse and what is its clinical significance?

The pulse quality with root is defined by two statements from the classics. The first says that the pulse with root can simply be felt in the proximal position. Two texts support this definition. The *Classic of Difficulties -- The Fourteenth Question* (難經。十四難) says: "The importance of the proximal portion of the pulse is just like that of the root of a tree. Although the leaves fade, the tree can live if the roots exist." While the pulse quality has root, the antipathogenic qi still exists, and so the patient can survive. The other text, the *Pulse Classic* (脈經) by Wang Shu-He, notes: "Even though the pulse is not felt in the distal and middle positions, if it can be felt at the proximal position, then we needn't worry about the patient dying."

The second definition of a pulse with root is one that can be felt at the deep depth of the *distal* and *middle* positions. Since the Kidney is the congenital root of the body and the fundamental resource of the source qi, the Kidney is to the body as the root is to the living tree. For this reason, the deep depth at any of the three positions of the pulse can be considered to reflect the health of the Kidney.

Based on these two definitions of root, a pulse that is easily felt at the deep depth of the distal and middle position, or any depth at the proximal position is considered to have root.

In the clinic, assessing the pulse quality for root can help to make a prognosis. Kidney qi is the congenital root of the body and the energetic resource for all the functional activities of the body. When the pulse quality has root, it means that the Kidney qi is abundant, and that the antipathogenic qi is sufficient and full of vitality. Even in severe illness, no matter what the morbid pulse quality, if the pulse quality is detectable with moderate to forceful pressing in at least the proximal position, then the disease can be cured. If the pulse disappears in the deep depth upon forceful pressing, or if it is forceless or indistinguishable in the proximal position, this is a pulse quality without root and the disease is critical.

11. What is the relationship in the pulse quality between the Stomach qi, spirit, and root?

The Stomach qi, spirit, and root in the pulse quality are closely related. All of them reflect the internal states of the qi, blood, essence, and spirit of the body. A gentle, mild, smooth, and stable pulse reflects healthy Stomach and Spleen functions. A moderately forceful pulse with regular rhythm in a supple blood vessel is considered to be full of spirit. It reflects abundant qi and blood as well as a good condition of the Heart. When the pulse is perceptible at the deep depth or in the proximal position it means that the pulse has root, which indicates sufficient Kidney essence and qi.

Overall, the presence of Stomach qi, spirit, and root in the pulse quality arise from different aspects of the mechanisms that create the pulse. The three aspects mutually complement and support each other. If the pulse quality lacks Stomach qi, it will lose spirit or root as well. Likewise with the other two: when one is missing, the other two will soon follow (see Table 4.1.4).

12. What are the major physiological variations for the normal pulse quality in an individual?

The first of two normal variations of the pulse deals with the location of the radial artery. Instead of being found in the usual *cùn kǒu* position located medial to the radius and roughly along the trajectory of the Lung channel, it is found elsewhere. Translating these normal deviations from Chinese, we have the "deviated angle pulse" and the "opposite middle pulse." In both cases, the radial artery bends away from the Lung channel to the dorsal side of the radius, closer to the Large Intestine channel. While the deep radial branch may remain palpable deeply in its usual *cùn kǒu* location, this is not the radial artery that is usually palpated there, and this can cause false findings of weak and deep qualities if the main radial artery is located closer to the Large Intestine channel.

Again, these are physiological variations and so do not indicate any particular pathology. It is, however, difficult to access the depth of the pulse when it is found atop the radius and thus examining the depth of a pulse should be avoided if this type of artery is found in a patient.

The second physiological variation deals with the pulse quality. Some people have pulse qualities that reflect a unique constitutional makeup that doesn't change over the course of their life. It does not indicate a pathological process; they were simply born this way. One of these physiological pulse quality variations is called the "six yang pulses." In this case, all six positions (distal, middle, and proximal on both the left and right sides) are flooding and large. In the other case, called "six yin pulses," all six positions are deep and thin. In both of these cases, these pulses do not indicate any particular illness.

13. How are the 28 pulses organized into six categories of pulses (六綱脈 *lìu gāng mài*)?

The "six categories of pulses" is the guiding principle used to classify and sort the pulse qualities based on similar features. The twenty-eight pathological pulse qualities are grouped into six categories for easy organization. These categories are superficial and deep, fast and slow, forceful and forceless.

Superficial Pulses		
The pulse is felt easily with a light touch but disappears with pressure.		
Pulse Name	**Pulse Characteristics**	**Indications**
浮 floating (*fú mài*)	easily felt with a light touch, grows faint when pressing deeper	exterior syndrome, yin deficiency
洪 flooding (*hóng mài*)	superficial, wide, and forceful upon arrival and gentle on departure	excessive heat
濡 soggy (*rú mài*)	superficial, thin, and forceless	deficiency or dampness
革 leather (*gé mài*)	superficial, wide, hollow, and taut giving the feeling of a drum skin	internal bleeding, essence deficiency
芤 hollow (*kōu mài*)	superficial, wide, forceless with a sense of emptiness when pressing lightly, like pressing on a green onion stalk	internal hemorrhage, yin collapse
散 scattered (*sàn mài*)	superficial, rootless, scattered, wide, uncountable, uneven in rhythm showing no sign of pause between pulsations	source qi collapse

Table 4.3.1 Superficial Pulses and their Indications

Deep Pulses

The pulse is distinct only with pressure.

	Pulse Name	Pulse Characteristics	Indications
沉	submerged (*chén mài*)	pulse can barely be felt with light touching, distinct only with heavy pressure	interior syndrome, or interior stagnation
伏	hidden (*fú mài*)	deeper than deep, found by pressing down to the bone where it is thin, forceless, and barely felt	syncope or excruciating pain
弱	frail (*ruò mài*)	deep, thin, and forceless, the pulse hits the fingers without strength	qi and blood deficiency
牢	confined (*láo mài*)	felt only at the deep level, stable, forceful, wide, taut, long	excess cold accumulation or hernia

Table 4.3.2 Deep Pulses and their Indications

Fast Pulses

The pulse rate is fast, more than five beats per breath or 90 beats per minute.

	Pulse Name	Pulse Characteristics	Indications
數	rapid (*shuò mài*)	pulse rate is fast, more than five beats per breath or ninety beats per minute	heat syndromes
促	rapid irregular (*cù mài*)	rapid with irregularly missed beats	yang excess, extreme heat; qi, blood, phlegm or food stagnation
疾	racing (*jí mài*)	pulse rate is very fast, seven to eight beats per breath or 140 to 180 beats per minute	hyperactivity of yang with exhaustion of yin, or source qi collapse
動	moving (*dòng mài*)	pulse is short and feels like beans spinning within the artery, rapid and forceful	pain or fright

Table 4.3.3 Fast Pulses and their Indications

Slow Pulses

The pulse rate feels slow, or less than four beats per breath or 60 beats per minute.

	Pulse Name	Pulse Characteristics	Indications
遲	slow (*chí mài*)	pulse rate is slow, less than four beats per breath or sixty beats per minute	cold syndromes
緩	moderate (*huǎn mài*)	slightly faster than the slow pulse, but still maintaining a retarded or sluggish feeling	dampness or spleen deficiency
澀	choppy (*sè mài*)	pulse arrives and departs unsmoothly giving an uneven or rough feeling	qi and blood stagnation, or essence deficiency
結	slow irregular (*jié mài*)	slow with irregularly missed beats	qi stagnation due to excess yin; blood stasis, phlegm

Table 4.3.4 Slow Pulses and their Indications

Forceful Pulses

The pulse is forceful with both light and heavy pressure.

	Pulse Name	Pulse Characteristics	Indications
實	excessive (*shí mài*)	forceful at all three positions and all three depths	excess syndromes
滑	slippery (*huá mài*)	pulse arrives and departs smoothly	phlegm or damp retention, food stagnation, excess heat
緊	tight (*jǐn mài*)	taut and forceful like a stretched twisted rope that vibrates left and right	cold syndrome or pain
弦	wiry (*xián mài*)	straight and long, like the string of a musical instrument	Liver and/or Gallbladder disorder, phlegm, pain or malaria

Table 4.3.5 Forceful Pulses and their Indications

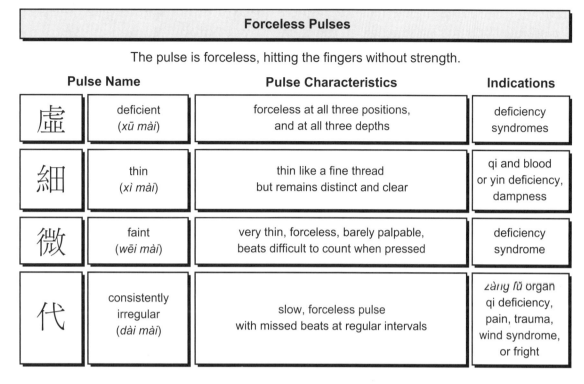

Forceless Pulses

The pulse is forceless, hitting the fingers without strength.

Pulse Name		Pulse Characteristics	Indications
虛	deficient (xū mài)	forceless at all three positions, and at all three depths	deficiency syndromes
細	thin (xì mài)	thin like a fine thread but remains distinct and clear	qi and blood or yin deficiency, dampness
微	faint (wēi mài)	very thin, forceless, barely palpable, beats difficult to count when pressed	deficiency syndrome
代	consistently irregular (dài mài)	slow, forceless pulse with missed beats at regular intervals	zàng fǔ organ qi deficiency, pain, trauma, wind syndrome, or fright

Table 4.3.6 Forceless Pulses and their Indications

14. Which pulse qualities not only indicate pathological change, but can also arise in a healthy person?

Floating, deep, slippery, wiry, thin, slow, and flooding pulses are all common pulse qualities that are frequently seen in the clinic. As we know, the floating pulse indicates an exterior pattern; the deep pulse indicates an interior pattern; the slippery pulse indicates the presence of phlegm, food retention, or excess heat patterns; the wiry pulse indicates dysfunction of the liver, and pain; the thready pulse indicates deficiency or dampness; the flooding pulse indicates excess heat in the qi level; and the slow pulse indicates a pattern of cold.

However, these pulse qualities do not only reflect the presence of illness; they can also appear in a healthy person. The physiological (normal) pulse can be affected by the age, gender, constitution, and season. In the clinic, we should carefully distinguish these physiological variations. For example, during the fall, the pulse quality can be slightly floating; a skinny person's pulse might also be slightly floating. During the winter, the pulse quality will be slightly deep; a heavy person's pulse may also be found at the deep depth. A young person's pulse quality is usually slightly slippery, which is also the case for pregnant women. During the spring, the pulse quality will be slightly wiry; an elderly person's pulse may also be slightly wiry. The pulse qualities in women and children tend to be thinner than those of the adult male. During the summer, the pulse will be slightly flooding. An athlete's pulse is commonly slow.

There are two criteria used to determine that a pulse quality does not indicate pathological change: (1) the pulse quality is full of Stomach qi, spirit, and root; (2) there are no other clinical signs or symptoms.

15. Why does the floating pulse not just reflect the presence of an exterior pattern, and why does the deep pulse not just reflect the presence of an interior pattern?

When exogenous pathogens attack the body, the antipathogenic qi rises against the pathogens. The yang pushes the qi and blood to the exterior; therefore the pulse is mostly felt at the superficial depth. Thus, the floating pulse usually indicates the presence of an exterior pattern, in which case it is most often floating and forceful.

However, the floating pulse may also be seen where there are yin deficiency patterns or in critical cases of declining yang. If the yin is deficient such that it cannot contain the yang, or the yang is too weak to match the yin, the yang will float to the body's surface. The pulse quality becomes floating without strength. In chronic endogenous diseases, the floating pulse is a critical portent of the exhaustion of antipathogenic qi. In *Lakeside Study of the Pulse* (瀕湖脈學), Li Shi-Zhen (李時珍) noted that "one should be very cautious when the patient with chronic illness appears with a floating pulse." Thus, although the floating pulse generally indicates an exterior pattern, it can also describe a floating yang condition.

When the antipathogenic qi is deficient, or when pathogenic factors obstruct the qi and blood, the qi and blood are prevented from rising to the surface to fight pathogens. The pulse is accordingly deep. This usually indicates an interior pattern. Deep and forceless qualities indicate a pattern of interior deficiency, while deep and forceful qualities indicate a pattern of interior excess.

However, a deep pulse also can be seen in an exterior pattern. When exogenous cold attacks the body surface, it impairs the opening and closing of the pores. Cold is characterized by contraction and stagnation, thus spasmodic contraction of the channels and blood vessels and impaired circulation of qi and blood can result. Qi and blood cannot rise to the surface of the body and so the pulse may appear at the deep level.

Thus, while a deep pulse generally indicates the presence of an interior pattern, it can also arise with an exterior pattern.

16. If the exterior heat pattern gives rise to a floating and rapid pulse quality, why then does an exterior cold pattern give rise to floating and tight qualities, rather than floating and slow?

The floating pulse reflects the presence of an exterior pattern and the rapid pulse reflects a heat pattern, so it is easy to understand how an exterior heat pattern can give rise to a pulse quality that is floating and rapid. In an exterior cold pattern, exogenous cold attacks the body surface and causes contraction of the skin, muscle, channels, and blood vessels. The pulse quality is tight due to the spasming and contraction of the blood vessels, thus a floating and tight pulse indicates the presence of an exterior cold pattern.

Why doesn't the exterior cold pattern present with a floating and slow pulse? As we know, the Heart stores the spirit. It controls the blood and blood vessels. The pulse and its rate depend on the Heart qi. A slow pulse is usually directly or indirectly related to the condition of the Heart qi, and is either due to obstruction of the Heart yang qi by cold, in which case the pulse is slow and forceful; or to Heart yang qi deficiency, where the driving force of the Heart is weak, which impedes circulation of the qi and blood, and the pulse is slow and forceless. The Heart is a fire organ and is sensitive to heat, but less so to cold. Hence the Heart doesn't slow down during the early stage of an attack of exogenous cold though it may speed up with an attack of exogenous heat. The cold just invades the body surface and doesn't affect the Heart; thus, the pulse will be floating and tight, and not floating and slow.

17. What is the "true visceral pulse" (真臟脈 *zhēn zàng mài*)?

The true visceral pulse is also called the death pulse, paradoxical pulse, or failure pulse. It is the quality that appears in a critical condition or final stage of disease. The quality of the true visceral pulse is characterized by the absence of Stomach qi, spirit, and root. It is a sign of failure of the source qi and exhaustion of the Stomach qi.

Basic Questions, Chapter 19 (素問。玉機真臟論) describes the true visceral pulses: "The true Liver pulse is extremely tense and cannot be bent. It is sharp, like touching the edge of a knife, or it is as taut as pressing the string of a musical instrument. The true Heart pulse is hard, short, and beating rigidly, like touching coix seeds (*yì yǐ rén*). The true Lung pulse is large and hollow. It feels like a feather on skin. The true Kidney pulse is extremely forceful. It feels as solid as if the fingers are flicking on a stone. The true Spleen pulse is alternately rapid and slow in an irregular fashion. All of these pulses imply death."

The following table describes the ten true visceral pulses that are commonly seen in ancient Chinese textbooks, but rarely seen in the modern acupuncture clinic.

Characters	Pulse Name	Pulse Image Description
偃刀脈	Knife pulse	Hard, taut, and tense, it feels like touching the edge of a knife.
轉豆脈	Bean-Rolling pulse	Plump and short, it beats rigidly like a bean.
彈石脈	Flick On Stone pulse	Hard and rapid, very deep, like a finger flicking on a stone.
釜沸脈	Bubble pulse	Extremely floating and rapid, this pulse feels like bubbles rising in boiling water which are numberless and float up but not down.
魚翔脈	Fish Swimming pulse	This vague pulse can only be identified on seeking. While touching, it is very faint. The pulse is irregular and not clear, like fish swimming in water.
蝦游脈	Shrimp Darting pulse	The pulse rate is unstable, sometimes rapid and sometimes slow at the superficial level. The pulse strength is also unstable, sometimes clear and sometimes vague. This pulse is like a shrimp in water which darts about irregularly, sometimes swimming to the water's surface and then diving into the deeper water to hide.
雀啄脈	Sparrow Pecking pulse	This pulse beat is very irregular, rapid and forceful with some three to five rapid beats occurring together. This is a deep pulse at the level of the tendons. It is like a sparrow pecking at food.
解索脈	Rope Untying pulse	This pulse is also very deep. It beats rapid, and then slow. The pulse changes irregularly like untying knots in a rope.
屋漏脈	Roof Leaking pulse	This pulse is very slow and irregular. The interval is long and unequal. It is like drops leaking from a roof after rain.

Table 4.3.7 True Visceral Pulses

Based on their characteristics, the true visceral pulses can be divided into three categories: those without Stomach qi, those without root, and those without spirit.

	Characteristics	Pulse Name	Clinical Significance
No Stomach qi	pulse beats hard, tense, and harsh beneath the fingers	Knife pulse	antipathogenic qi failure, Stomach qi is exhausted and can't match the functions of organs and thus allows Liver, Heart, or Kidney visceral pulses to appear alone
		Bean Rolling pulse	
		Flick On Stone pulse	
Rootless	extremely weak and vague, superficial	Bubble pulse	extreme heat in the three yang and absence of yin
		Fish Swimming pulse	extreme cold in the three yin with expiring yang floating outward
		Shrimp Darting pulse	
Lacking Spirit	irregular pulse rate, interval, and shape	Sparrow Pecking pulse	Spleen, Stomach and Kidney yang qi failure, spirit disappears and it is the sign of death
		Roof Leaking pulse	
		Rope Untying pulse	

Table 4.3.8 True Visceral Pulse Categories

18. What is agreement (順) and disagreement (逆) between the pulse quality and the symptoms?

Both the pulse qualities and the symptoms are outer manifestations of pathological changes that occur in the course of a disease. Under most circumstances, the pulse quality and the symptoms will match. If a certain pulse quality is present, certain associated symptoms will also appear; the two are both manifestations of a particular illness. Thus, the pulse quality "agrees" with the symptoms. This indicates a favorable pattern that is easily treated.

If the pulse and the symptoms do not match or are opposites, it is said that the pulse "disagrees" with the symptoms. This indicates that the pathological changes are complex, presenting an unfavorable pattern that is difficult to treat.

For example, when a patient has heat symptoms and the pulse is rapid, or a patient has cold symptoms and the pulse is slow, the pulse quality agrees with the symptoms. If a patient has symptoms of excess but the pulse is forceless and thin, or a patient with deficient symptoms has a flooding or firm pulse, then the pulse quality disagrees with the symptoms.

Zhang Jing-Yue (張景岳) gave an excellent explanation: "In all excess conditions, the pulse should be vigorous; if the pulse is faint, sluggish, thready, or feeble, it is a sign of a deteriorated condition. In all deficient conditions, the pulse should be soft and supple; if it is flooding, large, forceful, slippery, floating, or rapid, the prognosis is bad. In acute diseases, the floating, flooding, rapid, and forceful pulses agree with the pulse quality. The faint, moderate, soggy, and frail pulses in chronic diseases are also in agreement with the pulse quality. If the pulse disagrees, the condition is serious. Agreement between pulse quality and symptoms is good for the patient."

Disagreement between the pulse and the symptoms makes pattern differentiation difficult. Causes of disagreement include:

Sudden onset: When pathogens invade the body and cause a sudden onset of disease, although the symptoms have appeared, the pulse has not yet changed; in this case, the pulse and symptoms are not in agreement. Another example: sudden pain makes the qi and blood stagnate; thus, while the flow in the blood vessels reflects a superficial disease, it is unable to reflect the true condition of the body.

Mild illness: When an illness is mild, the qi and blood are not involved, hence the pulse quality does not change. For example, malaise may appear in the body but not in the pulse quality. Or, in some cases, the pulse quality has changed, but the patient has yet to feel any discomfort. This is a morbid pulse existing without disease in the body.

Internal obstruction: Sometimes phlegm, blood, and food stagnate in the body, which obstructs the flow of qi and blood. In this case, the pulse may become vague, which is like the pulse in a disease of severe deficiency.

Coexistence of disease: When many kinds of disease coexist in the same body, or a new disease occurs in a body with old disease, the pulse quality will not necessarily agree with the symptoms.

Constitutional difference: Overweight patients may have a deep pulse, even though the exogenous disease may be attacking the exterior of the body. Conversely, a slender patient's pulse quality may be floating even in the presence of interior disease. Or a floating and rapid pulse may be found in a yang-predominant body even when the disease is associated with yin.

19. What is the theory of retaining (從) and abandoning (捨) pulse qualities and symptoms, and when should it be done?

The pulse is in the blood vessels. The pulse beat, rhythm, and rate are manifestations of the movement of qi and blood. Reported symptoms are caused by the movement or blockage of qi and blood, or they are the external reflection of the excess or deficiency of qi and blood. Certain pulse qualities and symptoms appear when the body develops disease or when there are pathological changes in the qi and blood.

When the pulse quality and the symptoms are in agreement, this is a reflection of normal physiology or of a pathological change that is following normal behavior. But if there are manifestations that are not normal, such as when the pulse and the symptoms do not agree, then within each there is true and false, and it is necessary to differentiate clearly so as to eliminate the false and retain the true. This is known as the "theory of retaining and abandoning."

False appearances will arise when the pulse quality disagrees with the symptoms. The practitioner should comprehensively analyze the patient's pulse quality and symptoms and distinguish the true from the false to determine which data to retain and which to abandon. To keep the true and abandon the false is the process involved in retaining and abandoning. If a pulse quality reflects the true essence of an illness, and the symptoms present a false appearance, then keep the pulse and abandon the symptoms. The opposite may occur as well. If the symptoms are in accordance with pathological changes, but the pulse quality (whether due to the condition of the patient or the influence of the pathogens) is not following the normal rules, then it forms a false quality. The symptoms are then given precedence over the pulse quality.

According to Zhang Jing-Yue, the key is to identify the deficiency. Because the manifestations of excess are often changeable, manifestations of false excess are often seen. On the other hand, the manifestations of deficiency are usually true. If the pulse quality pertains to deficiency and the symptoms to excess, then the symptoms are false. When the pulse quality reflects excess and the symptoms show deficiency, the pulse quality is false. If a faint pulse is accompanied by restlessness, the fire is certainly deficient. Abdominal distention with a feeble pulse indicates Stomach deficiency. If the pulse is flooding and rapid, but fever and restlessness are absent, the pulse is false. A tight pulse without pain and distention would not be viewed as indicative of a pattern of internal excess.

20. Is pulse examination alone enough to make a clinical diagnosis?

Pulse examination is one of the most important diagnostic techniques in Chinese medicine. It was formed and developed through clinical observation and recorded in great detail in the *Yellow Emperor's Inner Classic* (黃帝內經), *Discussion of Cold-induced Disorders* (傷寒論), and *Essentials from the Golden Cabinet* (金匱要略). Through many years of clinical practice, it has evolved and improved, and has played a major role in TCM for the past two thousand years.

However, we cannot rely on pulse examination exclusively to complete the clinical diagnosis. As we know, inspection, listening and smelling, inquiry, and palpation are the four methods of diagnosis in Chinese medicine. Pulse diagnosis is only one part of this. The pulse quality reflects only one aspect of the pathological change, and it is not possible for it to reflect the patient's entire pathological condition. In some complicated cases, the pulse quality may not agree with the symptoms, such as exterior signs and symptoms appearing with a deep and thready pulse, or deficiency signs and symptoms appearing with a flooding and excessive pulse. In these cases we have to follow the symptoms and abandon the pulse. Clinically of course, we must take into consideration the other three examinations to arrive at a comprehensive and clear diagnosis when pulse signs disagree. This process must be based on a comprehensive analysis of the data gained from the four-pillared diagnosis (四診合參).

Although pulse examination is an important part of the four pillars, it still cannot replace the other examination methods. One should only use pulse examination to complete the clinical diagnosis, then base the treatment plan on this diagnosis; otherwise, one may bring unfavorable results to the patient or even endanger her life. Therefore, the clinical significance of pulse diagnosis should not be overemphasized. Clinically, the four pillars must be used together, and they must be investigated together. Only in this way can a correct diagnosis be made.

TCM Diagnosis
Comprehensive Examination

TCM Diagnosis
Comprehensive Examination

1)   Which of the following is the most important component in the observation of the spirit?

   a. Facial expression
   b. Mental state
   c. Physical activity
   d. Eye movement

2)   Which of the following patterns does *NOT* give rise to a pale facial complexion?

   a. Qi deficiency
   b. Blood deficiency
   c. Cold pattern
   d. Yin deficiency

3)   A female patient reports that her hair looks dull with a tendency to split. What do these symptoms indicate?

   a. Deficiency of Kidney yin
   b. Deficiency of Lung qi
   c. Deficiency of Liver blood
   d. Deficiency of Heart yang

4)   Hair that suddenly falls out in big clumps is due to:

   a. Kidney deficiency
   b. Blood deficiency with wind
   c. Lung qi deficiency
   d. Damp-heat

5)   Purplish sclera indicates:

   a. Liver fire
   b. Liver wind
   c. Dampness
   d. Blood stagnation

6)   When the eye's sclera is unclear, it indicates which of the following?

   a. Wind
   b. Heat
   c. Dampness
   d. Cold

7)   Which of the following does the eye reflect?

    a. The state of the spirit and essence
    b. The state of the qi and blood
    c. The state of the body fluids
    d. The state of the yin and yang

8)   Kidney essence exhaustion can cause which of the following?

    a. Exophthalmus
    b. Platycoria (dilation of the pupils)
    c. Sunken eyes
    d. Eyelid twitching

9)   Which of the following can cause eyelid twitching?

    a. Spleen deficiency with dampness
    b. Heart fire
    c. Qi and blood deficiency
    d. Kidney yin deficiency

10)   The condition of children sleeping with their eyes slightly open is due to which of the following?

    a. Spleen deficiency with qi and blood insufficiency
    b. Kidney deficiency with yin exhaustion
    c. Liver wind
    d. Excessive heat in the Liver channel

11)   A withered and parched helix is due to which of the following?

    a. Fire flaming up from the *shào yáng* channel
    b. Insufficiency of Kidney essence and Kidney yin
    c. Blood stagnation in the *shào yīn* channel
    d. Spleen deficiency

12)   A green or blue tip of the nose indicates which of the following?

    a. Blood deficiency
    b. Abdominal pain
    c. Damp heat
    d. Exterior wind cold

13)   Which of the following symptoms can be observed when excessive heat accumulates in the Lung?

    a. Purple lip color
    b. Red and swollen gums
    c. Red, swollen and purulent throat
    d. Nostrils flaring

14) Which of the following can cause involuntary drooling?

    a. Excess heat in the lung
    b. Lung qi deficiency
    c. Spleen qi deficiency with excessive dampness
    d. Kidney qi deficiency

15) Atrophic and pale gums indicate which of the following?

    a. Spleen qi deficiency
    b. Lung qi and yin deficiency
    c. Kidney deficiency with water retention
    d. Kidney qi deficiency

16) A chronic sore throat that is pink in color but isn't swollen can be caused by which of the following?

    a. Excess heat in the Lung and Stomach
    b. Kidney yin deficiency with heat
    c. Damp heat in the middle burner
    d. Wind phlegm accumulation in the throat

17) A blue infantile index finger vein indicates which of the following?

    a. Wind pattern
    b. Deficiency pattern
    c. Heat pattern
    d. Yin deficiency pattern

18) When observing the tongue coating, which of the following can help to distinguish whether the patient's condition is hot or cold in nature?

    a. Humidity
    b. Color
    c. Thickness
    d. Distribution

19) Which of the following tongue shapes can be seen in a normal healthy person?

    a. Tongue with prickles
    b. Tongue with cracks
    c. A swollen tongue
    d. A tender tongue

20) A patient's tongue body is short, blue purple, and moist. This appearance indicates which of the following?

    a. Pathogenic cold obstructing channels
    b. Qi and blood stagnation
    c. Excessive pathogenic heat
    d. Toxic heat attacking the Heart

21)   Which of the following tongue conditions can be seen in qi deficiency patients?

   a. Pink tongue with thin white coating
   b. Pale flabby tongue body with moist white coating
   c. Pale tongue with thin white coating
   d. Pale tongue with greasy white coating

22)   A thick dry white tongue coating indicates a pathogen on which of the following levels?

   a. *Wèi* level
   b. Qi level
   c. Blood level
   d. *Yíng* level

23)   A yellow greasy tongue coating indicates which of the following?

   a. Damp heat accumulation
   b. Body fluid injury due to excessive heat
   c. Cold damp accumulation
   d. Wind heat attack

24)   A deep red tongue with a white greasy tongue coating, indicates which of the following?

   a. Yin deficiency with damp phlegm
   b. Heat and phlegm accumulation
   c. Damp accumulation
   d. Yin deficiency with heat

25)   Which of the following tongue coating changes indicates that the pathogen is growing in strength?

   a. Tongue coating gets thicker
   b. Tongue coating gets thinner
   c. Tongue coating changes from moist to dry
   d. Tongue coating changes from yellow to white

26)   A deep red tongue body with big red spots on the tip indicates which of the following?

   a. Heat in the *yíng* level
   b. Toxic heat invading the Heart
   c. Excessive heat in the Lung and Stomach
   d. Blood stagnation

27)   A pale flabby tongue with a slightly yellow slippery coating indicates which of the following?

   a. Yang deficiency with dampness
   b. Qi and blood deficiency
   c. Damp heat accumulation
   d. Phlegm obstruction of the channels

28) When a pathogen moves from the exterior to the interior, which of the following tongue coatings would you expect to find?

    a. White on the tip and yellow at the root

    b. One half side white and one half side yellow

    c. Thinner on the tip and thicker at the root

    d. One half side thinner and one half side thicker

29) A pale tongue body with cracks on the edges most likely indicates which of the following?

    a. Internal cold accumulation

    b. Damp accumulation secondary to Spleen deficiency

    c. Deficiency of blood

    d. Deficiency of yin

30) According to the theory of warm diseases (*wēn bìng*), when a pathogenic factor invades the defensive level, the tongue condition should appear as which of the following?

    a. Pale tongue with a thin white coating

    b. Red tongue tip and borders with a thin white coating

    c. Deep red tongue body with little coating

    d. Crimson red tongue body without coating

31) A hoarse voice, gradually increasing and worsening at night, with an itching and slightly painful throat indicate which of the following symptoms?

    a. External dryness invasion

    b. Lung and Kidney yin deficiency

    c. Heat phlegm accumulation in the throat

    d. Qi stagnation

32) All of the following pathogenesis can cause aphonia, *EXCEPT*:

    a. Lung and Kidney yin deficiency

    b. Lung and Spleen qi deficiency

    c. Kidney and Liver yin deficiency

    d. Damp phlegm obstruction in Lung collaterals

33) Rude and incoherent speech with cursing and shouting in a loud voice is known as:

    a. Soliloquy *(dú yǔ)*

    b. Raving *(kuáng yán)*

    c. Delirium *(zhān yǔ)*

    d. Wrong speaking *(cuò yǔ)*

34) Which of the following has the symptoms of difficult, short and rapid respiration, with a sense of tightness, congestion, and breathlessness or constriction in the chest?

    a. Asthma *(chuǎn)*

    b. Wheezing *(xiào)*

    c. Upper stifling breath *(shàng qì)*

    d. Shortness of breath *(duǎn qì)*

35)   Which of the following is NOT caused by Lung qi failing to descend?

    a. Wheezing *(xiào)*

    b. Asthma *(chuǎn)*

    c. Upper stifling breath *(shàng qì)*

    d. Shortage of qi *(duǎn qì)*

36)   Which of the following types of cough are characterized by paroxysmal and uninterrupted cough, even leading to vomiting, and making the sound like the call of a crane, followed by recurrences:

    a. Diphtheria cough

    b. Whooping cough

    c. Chronic cough

    d. Asthma cough

37)   All of the following symptoms are caused by rebellious Stomach qi, *EXCEPT*:

    a. Vomiting

    b. Belching

    c. Sighing

    d. Hiccoughing

38)   A late stage lung cancer patient suddenly starts to hiccough. The hiccoughing is weak, interrupted, and recurs after long pauses. These symptoms indicate which of the following?

    a. Stomach qi exhaustion

    b. Stomach qi recovery

    c. Stomach yin increasing

    d. Yang qi increasing

39)   Which of the following is indicated by the following signs and symptoms: sour and stinking odor in the mouth like rotten eggs, belching with foul odor, and acid regurgitation?

    a. Gingivitis

    b. Stomach fire flaring up

    c. Food stagnation

    d. Damp heat in the middle burner

40)   Rotten apple odor in the ward (patient's room) indicates which of the following?

    a. Syphilis

    b. Later stage *xiāo kě* pattern

    c. Later stage of yin-water pattern (uremia)

    d. Profuse bleeding

41)   Which of the following information should be included as present history?

    a. The onset of the disease

    b. The characteristics of the main symptoms

    c. The development of a disease

    d. All of the above

42) Inquiring about chills and fever can help the practitioner to do which of the following?

   a. Infer the disease cause
   b. Distinguish the disease location
   c. Know the condition of yin and yang
   d. All of the above

43) Which of the following pathogenesis does *NOT* appear in low grade fever?

   a. Deficiency of antipathogenic qi
   b. Excess heat in the Stomach and Large Intestine
   c. Qi and yin deficiency
   d. Qi stagnation

44) Chills or cold sensations that are not relieved by covering up or putting on more clothes indicates which of the following:

   a. Yang deficiency
   b. Interior cold pattern
   c. Exterior pattern
   d. Yin deficiency

45) All of the following etiologies and pathogeneses can cause low grade fever (heat) or feverish sensations, *EXCEPT:*

   a. Blood stagnation
   b. Yin deficiency
   c. Yang deficiency
   d. Exopathogenic cold attack

46) Which of the following symptoms belong to *yáng míng fǔ* pattern?

   a. High fever
   b. Alternating chills and fever
   c. Low-grade fever in the afternoon and evening
   d. High fever in the afternoon

47) When do simultaneous chills and fever occur?

   a. Exterior pattern
   b. *Tài yáng* pattern
   c. Exopathogenic factor invading the defensive qi level
   d. All of the above

48) Which of the following is *NOT* a cause of continuous low-grade fever?

   a. Yin deficiency
   b. Qi deficiency
   c. Blood deficiency
   d. Stomach fire

49) Profuse sweating on the palms and soles indicates which of the following:

   a. Excessive heat in the Spleen and Stomach
   b. Gallbladder qi deficiency
   c. Excessive heat in the Lung
   d. Kidney yin deficiency

50) Sweat on only half of the body indicates which of the following

   a. Wind-phlegm obstructing the channels
   b. Yang qi deficiency
   c. Heat accumulating in the middle burner
   d. Yin deficiency

51) Sticky, warm yellowish sweating indicates which of the following?

   a. Yang exhaustion
   b. Yin exhaustion
   c. Heat in the Spleen and Stomach
   d. Yin deficiency

52) Which of the following headaches is caused by blood deficiency?

   a. Sharp and prickly pain on the left side of the head
   b. Migrating pain which moves without fixed location
   c. Distending pain with paroxysmal attack
   d. Dull pain with empty and light feeling

53) Which of the following can cause retraction pain?

   a. Blood stagnation
   b. Qi stagnation
   c. Malnutrition of tendons
   d. Essence, yin, blood, or yang deficiency

54) Which of the following are indicated by the following symptoms: epigastric pain with burning sensations, discomfort, hunger but no desire to eat, dry heaves or hiccoughing?

   a. Spleen and Stomach deficiency
   b. Excessive heat in the stomach
   c. Food stagnation
   d. Stomach yin deficiency

55) Which of the following are indicated by the following symptoms: chronic, persistent dizziness and vertigo with hollow and heavy sensations in the head that worsen during the afternoon and evening?

   a. Wind phlegm
   b. Liver yang rising
   c. Qi deficiency
   d. Kidney essence deficiency

56) Which of the following are indicated by the following symptoms: lingering headache with an empty sensation in the head accompanied by paroxysmal darkness before the eyes and blurred vision?

    a. Exopathogenic factor attack
    b. Liver qi stagnation
    c. Qi and blood deficiency
    d. Stagnation of blood

57) Which of the following are indicated by the following symptoms: palpitations that come and go, induced by anxiety or fright, with dizziness and vertigo?

    a. Phlegm disturbing the Heart
    b. Liver qi stagnation
    c. Heart qi deficiency
    d. Water rising up and disturbing the Heart

58) Numbness on one side of the arm indicates which of the following?

    a. Blood deficiency
    b. Liver yang rising
    c. Wind phlegm
    d. Kidney essence insufficient

59) Which of the following is the pathogenesis of photophobia (hypersensitivity to light)?

    a. Liver fire
    b. Kidney yin deficiency
    c. Wind heat attack
    d. Liver blood deficiency

60) Mild itching in both eyes indicates which of the following?

    a. Liver fire flaring up
    b. Blood deficiency
    c. Wind phlegm disturbing head
    d. Middle burner qi sinking

61) Thirst without a desire to drink or desire for only a small amount of fluid suggests which of the following?

    a. Dampness accumulation
    b. Phlegm retention
    c. Blood stagnation
    d. All of the above

62) Small, goat-sized stools indicate which of the following?

    a. Spleen qi deficiency
    b. Stomach fire
    c. Liver qi stagnation
    d. Kidney yin deficiency

63) Alternating attacks of dry and loose stools indicate which of the following?

    a. Liver qi stagnation with Spleen deficiency
    b. Food stagnation
    c. Stomach heat
    d. Damp heat in the Large Intestine

64) Which of the following is indicated by dark green watery diarrhea with a foul odor, severe abdominal pain that is resistant to pressure and not relieved after passage of the diarrhea?

    a. Heart fire pouring downward
    b. Blood stagnation in the Stomach
    c. *Yáng míng fǔ* pattern
    d. Damp-heat in the lower burner

65) Which of the following pathogenesis can cause fecal incontinence?

    a. Damp-heat in the lower burner
    b. Kidney yin deficiency
    c. Spleen and Kidney yang deficiency
    d. Spleen and Lung qi deficiency

66) Dripping after urination indicates which of the following?

    a. Spleen qi deficiency
    b. Kidney qi deficiency
    c. Damp-heat in the lower burner
    d. Heart fire transferring to Small Intestine

67) Which of the following pathogeneses can cause insomnia?

    a. Yin and yang imbalance
    b. Nutritive and defensive qi disharmony
    c. Heart spirit disturbed
    d. All of the above

68) Insomnia characterized by waking up repeatedly during the night indicates which of the following?

    a. Heart blood deficiency
    b. Kidney yin deficiency
    c. Gallbladder qi deficiency
    d. Heart fire blazing

69) Lower abdominal cramps after menstruation indicates which of the following?

    a. Excess
    b. Deficiency
    c. Heat
    d. Cold

70) Which of the following can cause both profuse and scanty menstrual bleeding?

a. Qi deficiency
b. Blood stagnation
c. Pathogenic heat
d. Phlegm obstruction

71) Season and weather can affect the normal pulse. In springtime, the normal pulse tends toward which of the following?

a. Wiry
b. Flooding
c. Superficial
d. Submerged

72) Which of the following emotional changes can temporarily cause the slow pulse?

a. Anger
b. Joy
c. Melancholy
d. Grief

73) The normal pulse condition should include which of the following?

a. Essence, qi, spirit
b. Stomach qi, spirit, and root
c. Qi, blood, and essence
d. Pectoral qi, blood, and spirit

74) A pulse that is full of spirit means which of the following?

a. The pulse can be felt at the deep level at the proximal position
b. The pulse is neither superficial nor submerged
c. The pulse is gentle but with force and a unified rhythm
d. The pulse is neither wide nor thin

75) Which of the following pulses is *NOT* considered deep in location?

a. Hidden
b. Confined
c. Leather
d. Frail

76) Which of the following components are different between a frail pulse and a soft pulse?

a. Strength
b. Depth
c. Rhythm
d. Rate

77)   A deep and choppy pulse can be caused by which of the following?

    a. Liver qi stagnation
    b. Water accumulation
    c. Blood stagnation due to pathogenic cold
    d. Spleen and Kidney yang deficiency

78)   The confined pulse is composed of which of the following groups of qualities?

    a. Deep, long, taut, forceful, and wide
    b. Deep, long, thin, taut, and forceful
    c. Middle depth, short, slippery
    d. Slippery, rapid, and forceful

79)   Which of the following conditions is *NOT* associated with the choppy pulse?

    a. Qi and blood stagnation
    b. Essence deficiency
    c. Threatened abortion
    d. Exterior wind cold

80)   Which of the following characteristic(s) are common to both the soggy and the frail pulses?

    a. Thready and forceless
    b. Superficial and forceless
    c. Deep
    d. Short

81)   A female patient suffers from profuse bleeding due to a miscarriage. Which of the following pulse conditions could be expected from her?

    a. Superficial
    b. Thin
    c. Choppy
    d. Hollow

82)   The slow irregular pulse can be caused by which of the following:

    a. Blood stagnation
    b. Excess cold
    c. Qi and blood deficiency
    d. All of the above

83)   Which of the following statements regarding the thin pulse is correct?

    a. Thin, but clear and distinct
    b. Thin, forceless, and indistinct
    c. Short and forceless
    d. Superficial and forceful

84)   The soggy pulse indicates which of the following?

    a. Blood deficiency
    b. Qi deficiency
    c. Dampness accumulation
    d. All of the above

85)   Which of the following is correct regarding the moderate pulse?

    a. Four beats per (practitioner's) breath
    b. Indicates cold pattern
    c. Only felt at the deep level
    d. Pulse hits the fingers without force

86)   Hidden pulse indicates which of the following?

    a. Pregnancy in women in absence of other pathological signs and symptoms
    b. Syncope
    c. Obstruction of excessive pathogens
    d. All of the above

87)   The flooding pulse indicates which of the following?

    a. Qi stagnation
    b. Food stagnation
    c. Excess heat
    d. Phlegm

88)   All of the following pulses are yin in nature *EXCEPT* which of the following?

    a. Tight pulse
    b. Submerged pulse
    c. Slow pulse
    d. Slow irregular pulse

89)   According to warm disease (*wēn bìng*) differentiation, a superficial rapid pulse indicates which of the following pathologies?

    a. Defensive level heat
    b. Qi level heat
    c. Nutritive level heat
    d. Blood level heat

90)   According to warm disease (*wēn bìng*) differentiation, which of the following pulses will be found with nutritive level heat?

    a. Superficial and rapid
    b. Excess
    c. Thin and rapid
    d. Wiry and rapid

91) Which of the following characteristics are common to the leather and hollow pulses?

   a. Superficial, wide, and empty in the middle
   b. Superficial and forceless
   c. Superficial and indistinct
   d. Superficial, thin, and forceless

92) All of the following pulse conditions are considered normal *EXCEPT*:

   a. A woman's pulse is generally thinner than a man's.
   b. The child's pulse is generally slower than the adult's.
   c. The elder patient's pulse is generally weaker than a younger patient.
   d. Pulses in the summer can feel slightly flooding.

93) According to *Shāng Hán Lùn* differentiation (six channel theory), which of the following pulses is associated with the *tài yīn* stage pattern?

   a. Thin and rapid
   b. Wiry or excessive
   c. Deep and slow
   d. Superficial and tight

94) Which of the following pulses is commonly found in a patient with a deep red tongue without coating?

   a. Thin and rapid
   b. Scattered
   c. Deep and frail
   d. Surging and rapid

95) Which of the following areas will be sensitive in the patient who has appendicitis?

   a. 1 to 2 *cùn* below ST-36
   b. 1 to 2 *cùn* below the GB-34
   c. 1 to 2 *cùn* below the ST-37
   d. 1 to 2 *cùn* below the sternum

96) "Pitting" edema is caused by:

   a. Water retention
   b. Blood deficiency
   c. Qi stagnation
   d. Pathogenic wind damp attack

97) Which of the following conditions would give rise to edema that pits when pressed, but immediately returns to level after releasing finger pressure?

   a. Water retention
   b. Qi stagnation
   c. Carbuncles and boils caused by heat toxin
   d. Blood stagnation

98) Which of the following patterns would you find in a patient whose forehead feels hot at first touch, but becomes mildly warm after prolonged contact?

    a. Heat from yin deficiency
    b. Exterior heat
    c. Interior heat
    d. Damp-heat

99) Which of the following patterns would be indicated when a patient's dorsal aspect of the hand (back of the hand) is hotter than the palm?

    a. Yin deficiency heat
    b. Exterior heat
    c. Interior heat
    d. Damp heat

100) A 34-year-old female patient complains of a stifling sensation in the chest and epigastrium, lassitude and heaviness of the body, poor appetite, lack of taste, no thirst, loose stools, and profuse white vaginal discharge. She has a pale tongue with a sticky thick white coating, and a slow slippery pulse. Which of the following facial colors would you expect to find in this patient?

    a. Bright orange yellow
    b. Hazy, smoky yellow
    c. Withered, dried-up yellow
    d. Dull pale yellow

101) A 52 year-old male patient was diagnosed as HIV-positive five years ago. Three days ago, he started feeling burning, tenderness, tingling and pain on his skin on the left side of his waist. Yesterday he found erythema and grouped vesicles in the area. Upon examination you find grouped, hard, deep-seated vesicles distributed unilaterally along a dermatome. Which of the following does this patient likely have?

    a. Measles
    b. German measles
    c. Boils and carbuncles
    d. Herpes zoster (shingles)

102) A 59-year-old male patient was diagnosed with bronchial pneumonia. The chief complaints are productive coughing and wheezing. He has a thin red tongue with a crack and little coating, and a weak pulse. The TCM diagnosis for him is a cough due to phlegm dryness. Which of the following phlegm appearances will this patient most likely see after he coughs?

    a. Scanty white thick sputum or white clots like rice, very difficult to expectorate or blood-streaked sputum
    b. Profuse thin white sputum, easy to expectorate, worse at night
    c. Sticky yellow sputum, may accumulate into clots, difficult to expectorate
    d. The phlegm shape looks like dirty cotton balls with a dark black color, or sticky sputum that looks like glue. It is difficult to expectorate.

103) A 32-year-old female suffers from a UTI for two days. The symptoms include painful and hesitant urination. She also complains of irritability, insomnia, thirst, and a desire to drink cold water. Her tongue is red and her pulse is rapid. With which of the following indications might she also present?

    a. Loose stools
    b. Red color in the canthus area of the eye
    c. Yellow facial complexion
    d. Flabby tongue body

104) A 42-year-old male has an earth type constitution. Clinically, he presents with dizziness, fatigue, palpitation and depression, a greasy tongue coating, and slippery pulse. Which of the following physical traits would he most likely present?

    a. Emaciated
    b. Obese
    c. Tall
    d. Short

105) A 56-year-old male diabetes mellitus patient was also diagnosed with chronic renal failure. Manifestations include general fatigue, weakness, and malaise. He also reports low back pain, weak knees, nocturia, and impotence. Upon examination you discover pitting edema on his ankles. He has a pale tongue with a slightly greasy white coating. His pulse is deep and deficient. Which of the following colors would you most likely see in his facial complexion?

    a. Green-blue
    b. Red
    c. Yellow
    d. Sallow dark

106) A 43-year-old male HIV-positive patient has suffered from chronic sinusitis for the past ten years. The sinus infection comes and goes. It is usually induced by exertion or when he catches a cold, which occurs three or four times per year. He also complains of fatigue and loose stools. He has a pale tongue with a slightly thick greasy coating and a deficient pulse. Which of the following types of nasal discharge would you expect in this patient?

    a. Profuse and turbid pus, dark yellow or green yellow discharge with a foul smell
    b. Scanty yellow discharge, possibly with blood and pus
    c. Profuse watery discharge, alternating between white and green or a light yellow color
    d. Profuse and watery

107) A 43-year-old female patient was diagnosed with carcinoma of the pancreas two months ago. She has since begun radiation and chemotherapy. Currently, she suffers from the side effects of the chemotherapy which include fatigue, nausea, vomiting, and anorexia. The vomitus is frequent though only in small amounts. The vomitus contains undigested food and does not have a strong odor. Which of the following pathogeneses is most likely to have caused her current condition?

a. Damp heat in the middle burner

b. Stomach and Spleen yang deficiency with cold

c. Food stagnation

d. Liver attacking Stomach

108) A young man woke up one morning to see a patch of hair fall from his head. The night before, he had slept beneath an open window. Which of the following best describes the cause of his condition?

a. Blood deficiency with invasion of wind

b. Premature senility

c. Insufficiency of the Kidney essence

d. Insufficiency of the Heart qi

109) A patient suffers from palpitations, dream-disturbed sleep, forgetfulness, and anorexia. The abdomen is distended and the stools are loose. The patient appears listless and has a sallow complexion. There are numerous subcutaneous hemorrhages on the arms and legs. She has not had her period in three months. The pulse is thin and forceless. Which of the following represents the most likely appearance of her tongue?

a. Pale and tender tongue body with a white coating

b. Pale white coating

c. Pink body with a red tip

d. Pale tongue body with red tip

110) A 28-year-old female complains of chest pain, insomnia, palpitations, migraine headaches, lower abdominal pain and distention before and during her period, and heavy menstrual flow that is dark red in color with numerous clots. There is also a mass on her neck. Her conventional medical diagnosis is thyroiditis. Which is the most likely tongue appearance this patient will present?

a. Purple tongue with a red tip

b. Purple red tongue with petechiae (purple dots) on the tongue's edges

c. Purple tongue with a thin yellow tongue coating

d. Pale tongue with petechiae on the tongue's edge

111) A female patient has a history of acute nephritis and a duodenal ulcer. For five years she has been symptom-free, however she still has weakness in the limbs, a pale yellowish complexion, abdominal bloating, poor appetite, shortness of breath, loose stools, and sweating after even slight physical exertion. Her pulse is submerged and deficient. What is the most likely tongue appearance this patient would present?

a. Pale, with a slippery thin white coating

b. Pale, with teeth marks and a thin white coating

c. Pale, with a white greasy coating

d. Pale, with a yellow greasy coating

112) A patient comes to you with a diagnosis of cardiac edema. His primary symptoms are scanty urinary output, whole body edema that makes it difficult for him to sleep lying down horizontally at night, a feeling of general heaviness in his head and body, coldness in his extremities, and no thirst. His pulse is deep, his face is pale and slightly cyanotic, as are his fingers. Which of the following represents the most likely tongue appearance that this patient will have?

    a. Red body with a yellow greasy coating
    b. Pale body with a white greasy coating
    c. Pale and flabby body with a moist white coating
    d. Pale purple body with dark spots on the edge and a thin white coating

113) Shari, a 20-year-old female, has not had her period in the 40 days since she had a miscarriage. At the time of the miscarriage, there was hemorrhaging but the bleeding has long since stopped. Now she reports a dull ache with occasional sharp, paroxysmal pain. How do you expect her tongue to appear?

    a. Red tip, normal shaped body and a yellow coating
    b. Pale body with a thin white coating
    c. Hypoglossal vein engorgement with a red body and a thin yellow coating
    d. Hypoglossal vein engorgement with a pale, dusky body and a thin coating

114) A 45-year-old smoker who has a history of dry hacking cough also complains of being chronically tired. For a week before coming in for treatment his coughing was especially bad. Two days before coming in, his coughing had lessened but he began to experience continual nausea along with occasional dry vomiting. His mouth is dry and he is thirsty. Which of the following is the most likely appearance of his tongue?

    a. Red with yellow greasy coating
    b. Red with white gray coating
    c. Red with dry coating
    d. Pale with red tip and thin yellow coating

115) A 32 year-old male patient complains of low back pain. He experiences stiffness, especially in the mornings when he goes for a run on the beach. He says he always stretches before and after his run, but his back remains stiff and sometimes feels cold. Sometimes the pain radiates down to his legs. How do you expect his tongue to appear?

    a. White and sticky tongue coating
    b. Red body with scanty coating
    c. Red body with yellow coating
    d. Pale body with thin yellow coating

116) Symptoms such as mental depression, dullness of thought, incoherent speech, weeping and laughing without reason, or sudden collapse, coma, and gurgling with sputum in the throat would likely present with which of the following signs?

    a. Pale tongue with a moist thin white coating; submerged and slippery pulse
    b. Purple tongue with a thin white coating; choppy and wiry pulse

c. Deep red tongue without coating; thin and rapid pulse

d. White, greasy tongue coating; wiry and slippery pulse

117) A patient complains of feeling something stuck in her throat that won't move up or down. You diagnose plum-pit pattern. Which of the following tongue appearances would you expect to see in this patient?

a. Dry, yellow coating

b. White, moist or greasy coating

c. Yellow, greasy coating

d. Thin yellow coating

118) A young woman comes to your office complaining of a cough that does not go away. As you question her, you discover that her cough began four months ago with a flu that kept her in bed for three weeks with a high fever, constipation, and a red rash. All of her symptoms are now gone except for this cough, which is very painful for her. She complains of feeling "globs" of sputum stuck in her throat and chest, but she can't seem to cough them up. Her face appears slightly flushed and she gets thirsty easily. Her pulse is slightly rapid and slightly thready. Which of the following tongue appearances would you expect to find in this case?

a. Red body with a white moist greasy coating

b. Pale swollen body with a white greasy coating

c. Red body with a thick dry yellow coating

d. Pink body with a dry white coating

119) A 35-year-old male has suffered from chronic colitis over the past six years. His symptoms include loose stools, poor appetite, bloating after eating, and periodic nausea. Which of the following tongue conditions would you expect to find in this patient?

a. Prickled tongue with a yellow coating

b. Red cracked tongue with a thin yellow coating

c. Thin and small tongue body with a thin white coating

d. Slightly pale tongue with teeth marks and a greasy white coating

120) Simon, age 31, complains of impotence and inability to maintain an erection for more than one minute. He also complains of exhaustion, cold hands and feet, and loose stools. Upon examination, you notice that he has beads of sweat on his forehead. He says he sweats very easily during the day with the slightest exertion. He also complains of diarrhea in the early hours of the morning at least twice a week. Additionally, he is being treated by Western doctors for bronchial asthma. He currently uses a steroidal inhaler because of his difficulty inhaling. What kind of tongue and pulse would you expect to find in Simon at this time?

a. Red tongue body with a yellow coating, wiry and rapid pulse

b. Pale tongue body with a yellow coating, slippery and wiry pulse

c. Pale tongue body with a thin white coating, deep and deficient pulse

d. Pale tongue body without coating, soft and deficient pulse

121) Steve, a 29-year-old man, presents with excruciating epigastric and abdominal pain that is so severe that he cannot tolerate being touched. There is a strong sensation of coldness in the epigastrium. He is vomiting and unable to eat. There are big lumps or knots in the abdominal skin that look like worms. Which of the following tongue presentations would you expect to see in this patient?

    a. Red tongue body with a greasy yellow coating
    b. Red tongue body with a thin white coating
    c. Pale tongue body with a moist white tongue coating
    d. Pale tongue body with teeth marks and no coating

122) Marianne is a 52-year-old woman has been suffering from headaches for the past three years. The headaches occur mostly in the forehead and facial areas, but also on the top of the head. The headaches started after a fast and are worse during the daytime. They are accompanied by a feeling of fuzziness in the head. She reports that she has also been suffering from chronic catarrh and rhinitis for the past 25 years. She suffers with chronic low back pain and frequent urination. She feels tired. She is also constipated and does not move her bowels every day. When she does have a bowel movement, the stools are loose. She generally feels cold. With which of the following tongue and pulse signs will this patient most likely present?

    a. Deep and frail pulse; pale and stiff tongue with a thin white coating
    b. Deep and frail pulse; pale and swollen tongue with a sticky white coating
    c. Deep and frail pulse; pale and swollen tongue with a sticky yellow coating
    d. Thin and wiry pulse; pale and stiff tongue with a sticky yellow coating

123) Sarah, a 35-year-old female patient, suffers from insomnia during the past three years since she had her second baby. She took *Guī pí tāng* (Restore the Spleen Decoction) for two months, but her insomnia symptoms did not improve at all. Two weeks ago she started taking *Suān zǎo rén tāng* (Sour Jujube Decoction) and her sleep has improved greatly. What kind of tongue and pulse presentation would you expect in this patient?

    a. Pale tongue with a thin white coating; thin and deficient pulse
    b. Flabby tongue with teeth marks and a thin white coating; slippery and deficient pulse
    c. Red tongue with little coating; thin and rapid pulse
    d. Dry red tongue with little coating; thin, wiry, and rapid pulse

124) Doug, a 35-year-old male patient, was diagnosed with hepatitis C two years ago. He complains of epigastric focal distention, fullness and tightness but without pain, and frequent dry heaves, periodic diarrhea, and anorexia. For one month he has taken *Bàn xià xiè xīn tāng* (Pinellia Decoction to Drain the Epigastrium) and now reports that he feels his symptoms are much improved. What kind of tongue coating would you expect this patient to have prior to taking the formula?

    a. Thin greasy yellow
    b. Thick moist white
    c. Thin greasy
    d. No tongue coating

125) A 32-year-old male suffers from acute hepatitis. His TCM doctor suggests that he take *Xiǎo chái hú tāng* (Minor Bupleurum Decoction) because, according to TCM diagnosis, this patient will likely have a *shào yáng* pattern. What kind of tongue coating is this patient likely to have at this stage?

   a. Dry and yellow
   b. White and moist
   c. Thick and white
   d. Thin and white

126) A 58-year-old male has suffered from chronic bronchitis for over ten years. Five days ago, his cough worsened when he caught a cold. Now he coughs all day with profuse thick yellow sputum that is difficult to expectorate. He reports fullness and distention in the chest and hypochondriac region as well as chest pain induced by cough. Other symptoms include shortness of breath and sonorous breathing, a red face, thirst with a desire to drink water, and a slippery rapid pulse. Which of the following tongue descriptions would you most likely find in this patient?

   a. Red tongue with thin yellow coating
   b. Red tongue with a thin greasy yellow coating
   c. Red tongue without coating
   d. Red tongue with a thick turbid greasy coating

127) A 55-year-old male has suffered from hemiplegia (post-stroke sequellae) on his left side for the past five months. It is difficult for him to speak clearly, and he also has a deviated mouth and eyes. His face looks withered yellow without sheen. His limbs are slightly swollen. His pulse is thin, choppy, and forceless. With which of the following tongue appearances might he present?

   a. Red tongue with a greasy yellow coating
   b. Pale tongue with a thin white coating
   c. Red tongue with a yellow coating
   d. Pale tongue with a white greasy coating

128) Lily is a 35-year-old female who was diagnosed with uterine fibromyomas. Over the past five years she has experienced profuse menstrual bleeding and severe cramping, the menses is dark red and with clots. The abdominal cramps are worse with pressure, but relieved by warmth. Which of the following signs might she also have?

   a. Dry lips
   b. Red tongue tip
   c. Scanty coating
   d. Purplish spots on the tongue border

129) Cherie is a 68-year-old female who was diagnosed with emphysema five years ago with symptoms aggravated during the winter. She complains of shortness of breath, wheezing, coughing with copious watery sputum, and a heavy, tight feeling in the chest. She also complains of weakness in the legs and low back. Which of the following signs might she also have at this time?

    a. Red tongue with greasy yellow coating; rapid and slippery pulse
    b. Greasy white coating; frail and slippery pulse
    c. Pale tongue with a moist white coating; submerged and slow pulse
    d. Purple tongue with a thin coating; choppy and wiry pulse

130) A 50-year-old male patient complains of a dry and sore throat with hoarseness for over two months. Last week he also found a small hard nodule in the throat area and his hoarseness is still getting worse. He has a dry, purple tongue, and a choppy pulse. What is the pathogenesis that is causing his hoarseness?

    a. Heat phlegm obstructing throat
    b. Exterior dryness attack
    c. Blood stagnation
    d. Lung and Kidney yin deficiency

131) Linda told you that her 76-year-old father is always murmuring to himself with repetitions and interruptions. The content is incoherent, but it stops when he meets with people. His consciousness is clear, but his thinking and reactions are slow. What is the pathogenesis?

    a. Heart qi and/or blood deficiency
    b. Heat disturbing the Heart
    c. Kidney yin deficiency
    d. Blood stagnation

132) A 56-year-old male patient was diagnosed with asthma over the past 15 years. Symptoms and signs include shallow and difficult breathing, or shortness of breath, inhalation more difficult than exhalation, and symptoms worsen with exertion. Which of the following patterns apply to him?

    a. Lung qi deficiency
    b. Heat phlegm accumulation in the Lung
    c. Kidney deficiency
    d. Spleen yang deficiency

133) A male patient suffers from bronchial asthma for over 15 years, usually worse during the wintertime. The symptoms include difficulty exhaling, a heavy and full sensation in the chest, and cough with profuse thick white phlegm. He has a light pale tongue covered by a thick white coating, and a slippery pulse. Which of the following patterns apply to him?

    a. Wind cold attacking the Lung
    b. Kidney yang deficiency
    c. Cold phlegm obstructing the Lung
    d. Lung qi deficiency

134) A 67-year-old male patient currently under chemotherapy for his lung cancer seeks out your help. He suffers from severe nausea and violent vomiting, especially after eating. The vomiting has a sharp and crisp sound. The vomitus is made up of food followed by clear fluids or green mucus. What is the pathogenesis for his condition?

    a. Food stagnation
    b. Cold dampness attacking the Stomach
    c. Spleen and Stomach qi deficiency
    d. Stomach yin deficiency

135) A 65-year-old female patient has been hiccoughing for over three months. The hiccoughs are intermittent and sound slow and forceless. It is induced or aggravated by eating or drinking something cold. Her appetite is very poor. Her tongue is flabby and pale with a moist white coating, and her pulse is submerged, slow, and forceless. What is the pathogenesis of this condition?

    a. Pathogenic cold attacking the Stomach
    b. Spleen and Kidney yang deficiency
    c. Stomach yin deficiency
    d. Liver attacking Stomach

136) A 35-year-old male patient complains of loose stools over the last two months; the stools look like "duck droppings." He also has dull abdominal pain, frequent loud borborygmi, pale urine, and cold limbs. His tongue is pale and his pulse is submerged and thin. What is the *zàng fǔ* diagnosis for this patient?

    a. Interior cold in the Large Intestine
    b. Damp heat in the lower burner
    c. Liver attacking Spleen
    d. Exterior cold invading the Large Intestine

137) What do the following symptoms indicate: depression, sighing, poor appetite, belching, plum-pit sensation, irritability, distending pain in the hypochondriac and costal regions, chest stuffiness, irregular menses, dysmenorrhea, thin, white tongue coating with a wiry pulse?

    a. Liver yang rising
    b. Liver qi stagnation
    c. Kidney and Liver yin deficiency
    d. Damp phlegm obstructing the Lung

138) A 38-year-old man with a five-year history of diabetes mellitus presents with anorexia, nausea, and vomiting. His urine output has increased significantly over the past 24 hours and he is now starting to experience a vague abdominal discomfort. His breathing is deep and rapid and his breath has a rotten fruity odor. Random blood glucose level is high. What is the diagnosis?

a. Acute hypoglycemic episode
b. Diabetic ketoacidosis
c. Acute renal failure from diabetic nephropathy
d. Insulin overdose

139) A 43-year-old female complains of excessive vaginal discharge. A thin and transparent white liquid is profuse and continuous. She also reports frequent and copious urinary output, loose stools, and a cold feeling in the abdomen. Her tongue is pale with a thin white coating and her pulse is submerged. What is her diagnosis?

a. Leukorrhea due to damp cold in the lower burner
b. Leukorrhea due to deficiency of the Kidney
c. Leukorrhea due to deficiency of the Spleen
d. Leukorrhea due to damp heat in the lower burner

140) A 40-year-old female has had a low grade fever for three months. It usually occurs in the morning or is induced by exertion. Other symptoms included emaciation, shortness of breath, general weakness and lack of spirit, dryness in the mouth without desire to drink, sweating on exertion, poor appetite, and 2–3 daily soft bowel movements. Her body temperature is 99.5–100.4° F and she has a pale face and tongue. What is the pathogenesis?

a. Damp heat in middle burner
b. Kidney yin deficiency with empty heat
c. Spleen qi deficiency
d. Blood stagnation

141) A 67-year-old female patient's hearing has declined rather suddenly and she has a constant ringing in her ears that cannot be alleviated by pressing her hand over her ears. She has a bad temper and often has headaches. Her face is flushed and her pulse is forceful and wiry. What is the pathogenesis?

a. Kidney yin deficiency with deficiency heat
b. Liver fire flaring up
c. Liver blood deficiency wind
d. Phlegm heat in the Gallbladder channel

142) A 34-year-old female patient suffers from chronic fatigue pattern for three years. Her tongue is slightly pale with teeth marks and there is a thin white coating. Her pulse is deficient. TCM diagnosis is qi deficiency. Which of the following symptoms might she also have?

a. Irregular menstruation
b. Thirst
c. Spontaneous sweating
d. Dream-disturbed sleep

143) A 43-year-old woman complains of a low-grade fever that persists throughout the day. She also experiences a heavy sensation in her head, limbs, and trunk; the stifling sensation in her chest especially bothers her. Her appetite is poor, associated with abdominal distention and lethargy after meals. Her pulse is soggy and slippery, and her tongue has a sticky slightly yellow coating. What is the diagnosis?

   a. Kidney yin deficiency
   b. Damp heat in the upper burner
   c. Spleen qi deficiency with dampness
   d. Spleen qi deficiency

144) A female patient has a history of acute nephritis and duodenal ulcer. For five years she has had no kidney or ulcer symptoms, but she does have weakness in the limbs, a pale and yellowish complexion, abdominal bloating, poor appetite, shortness of breath, loose stools, and sweating after slight physical exertion. What is the pathogenesis?

   a. Kidney essence insufficiency
   b. Kidney qi deficiency
   c. Spleen qi deficiency
   d. Spleen yang deficiency

145) A 38-year-old man has been suffering from headaches for the past five years. The headaches occur over the whole head and are dull but intense in character. They improve when lying down, and worsen with stress or exposure to light. The headaches are accompanied by nausea, vomiting, and a feeling of cold. He also has hypochondriac pain and is prone to constipation. The tongue is slightly dusky and swollen, with a dirty coating. What is the correct diagnosis for this patient?

   a. Liver yang rising due to Liver yin deficiency
   b. Liver yang rising due to Liver blood deficiency
   c. Liver yang rising due to Liver and Kidney yin deficiency
   d. Liver fire

146) A 21-year-old male suffered from palpitations with anxiety for two years. He has palpitations 5–8 times a day. He also complains of poor memory, dizziness when studying hard, and insomnia with dream-disturbed sleep. He has a pale face, a pale tongue with a thin white coating, and a frail pulse. What is the diagnosis?

   a. Heart qi deficiency
   b. Heart blood deficiency
   c. Fire disturbing the Heart spirit
   d. Phlegm obstructing the orifices

147) Ralph is a timid person who gets palpitations when he is surprised. He is easily frightened, especially by strange noises. He suffers from restlessness, dream-disturbed sleep, irritability, and anorexia. His tongue coating is thin and white. What is the most appropriate diagnosis for this patient?

   a. Gallbladder qi deficiency
   b. Hyperactivity of fire due to yin deficiency
   c. Heart and Spleen qi deficiency
   d. Liver qi stagnation

148) Linda, a 48-year-old female, has complained of palpitations and insomnia for about a month. She also feels dizzy and nauseated. She has a bitter taste in her mouth and likes drinking cold water. Her menstrual cycle has been irregular for one year. Her tongue has a yellow greasy coating. The pulse is wiry and slippery. What is the correct diagnosis for her?

   a. Lack of coordination between the Gallbladder and Stomach, with stirring up of phlegm heat
   b. Heart qi and blood deficiency
   c. Hyperactivity of the Liver yang and Spleen qi deficiency
   d. Pathogenic cold in the Stomach

149) A 32-year-old female suffers from persistent, severe headaches with repeated attacks and a fixed location. Her symptoms are caused by which of the following?

   a. Blood stagnation
   b. Wind cold attack
   c. Qi stagnation
   d. Yin deficiency

150) An 18-year-old female complains of chest pain, insomnia, palpitations, migraine headaches, lower abdominal pain and distention before and during her period, and an excessive menstrual flow with a dark red color and clots. There is a mass on her neck. The Western medical diagnosis is thyroiditis. What is the pathogenesis?

   a. Heart blood stagnation
   b. Kidney yin deficiency
   c. Liver blood stagnation
   d. Liver qi stagnation

151) A 32-year-old male has excruciating pain in his left first metatarsophalangeal joint. It is red, warm, shiny, and extremely tender. He also has chills, fever, malaise, and tachycardia. His laboratory test results shows uric acid above 7.0 mg/dL. His tongue is red with a greasy yellow coating, and his pulse is rapid and slippery. What is the TCM diagnosis?

   a. Wind heat *bi* pattern
   b. Damp heat *bi* pattern
   c. Blood stagnation
   d. Qi stagnation

152) A 50-year-old female patient has had pain in her left elbow for six months. The pain is severe and worsens with movement or when trying to grip an object with her hand. She is unable to work or carry out her daily household chores. A surgeon diagnosed the condition as lateral humeral epicondylitis. Heat therapy provides temporary relief from the pain. Examination shows local tenderness over the left lateral humeral epicondyle. Pain is also elicited by resisting dorsiflexion of the patient's left hand. What is the pathogenesis?

   a. Wind cold
   b. Damp heat with blood stagnation
   c. Cold dampness with blood stagnation
   d. Blood stagnation

153) A 25-year-old male patient complains of a headache lasting two days. He says that two days ago he started to feel the headache in the occipital region. The pain is violent, boring, and tight. It extends to the nape of the neck and upper back. His headache gets worse when exposed to wind or cold. He has had chills for the past two days and his body temperature is 100.4° F. Which of the following symptoms might this patient also have?

   a. Sore throat
   b. Red eyes
   c. Constipation
   d. Nasal discharge

154) A 30-year-old woman comes to your office with a chief complaint of dizziness. When she stands up from her chair she feels dizzy and sometimes blacks out. She also has numbness of the limbs and muscle twitching. Her menstrual cycle is delayed and her sleep is very light. Sunlight makes her eyes hurt. Her face and tongue are pale, and her pulse is forceless. Which of the following signs and symptoms are consistent with her condition?

   a. Lack of appetite
   b. Lumbar and knee pain
   c. Emotional instability
   d. Brittle and pale nails

155) A 43-year-old female complains of dizziness, fatigue, loose stools, loss of appetite, blurred vision, and a numb, tingling sensation in the limbs. Her face looks sallow and she has a pale tongue and a choppy pulse. According to *zàng fǔ* diagnosis, what do these indications suggest?

   a. Kidney and Spleen yang deficiency
   b. Spleen and Liver blood deficiency
   c. Lung and Heart qi deficiency
   d. Kidney and Liver yin deficiency

156) A 43-year-old male patient complains of constipation over four weeks. The stools are not dry, but small, like a goat's stools, and difficult to evacuate. He was diagnosed with IBS two years ago and suffers from alternating constipation and diarrhea. His symptoms indicate which of the following?

   a. Heart fire
   b. Spleen qi deficiency

c. Kidney yin deficiency

d. Liver qi stagnation

157) A 45-year-old female complains of constipation and fatigue after bowel movements. Her stools are soft. She also perspires easily and has a pale tongue. What is the diagnosis?

a. Heat in the intestines

b. Qi stagnation

c. Qi blocked by cold

d. Qi deficiency

158) A patient complains that he has thirst, drinks a lot of water, has excessive appetite, bad breath, swollen and painful gums, and a burning sensation in the epigastrium. What is the diagnosis?

a. Stomach fire blazing

b. Stagnation of the Stomach qi

c. Deficiency of Spleen qi

d. Liver fire invading Stomach

159) A 32-year-old male presents with burning epigastric pain. He also has an empty and uncomfortable sensation in the stomach with hunger but no desire to eat, hiccoughs, thirst, and constipation. His tongue is red and dry with little coating and he has a thin, rapid pulse. What is the most appropriate TCM diagnosis for him?

a. Stomach yin deficiency

b. Stomach fire

c. Stomach qi deficiency

d. Food stagnation

160) A 40-year-old female has had dull epigastric pain for over 20 years. Two years ago she was diagnosed with an ulcer in the duodenal bulb with chronic superficial gastritis. The pain radiates to her back and is accompanied by nausea and regurgitation of clear fluids. She has a poor appetite, a dulled sense of taste, and a preference for hot beverages. The pain is alleviated with local pressure. Her stools are sticky and loose. She has a pale tongue with a thin, white coating and a deficient pulse. What is the pathogenesis?

a. Exogenous cold attack on the Stomach

b. Stomach and Spleen yang deficiency with cold

c. Stomach yin deficiency

d. Damp and cold accumulation in the middle burner

161) A patient has had diarrhea and fever for two days. The symptoms include abdominal pain, tenesmus, blood and mucus in the stools, and a burning sensation in the anus. He is thirsty and passes scanty, deep-yellow urine. His tongue has a yellow sticky coating and his pulse is slippery and rapid. What is the diagnosis for this patient?

a. Spleen damp heat

b. Large Intestine damp heat

c. Bladder damp heat

d. Heart fire transferring to the Small Intestine

162) A 30-year-old male patient has not had a bowel movement for four days. Before that, he also had constipation with dry stools. He tells you that he is passing dark and scanty urine. You also witness restlessness, a red face, dry mouth, foul breath, and abdominal fullness. His tongue is red with a yellow dry coating, and the pulse is slippery and rapid. What is the diagnosis for this patient?

    a. Excess heat in the Stomach and Large Intestine
    b. Lung heat transmitting to the Large Intestine
    c. Dryness of the Large Intestine
    d. Spleen qi deficiency

163) A 54-year-old male patient has suffered from insomnia for six months, accompanied by dizziness, tinnitus, irritability, low back pain, and seminal emission. His pulse is rapid and frail. What is the diagnosis?

    a. Spleen qi deficiency with blood deficiency
    b. Upward disturbance of Liver fire
    c. Disharmony of Heart and Kidney
    d. Liver and Kidney yin deficiency

164) A 32-year-old male complains of insomnia for three weeks, waking during the night, with nightmares and dreams of flying. He has a bitter taste in his mouth, thirst, mental restlessness, and palpitations. He also has facial acne, canker sores, and is constipated. What is the TCM diagnosis?

    a. Liver qi stagnation with heat
    b. Kidney and Heart disharmony
    c. Heart fire blazing
    d. Heart blood and Spleen qi deficiency

165) A 17-year-old girl was at the scene of a terrorist attack half a year ago. Since then, she has become highly sensitive to any noise around her. She gets palpitations and anxiety from any sudden noise. Other symptoms include tinnitus, nightmares, and difficulty making decisions. She has a slightly pale tongue with a thin white coating, and a wiry and thin pulse. What other symptom(s) may she have?

    a. Shortness of breath
    b. Extremely cold limbs
    c. Sensations of heat in the palms and soles
    d. Insomnia

166) A 32-year-old female patient comes to your office because she suffers from irregular menstruation. She states that her menstrual cycle has gradually become more irregular over the past four years since she divorced her husband. She has a wiry pulse. Which of the following symptoms might she also have?

    a. Sweating
    b. Chills and fever
    c. Frequent sighing
    d. Cough

167) Barbara, age 34, complains of infertility and has had three miscarriages during the past eight years. Since her first miscarriage, she has had an irregular menstrual cycle and lower abdominal pain during menstruation, which is aggravated by pressure and relieved by warmth. Her tongue is pale purple with a dry thin coating, and her pulse is thin, submerged, and frail. What is her diagnosis?

    a. Deficiency cold of the Penetrating Vessel *(chōng mài)* and Conception Vessel *(rèn mài),* with blood stagnation

    b. Kidney essence insufficiency

    c. Spleen yang deficiency

    d. Blood stagnation with heat

168) A 16-year-old girl comes in because of menstrual problems. Her period started when she was 14 and has a 21-day cycle. The blood is bright red and she bleeds heavily. She has cramps during the first two days of the flow. She drinks a lot of cold water and likes to eat ice cream. What other symptom(s) would you expect?

    a. Constipation

    b. Thirst

    c. Scanty urination

    d. All of the above

169) A 37-year-old woman complains of mild, persistent uterine bleeding, irregular menstruation (either early or late), extended or continuous menstrual flow, spotting between periods, abdominal pain and distention, and coldness in the lower abdomen. Her lips and mouth are dry, and she has a low-grade fever in the evenings along with warm palms and soles. What is the best diagnosis for this patient?

    a. Deficiency heat of the Penetrating Vessel *(chōng mài)* and Conception Vessel *(rèn mài)* with blood stagnation

    b. Deficiency cold of the Penetrating Vessel *(chōng mài)* and Conception Vessel *(rèn mài)* with blood stagnation

    c. Kidney yin deficiency with Liver yang rising with blood stagnation

    d. Downward flow of damp heat with blood stagnation

170) A 6-year-old boy has been diagnosed with lobar pneumonia. His body temperature is 110°F. He presents with tachypnea, profuse sweating, red face, dry lips, severe thirst, and irritability. Which of the following pulses will he likely have?

    a. Superficial and rapid

    b. Surging and rapid

    c. Thready and rapid

    d. Submerged and excessive

171) A 31-year-old female patient gave birth two days ago. She is bleeding a lot because of metratonia (atony of the uterine walls after childbirth). She also suffers from post-partum depression. She may present with any of the following pulses, *EXCEPT*:

    a. Thready

    b. Leather

    c. Hollow

    d. Wiry

172) A 32-year-old female has difficulty controlling herself and cries a lot. The TCM diagnosis is restless organ disorder (*zàng zào*). Which of the following is the most likely pulse for her?

    a. Thin and rapid
    b. Wiry and slippery
    c. Submerged and frail
    d. Choppy and slow

173) A patient complains of a feeling that something is stuck in her throat and it won't move up or down. You diagnose plum-pit pattern. Which of the following is her likely pulse?

    a. Wiry and slow, or wiry and slippery
    b. Wiry and thin, or wiry and tight
    c. Slippery and rapid, or slippery and thin
    d. Rapid and thin, or thin and frail

174) A patient presents with palpitations, pain in the heart region which may radiate to the medial aspect of the left arm or shoulder, discomfort, feeling of oppression or constriction of the chest, cyanosis of lips and nails, and cold hands. Which of the following is the most likely pulse?

    a. Slippery
    b. Thin
    c. flooding
    d. Slow-irregular

175) A 45-year-old male construction worker had been suffering from chronic low back pain accompanied by insomnia and seminal emission for over ten years. Yesterday his low back was struck by a ladder while at work. Today, he feels severe pain at the site of the injury. The pain is made worse with massage and acupressure. His tongue is red with little coating. What kind of pulse might you expect for him at this time?

    a. Thin and rapid
    b. Thin and choppy
    c. Wiry and rapid
    d. Slippery and rapid

176) A 40-year-old female has had a low-grade fever for more than three months. It usually occurs in the morning or is induced by fatigue. Other symptoms include emaciation, shortness of breath, general weakness with a lack of spirit, dryness in the mouth with no desire to drink, sweating on exertion, poor appetite, and two to three daily soft bowel movements. Upon examination, you find that her body temperature is 99.7 F., and she has a pale face and tongue. Which is her most likely pulse?

    a. Flooding
    b. Frail
    c. Submerged
    d. Slippery

177) A 35-year-old male has been married for about two years. He complains that his erection is now weak and cannot be sustained. He also suffers from dizziness, blurred vision, disturbed sleep, soreness and weakness in the lower back and knees, and occasional involuntary nocturnal emissions. He has a pale face and tongue. Which of the following pulses will he most likely have?

   a. Deep and thin
   b. Deep and excessive
   c. Wiry and slippery
   d. Choppy and frail

178) A 30-year-old male has suffered from lower abdominal pain for three days. The pain is located on the left side below the level of the umbilicus. It is a severe contracting pain that radiates to the testicles. He applied an ice pack to the area but it made the pain worse. His tongue is pale with a white coating. Which is the most likely pulse that he will have?

   a. Choppy and slippery
   b. Submerged, slow, and wiry
   c. Wiry and slippery
   d. Slow and frail

179) A 65-year-old male has suffered from hand tremors for about two years. He was diagnosed by a neurologist with Parkinson's disease. Other symptoms and signs include dizziness, tinnitus, and numbness of the limbs. He also complains of dream-disturbed sleep, night sweats, blurred vision, and night blindness. He has a pale face and tongue. Which of the following pulses will you likely find in this patient?

   a. Wiry and rapid
   b. Wiry and excessive
   c. Thin
   d. Flooding

180) A 48-year-old female complains of insomnia. She said that during the past couple months she has had a hard time falling asleep. She also feels irritable and hot at night. Other signs and symptoms include palpitations, dizziness, tinnitus, memory loss, dry mouth and thirst, night sweats, and weak and achy low back and knees. She has a red tongue. Which of the following pulses will likely be found in this patient?

   a. Submerged and slow
   b. Wiry and thin
   c. Slippery and excessive
   d. Thready and rapid

181) A 35-year-old female comes in for treatment of her chronic loose stools that have lasted over three years. She was diagnosed with irritable bowel syndrome. The diarrhea is usually accompanied with abdominal pain which is relieved somewhat after the bowel movement. She has episodes of loose stools five to six times per day. It is often induced by emotional depression or anger. She is currently going through a divorce. She also suffers from hypochondriac pain and distention, retching, and lack of appetite. Her tongue is dusky purple with teeth marks and a thin white coating. Which of the following pulses will most likely be found in this patient?

   a. Slippery and rapid
   b. Frail and thin
   c. Soggy and rapid
   d. Wiry and moderate

182) A 30-year-old male has suffered from asthma for over 20 years. He has asthma attacks five to eight times per year. These attacks are induced by weather changes or when he catches a cold. He had a flu last week with chills and fever, headache, body aches, and cough. Now he experiences shortness of breath and cough with watery sputum. He looks very skinny and pale, has a weak voice, and sweats easily. His tongue is pale with a thin coating. What is the most likely pulse one would find in this patient?

   a. Superficial and rapid
   b. Submerged and slow
   c. Superficial and deficient
   d. Slippery and wiry

183) A 32-year-old female has been pregnant for over 25 weeks. Last week she began to experience some uterine bleeding. The blood is dark purple in color and accompanied by abdominal pain that is aggravated by pressure. She was diagnosed with uterine fibroids over eight years ago, and she has had three miscarriages prior to her current pregnancy. Which of the following pulses will most likely be found in this patient?

   a. Wiry
   b. Leather
   c. Hollow
   d. Choppy

184) A 58-year-old African American male patient had a CVA two weeks ago. He now suffers from hemiplegia on his right side. During the physical examination you find that there are big scars on his chest and right inner leg, the result of a bypass surgery three years ago. His right hand and ankle are swollen. Blood pressure is 180/90 mmHg. His tongue is swollen with a purplish color and there is a thick yellow greasy coating. His hypoglossal veins are purple and extended. Which of the following pulses will most likely be found in this patient?

   a. Flooding and rapid
   b. Submerged, wiry, and thin
   c. Wiry, slippery, and choppy
   d. Slippery and wiry

185) Mr. Hong, a 58-year-old male, was admitted to the hospital six days ago because of a stroke that left his right side paralyzed. He also suffers from dizziness, headache, insomnia, irritability, dry mouth, and thirst. He worries a lot and is afraid he will not walk again. His blood pressure is 160/95mmHg and he has a red cracked tongue with little coating. Which of the following pulses will most likely be found in Mr. Hong?

    a. Wiry and thin
    b. Choppy and wiry
    c. Slippery and rapid
    d. Surging and rapid-irregular

186) A 34-year-old female has suffered from migraine headaches for over 12 years. The pain is on the top of the head with a dull, achy, cold sensation. The pain is accompanied by nausea, dry heaves or spitting of clear fluids, as well as photosensitivity. The pain usually occurs just after her menstrual period. Her cycle is 34 days. Upon examination, you find that she is 5'4" tall and weighs 95 lbs. Her tongue is slightly pale with a white, moist coating. Which of the following is the pulse most likely to be found in this patient?

    a. Choppy and thin, or choppy and wiry
    b. Thin and slow, or thin and wiry
    c. Slippery and slow, or slow and submerged
    d. Tight and wiry, or soggy and wiry

187) A 36-year-old female had an abortion to terminate her three month pregnancy. That was four months ago, and since then she hasn't had a menstrual period. She also suffers from constant low abdominal pain and complains of fatigue, dizziness, and periodic blurred vision. Physical examination finds that there are tender spots on her lower abdomen that are sensitive to pressure. Her tongue is pale purple with a thin coating. Which of the following pulses will most likely be found in this patient?

    a. Thin and frail
    b. Choppy and wiry
    c. Choppy and thin
    d. Faint and choppy

188) A 44-year-old female was diagnosed with mitral stenosis. She suffers from dyspnea on exertion, paroxysmal nocturnal dyspnea, orthopnea, weakness, fatigue, and palpitations. Her ankles are swollen. The TCM diagnosis is Lung and Heart qi deficiency with water retention. Which of the following pulses will you likely find in this patient?

    a. Confined
    b. Submerged, slow, and slippery
    c. Frail, consistently irregular
    d. Slippery

189) A 6-year-old boy is experiencing excruciating epigastric and abdominal pain. He won't allow you to examine his abdomen because pressure will increase the pain. You find the boy's lips and face are pale and he is sweating a lot. His hands and feet are extremely cold. Which of the following pulses will most likely be found in this patient?

   a. Excessive and slippery
   b. Thin and submerged
   c. Choppy and wiry
   d. Tight and slow

190) A 35-year-old female has experienced UTI symptoms three to four times per year for the past six years. She uses antibiotics each time to control the symptoms until last year, when she developed a yeast infection. Her UTIs are usually induced by exertion and in general her energy level is very low. She urgently needs to urinate every hour, and it is painful and burning. Her tongue has teeth marks, and is slightly pale with a greasy yellow coating. Which of the following pulses will most likely be found in this patient?

   a. Deficient
   b. Slippery
   c. Rapid
   d. All of the above

191) A 6-year-old boy is brought to your office by his mother because he has scarlet fever. You learn that he has had a high fever for the past 24 hours. The fever is worse at night. He also suffers from severe irritability and restlessness. You find there are some faint and indistinct erythema and purpura on his body. Which of the following pulses would you expect to find in this patient at the time of this evaluation?

   a. Wiry and rapid
   b. Thin and rapid
   c. Excessive and slippery
   d. Hollow

192) Joe is a 51-year-old male Wall Street broker who has been diagnosed with hypertension over the past ten years. He experiences dizziness, distending headache, insomnia, dream-disturbed sleep, and occasional tinnitus which is high pitched. Three days ago, after returning home from work, he suddenly felt numbness in his limbs and stiffness along his left side. This was accompanied by inability to speak and facial hemiplegia on the left side. His tongue is red with a thin yellow coating. Which of the following pulses will you find in Joe at this time?

   a. Thin and wiry
   b. Slippery and rapid
   c. Choppy and excessive
   d. Wiry and excessive

193) A 33-year-old female patient had a miscarriage three years ago. Since then, she has suffered from persistent mild headaches that have a dull, empty feeling. This headache is worse in the morning and is aggravated by exertion. It is even worse during or after her menstrual period. Other signs and symptoms include low energy, shortness of breath, palpitations, and insomnia. Her tongue looks pale and has a thin white coating. Which of the following pulses are most likely to be found in this patient?

    a. Choppy and wiry
    b. Submerged and slow
    c. Slippery and choppy
    d. Frail and thin

194) A 31-year-old woman has been pregnant for four months and complains of frequent uterine bleeding, which is spotty and dark red in color, with abdominal pain and slight spasms. According to the results of several ultrasounds, she has a fibroid tumor that is increasing in size. She also told you that she has suffered from dysmenorrhea over the past 15 years and that her menstrual periods are always overflowing, with dark purple blood and clots. She has had four miscarriages and she wants you to help her carry this baby to full-term. Which of the following pulses would you expect to find in this patient?

    a. Slippery, wiry, and rapid
    b. Slippery, rapid, and choppy
    c. Hollow, rapid
    d. Tight, rapid, and superficial

195) A 24-year-old female complains of hand tremors and nervousness. She said that over the past couple weeks she has been emotionally unstable and has experienced palpitations, restlessness, and insomnia. She also has loose stools and is losing weight. She sweats a lot, is intolerant of heat, and has muscle weakness. Laboratory studies show increased serum T_3 and serum T_4. Pulse rate is 120bpm, and her blood pressure is 120/83 mmHg. She has a red tongue with a thready yellow coating. Her Western diagnosis is hyperthyroidism. Which of the following pulses will most likely be found in her?

    a. Choppy and rapid
    b. Wiry and rapid
    c. Superficial and thin
    d. Wiry and slippery

196) A 16-year-old boy was sent to the ER because of perforating appendicitis. He suffers from wandering pain. Which of the following pulses might he currently have?

    a. Tight
    b. Moving
    c. Hidden
    d. Any of the above are possible

197) A patient complains of weak limbs. He is thirsty but has no desire to drink. He will occasionally drink a little hot beverage. His head and body feel heavy. His stools are loose, and his pulse is soggy. Which of the following is the most likely diagnosis?

    a. Spleen blood deficiency

    b. Gallbladder qi deficiency

    c. Damp heat in the *yáng míng fŭ*

    d. Spleen qi deficiency with dampness

198) Sita is a 65-year-old female who was diagnosed with glaucoma two years ago. She suffers from spots before her eyes, blurry vision, mild headaches, and vertigo. She also complains of hot palms and soles as well as depression. What kind of pulse would you expect to find in her left middle pulse position?

    a. Thin and wiry

    b. Wiry and slippery

    c. Frail and slow

    d. Faint

199) A patient suffers from palpitations, dream-disturbed sleep, forgetfulness, and anorexia. The abdomen is distended and there are loose stools. The patient appears listless and has a sallow complexion. There are numerous subcutaneous hemorrhages on the arms and legs. The patient's tongue is pale with teeth marks. Which of the following pulses will most likely be found in this patient?

    a. Thin

    b. Thin and deficient

    c. Submerged and slow

    d. Confined

200) A patient reports having diarrhea and fever for the past two days. The symptoms include abdominal pain, tenesmus, and blood and mucus in the stools, with a burning sensation in the anus. The patient is thirsty and is passing scanty, deep-yellow colored urine. The tongue coating is yellow and sticky. Which of the following pulses will this patient likely have?

    a. Deficient

    b. Soggy

    c. Frail

    d. Rapid and slippery

TCM Diagnosis
Comprehensive Examination

ANSWER KEY: TCM DIAGNOSIS COMPREHENSIVE EXAMINATION

1)   d.   Eye movement

2)   d.   Yin deficiency

3)   b.   Deficiency of Lung qi

4)   b.   Blood deficiency

5)   b.   Liver wind

6)   c.   Dampness

7)   a.   The state of the spirit and essence

8)   b.   Platycoria (dilation of the pupils)

9)   c.   Qi and blood deficiency

10)   a.   Spleen deficiency with qi and blood insufficiency

11)   b.   Insufficiency of Kidney essence and Kidney yin

12)   b.   Abdominal pain

13)   d.   Nostrils flaring

14)   c.   Spleen qi deficiency with excessive dampness

15)   d.   Kidney qi deficiency

16)   b.   Kidney yin deficiency with heat

17)   a.   Wind pattern

18)   b.   Color

19)   b.   Tongue with cracks

20)   a.   Pathogenic cold obstructing channels

21)   c.   Pale tongue with thin white coating

22)   b.   Qi level

23)   a.   Damp heat accumulation

24)   a.   Yin deficiency with damp phlegm

25)   a.   Tongue coating gets thicker

26)   b.   Toxic heat invading the Heart

27)   a.   Yang deficiency with dampness

28) a. White on the tip and yellow at the root

29) b. Damp accumulation secondary to Spleen deficiency

30) b. Red tongue tip and borders with a thin white coating

31) b. Lung and Kidney yin deficiency

32) c. Kidney and Liver yin deficiency

33) b. Raving (*kuáng yán*)

34) a. Asthma (*chuǎn*)

35) d. Shortage of qi (*duǎn qì*)

36) b. Whooping cough

37) c. Sighing

38) a. Stomach qi exhaustion

39) c. Food stagnation

40) b. Later stage *xiāo kě* pattern

41) d. All of the above

42) d. All of the above

43) b. Excess heat in the Stomach and Large Intestine

44) c. Exterior pattern

45) d. Exopathogenic cold attack

46) d. High fever in the afternoon

47) d. All of the above

48) d. Stomach fire

49) a. Excessive heat in the Spleen and Stomach

50) a. Wind-phlegm obstructing the channels

51) b. Yin exhaustion

52) d. Dull pain with empty and light feeling

53) c. Malnutrition of tendons

54) d. Stomach yin deficiency

55) d. Kidney essence deficiency

56) c. Qi and blood deficiency

57) a. Phlegm disturbing the Heart

58) c. Wind-phlegm

59) d. Liver blood deficiency

60) b. Blood deficiency

61) d. All of the above

62) c. Liver qi stagnation

63) a. Liver qi stagnation with Spleen deficiency

64) c. *Yáng míng fǔ* pattern

65) c. Spleen and Kidney yang deficiency

66) b. Kidney qi deficiency

67) d. All of the above

68) b. Kidney yin deficiency

69) b. Deficiency

70) b. Blood stagnation

71) a. Wiry

72) b. Joy

73) b. Stomach qi, spirit and root

74) c. The pulse is gentle but with force and a unified rhythm

75) c. Leather

76) b. Depth

77) c. Blood stagnation due to pathogenic cold

78) a. Deep, long, taut, forceful, and wide

79) d. Exterior wind cold

80) a. Thready and forceless

81) d. Hollow

82) d. All of the above

83) a. Thin, but clear and distinct

84) d. All of the above

85) a. Four beats per (practitioner's) breath

86) d. All of the above

87) c. Excessive heat

88)   a.   Tight pulse

89)   a.   Defensive level heat

90)   c.   Thin and rapid

91)   a.   Superficial, wide, and empty in the middle

92)   b.   The child's pulse is generally slower than the adult's.

93)   c.   Deep and Slow

94)   a.   Thin and rapid pulse

95)   a.   1 to 2 *cùn* below Stomach 36

96)   a.   Water retention

97)   b.   Qi stagnation

98)   b.   Exterior heat

99)   b.   Exterior heat

100)   d.   Dull pale yellow

101)   d.   Herpes zoster (shingles)

102)   a.   Scanty white thick sputum or white clots like rice, very difficult to expectorate or blood-streaked sputum

103)   b.   Red color in the canthus area of the eye

104)   b.   Obese

105)   d.   Sallow Dark

106)   c.   Profuse watery discharge, alternating between white and green or a light yellow color

107)   b.   Stomach and Spleen yang deficiency with cold

108)   a.   Blood deficiency with invasion of wind

109)   d.   Pale tongue body with red tip

110)   b.   Purple red tongue with petechiae (purple dots) on the tongue's edges

111)   b.   Pale, with teeth marks and a thin white coating

112)   c.   Pale and flabby body with a moist white coating

113)   d.   Hypoglossal vein engorgement with a pale, dusky body and a thin coating

114)   c.   Red with dry coating

115)   a.   White and sticky tongue coating

116)   d.   White, greasy tongue coating; wiry and slippery pulse

117)   b.   White, moist or greasy coating

118)   c.   Red body with a thick dry yellow coating

119)   d.   Slightly pale tongue with teeth marks and a greasy white coating

120)   c.   Pale tongue body with a thin white coating, deep and deficient pulse

121)   c.   Pale tongue body with a moist white tongue coating

122)   b.   Deep and frail pulse; pale and swollen tongue with a sticky white coating

123)   d.   Dry red tongue with little coating, and a thin, wiry, and rapid pulse

124)   a.   A thin greasy yellow tongue coating

125)   d.   Thin and white

126)   b.   Red tongue with a thin greasy yellow coating

127)   b.   Pale tongue with a thin white coating

128)   d.   Purplish spots on the tongue border

129)   c.   Pale tongue with a moist white coating, submerged and slow pulse

130)   c.   Blood stagnation

131)   a.   Heart qi and/or blood deficiency

132)   c.   Kidney deficiency

133)   c.   Cold phlegm obstructing the Lung

134)   d.   Stomach yin deficiency

135)   b.   Spleen and Kidney yang deficiency

136)   a.   Interior cold in the Large Intestine

137)   b.   Liver qi stagnation

138)   b.   Diabetic ketoacidosis

139)   b.   Leukorrhea due to deficiency of the Kidney

140)   c.   Spleen qi deficiency

141)   b.   Liver fire flaring up.

142)   c.   Spontaneous sweating

143)   b.   Damp-heat in the upper burner

144)   c.   Spleen qi deficiency

145)   b.   Liver yang rising due to Liver blood deficiency

146)   b.   Heart blood deficiency

147)   a.   Gallbladder qi deficiency

148)   a.   Lack of coordination between the Gallbladder and
             Stomach with stirring up of phlegm-heat

149)   a.   Blood stagnation

150)   c.   Liver blood stagnation

151)   b.   Damp heat *bì* pattern

152)   c.   Cold damp with blood stagnation

153)   d.   Nasal discharge

154)   d.   Brittle and pale nails

155)   b.   Spleen and Liver blood deficiency

156)   d   Liver qi stagnation

157)   d   Qi deficiency

158)   a   Stomach fire blazing

159)   a.   Stomach yin deficiency

160)   b.   Stomach and Spleen yang deficiency with cold

161)   b.   Large Intestine damp heat

162)   a.   Excess heat in the Stomach and Large Intestine

163)   c.   Disharmony of Heart and Kidney

164)   c.   Heart fire blazing

165)   d.   Insomnia

166)   c.   Frequent sighing

167)   a.   Deficiency cold of the Penetrating Vessel *(chōng mài)* and Conception Vessel
             (rèn mài), with blood stagnation

168)   d.   All of the above

169)   b.   Deficiency cold of the Penetrating Vessel *(chōng mài)* and Conception Vessel
             (rèn mài) with blood stagnation

170)   b.   Surging and rapid

171)   d.   Wiry

172)   a.   Thin and rapid

173)   a.   Wiry and slow or wiry and slippery

174)   d.   Slow-irregular

175)   b.   Thin and choppy

176)   b.   Frail

177)   a.   Deep and thin

178)   b.   Submerged, slow and wiry

179)   c.   Thin

180)   d.   Thready and rapid

181)   d.   Wiry and moderate

182)   c.   Superficial and deficient

183)   d.   Choppy

184)   c.   Wiry, slippery and choppy

185)   a.   Wiry and thin

186)   b.   Thin and slow or thin and wiry

187)   c.   Choppy and thin

188)   c.   Frail, consistently irregular

189)   d.   Tight and slow

190)   d.   All of the above

191)   b.   Thin and rapid

192)   d.   Wiry and excessive

193)   d.   Frail and thin

194)   b.   Slippery, rapid, and choppy

195)   b.   Wiry and rapid

196)   d   Any of the above are possible

197)   d   Spleen qi deficiency with dampness

198)   a   Thin and wiry

199)   b   Thin and deficient

200)   d.   Rapid and Slippery

BIBLIOGRAPHY

■ Premodern Texts

Ao's Golden Mirror Collection [for Cold Damage] (敖氏[傷寒] 金鏡錄
Ào shì [shāng hán] jīn jìng lù): Du Qing-Bi, 1341.

Case Records as a Guide to Clinical Practice (臨證指南醫案 *Lín zhèng zhǐ nán yī àn*):
Ye Tian-Shi, 1746.

Classic of Difficulties   (難經 *Nàn Jīng*): [attributed to] Bian Que, 407–310 BCE.

Classic on the Principles of Observation (望診遵經 *Wàng zhěn zūn jīng*): Wang Hong , 1875.

Discussion of Blood Patterns (血證論 *Xuè zhèng lùn*): Tang Rong-Chuan, 1884.

Discussion of Cold Damage (傷寒論 *Shāng hán lùn*): Zhang Zhong-Jing, 200 CE.

Discussion of the Origins of the Symptoms of Disease (諸病源侯論 *Zhū bìng yuán hòu lùn*):
Chao Yuan-Fang, 605–616.

Essential Pivot of Diagnosis (診家樞要 *Zhěn jiā shū yào*): Hua Shou, 1359.

Essentials from the Golden Cabinet (金匱要略 *Jīn guì yào lùe*): Zhang Zhong-Jing, 200 CE.

Golden Mirror of the Medical Tradition (醫宗金鑑 *Yī zōng jīn jiàn*): Wu Qian, 1739.

Guidance to Examination (察病指南 *Chá bìng zhī nán*): Shi Fa, 1241.

Lakeside Study on Pulse (瀕湖脈學 *Bín hú mài xué):* Li Shi-Zhen, 1564.

Master Cui's Pulse Rhymes (崔氏脈訣 *Cuī shì mài jué*): Cuï Jia-Xu, 1111–1191.

Pulse Classic (脈經 *Mài jīng*): Wang Shu-He, 254–316.

Rhymes of the Four Examinations (四診抉微 *Sì zhěn jué wēi*): Lin Zhi-Han, 1723.

Three Finger Meditation (三指禪 *Sān zhǐ chán*): Zhou Xue-Teng, 1827.

Thorough Understanding of Cold Damage (傷寒指掌 *Shāng hán zhǐ zhǎng)* Wu, Kun-An, 1796.

Treasury Classic (中藏經 *Zhōng càng jīng*): [attributed to] Hua Tuo, 145–208.

Treatise on the Spleen and Stomach (脾胃論 *Pǐ wèi lùn*): Li Dong-Yuan, 1180–1251.

True Eye of Diagnosis (診家正眼 *Zhěn jiā zhèng yǎn*): Li Zhong-Zi, 1642.

Yellow Emperor's Inner Classic: Basic Questions (黃帝內經素問 *Huáng dì nèi jīng sù wèn*):
Anonymous, 200 CE

Yellow Emperor's Inner Classic: Divine Pivot (黃帝內經靈樞 *Huáng dì nèi jīng líng shū*):
Anonymous, 200 CE

■ Contemporary Texts

Beinfield, Harriet and Efrem Korngold. *Between Heaven and Earth: A Guide to Chinese Medicine.* New York: Ballentine Books, 1992.

Cheng Xin-Nong. *Chinese Acupuncture and Moxibustion.* Beijing: Foreign Languages Press, 1987.

Deng Tie-Tao. *A Study of Diagnosis in Chinese Medicine* (中醫診斷學 *Zhōng yī zhén duàn xué*). Beijing: People's Medical Publishing House, 1987.

Kaptchuk, Ted J. *The Web That Has No Weaver,* New York: Congdon & Weed, 1983.

Liu Guan-Jun. *Pulse Diagnosis* (脈診 *Mài zhěn*), Shanghai: Science and Technology Press, 1979.

Long Zhi Xian. *Basic Theories of Traditional Chinese Medicine* (中醫基礎理論 *Zhōng yī jī chǔ lǐ lùn*). Beijing. Academy Press, 1998.

Long Zhi Xian. *Diagnostics of Traditional Chinese Medicine* (中醫診斷學 *Zhōng yī zhén duàn xué*). Beijing: Academy Press, 1998.

Maciocia, Giovanni. *The Foundations of Chinese Medicine.* Edinburgh: Churchill Livingstone, 1989.

Qi Nan and Yang Fu Gou. *Zang Fu and Clinical Practice in Chinese Medicine* (中醫藏象与临床 *Zhōng yī zàng xiàng yǔ līn chuáng*). Beijing: Chinese Medicine Ancient Book Publishing House, 2001.

Song Tian Bin. *Tongue Diagnosis in Chinese Medicine* (中醫舌診 *Zhōng yī shé zhén*). Beijing: People's Medical Publishing House, 2005.

Wiseman, Nigel and Feng Ye. *A Practical Dictionary of Chinese Medicine.* Brookline, MA.: Paradigm Publications, 1998.

Xiao Xiang-Ru. *Encyclopedia of Smelling and Listening Method in Chinese Medicine* (中華醫學聞診大全 *Zhōng huá yī xué wèn zhèn dà quán*). Shanxi: Science and Technology Press, 1998.

Xiao Xiang-Ru. *Encyclopedia of Observation Method in Chinese Medicine* (中華醫學望診大全 *Zhōng huá yī xué wàng zhèn dà quán*). Shanxi: Science and Technology Press, 1998.

Zhang Zhong-Fan. *Encyclopedia of Inquiring Method in Chinese Medicine*

(中華醫學問診大全 *Zhōng huá yī xué wèn zhèn dà quán*). Shanxi: Science and Technology Press, 1999.

Zhao En-Jian. *Pulse Diagnosis in Chinese Medicine* (中醫脈診學 *Zhōng yī mài zhén xué*). Tianjing: Science and Technology Press, 1988.

Zhao Jin-Ze. *A Study of Symptom Identification in Chinese Medicine Diagnosis*

(中醫證狀鑒別診斷學 *Zhōng yī zhèn zhuàng jiàn bié zhén duàn xué*). Beijing: People's Medical Publishing House, 1984.

Zhu Wen-Feng. *A Study of Diagnosis in Chinese Medicine* (中醫診斷學 *Zhōng yī zhén duàn xué*). Beijing: People's Medical Publishing House, 1999.

AUTHORS

■ Authors

Qiao Yi, M.D. (China), M.P.H., L.Ac.

Dr. Qiao graduated from Beijing University of TCM in 1987 where she also received her medical degree. She received her Masters degree in public health from U.C.L.A. She has served as the clinical director at both Emperor's College and SAMRA University; and as Associate Dean and Academic Dean at Yo San University and Emperor's College, respectively.

Dr. Qiao has been teaching TCM courses since 1991 at schools in Southern California, where she was also involved with curriculum development. She served as commissioner for the Accreditation Commission for Acupuncture and Oriental Medicine (ACAOM) for eight years.

In addition to her teaching duties, Dr. Qiao performs acupuncture research at Cedar Sinai Hospital, and maintains a private practice in Los Angeles. She is also the proud mother of Erick, who is almost as old as the time in which it took to complete this textbook.

Dr. Qiao and Al Stone published their first textbook (on Chinese herbal formulas) with Snow Lotus Press in 1999.

Al Stone, L.Ac., D.A.O.M.

Dr. Stone graduated from Emperor's College with a Masters in TCM in 1997. Ten years later, he earned his Doctorate in acupuncture and Oriental medicine (D.A.O.M.), also from Emperor's College. Dr. Stone is best known as the founder of the website *acupuncture.com*. He maintains a significant online presence at *gancao.net*, and an internal medicine practice that focuses on Chinese herbal medicine in Santa Monica, California. Dr. Stone also teaches classes and supervises in the clinic at Emperor's College.

Dr. Stone has been editing TCM texts since 1995, including *The Treatment of Lupus, Scleroderma, and Dermatomyositis with TCM*, published by People's Medical Publishing House in Beijing.

■ Peer-Review Committee

John Nei-Qiang Gu, L.Ac., M.D. (China): Nei-Qiang Gu is from the famous Gu family lineage of Shanghai. His father and grandfather practiced dermatology, which includes the surgical procedures of TCM. Dr. Gu graduated from Shanghai University of TCM in 1962. With forty years of experience, Dr. Gu has published more than thirty research papers and books. He is currently a faculty member at both Emperor's College and Yo San University.

Hua-Bing Wen, L.Ac., M.D. (China): Dr. Wen graduated from Beijing University of TCM with Bachelor's and Master's degrees specialized in nephrology and endocrinology. He has been an instructor and clinic supervisor at schools in China and the U.S. He has conducted research in stroke and diabetes treatment with TCM and has had several papers published. He is a faculty member at both Emperor's College and Yo San University, and maintains a private practice in Beverly Hills, California.

Joseph Chang-Qing Yang, Ph.D., L.Ac. , M.D. (China): Dr. Yang graduated from Heilongjiang University of TCM where he was awarded his Bachelor's and Master's degrees with a specialization in TCM diagnosis. He also received a Ph.D. in Psychiatry from Kobe University in Japan. Dr. Yang has considerable experience as a faculty member and clinic supervisor in TCM schools in Harbin, China and in the U.S., including at Emperor's College and Yo San University. He maintains a private practice in Santa Monica, California.

Tiende Yang, L.Ac., M.D. (China): Dr. Yang has been officially entitled and registered as an Asian academic heir of the *Most Distinguished Acupuncturists and Traditional Chinese Specialists*, the highest rank for Traditional Chinese Medical Doctors in the People's Republic of China. To preserve the heritage of Chinese Medicine, five hundred of the most respected Chinese doctors selected two pupils each to pass on their time-honored medical knowledge and skills. Dr. Yang is one of those selected. He started his apprenticeship under his father at the age of 16. As an assistant professor of Traditional Chinese Medicine at Beijing University of Traditional Chinese Medicine since 1988, he was the physician in charge of the department of acupuncture and moxibustion at the Beijing Dongzhimen Hospital. Dr. Yang is a clinic supervisor at Emperor's College and maintains a private practice in Beverly Hills, California.

Chun Yi "Meredith" Qian, L.Ac., M.D. (China), : Dr. Qian received her M.D. degree in 1983 in China. She then earned her Master's Degree of Acupuncture Science in 1986 at the distinguished China Academy of TCM at the Institute of Acupuncture in Beijing. From 1993 to 1998, she was a visiting physician and served as the head of the integrative medicine department at the esteemed Chaim Sheba Medical Center at Tel-Hashomel in Israel. In 1998, Dr. Qian was invited to give medical assistance to world leaders in Washington, D.C. and administered acupuncture and herbal medicine to the late king of Jordan at the renowned Mayo Clinic in Rochester, Minnesota. Since 1998, Dr. Qian has been a professor and clinic supervisor at a university of Oriental medicine in Los Angeles, California.

Qi Wei Zheng, L.Ac., M.D. (China): Dr. Zheng earned his M.D. degree in 1976 in China. He then received his Master's Degree of Acupuncture Science in 1981, at the prestigious China Academy of TCM, Institute of Acupuncture, in Beijing. In 1995, Dr. Zheng earned tenure as a professor at the China Academy of TCM. Dr. Zheng also became the vice director of the Beijing International Acupuncture Training Center and became chief of its teaching department in the same year. Since 1998, Dr. Zheng has been a professor and clinic supervisor at a university of Oriental medicine in Los Angeles, California.

Zhen Hao, L.Ac., M.D. (China): Dr. Hao graduated from Beijing University of TCM where she received her Bachelor's and Master's degrees, specializing in TCM pediatrics. She has taught at TCM schools in the U.S. and China in such subjects as TCM diagnosis, fundamental theory, and Chinese herbal medicine. Dr. Hao currently practices in Mission Viejo, California.

Index